Contents

Medical Masterclass third edition

Editor-in-Chief

Dr John D Firth DM FRCP
Consultant Physician and Nephrologist
Addenbrooke's Hospital
Cambridge
UK

Neurology, medical ophthalmology and psychiatry

Editors

Dr Sivakumar Sathasivam PhD MRCP(UK)
Consultant Neurologist
The Walton Centre for Neurology and Neurosurgery NHS Trust
Liverpool
UK

Dr Greg Heath BSc MBBS MRCOphth MRCP(UK) MCOptom DipClinOptom FHEA
Consultant Medical Ophthalmologist
York Teaching Hospital NHS Foundation Trust
York
UK

Dr David Horton BA Hons (Oxon) BM BCh MRCPsych
Specialty Trainee in Child and Adolescent Psychiatry
Solent NHS Trust
Southampton
UK

Third edition

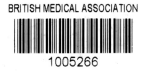

Disclaimer

Although every effort has been made to ensure that drug doses and other information are presented accurately in this publication, the ultimate responsibility rests with the prescribing physician. Neither the publishers nor the authors can be held responsible for any consequences arising from the use of information contained herein. Any product mentioned in this publication should be used in accordance with the prescribing information prepared by the manufacturers.

The information presented in this publication reflects the opinions of its contributors and should not be taken to represent the policy and views of the Royal College of Physicians of London, unless this is specifically stated.

Every effort has been made by the contributors to contact holders of copyright to obtain permission to reproduce copyrighted material. However, if any have been inadvertently overlooked, the publisher will be pleased to make the necessary arrangements at the first opportunity.

List of contributors

Dr Alice Ashby MBChB MA MRCPsych
Consultant Liaison Psychiatrist
St Thomas' Hospital
London
UK

Dr Harry Costello MBBS BSc
Academic Clinical Fellow Core Psychiatry
Trainee
St Pancras Hospital
Camden and Islington NHS Foundation
Trust
London
UK

Dr Greg Heath BSc MBBS MRCOphth
MRCP(UK) MCOptom DipClinOptom
FHEA
Consultant Medical Ophthalmologist
York Teaching Hospital NHS Foundation
Trust
York
UK

Dr David Horton BA Hons (Oxon)
BM BCh MRCPsych
Specialty Trainee in Child and
Adolescent Psychiatry
Solent NHS Trust
Southampton
UK

Dr Andrew J Larner MD MRCP(UK)
Consultant Neurologist
The Walton Centre for Neurology and
Neurosurgery NHS Trust
Liverpool
UK

Dr Ranjith K Menon MD FRCP MD
(Res) MRCP Neuro Stroke Fellowship
Consultant Vascular Neurologist
The Walton Centre for Neurology and
Neurosurgery NHS Trust
Liverpool
UK

Dr S Neil Sarkar BSc AKC MBBS
MRCPsych PGDipAP FHEA
Consultant Psychiatrist (General Adult,
Acute and Primary Care Psychiatry)
Camden and Islington NHS Foundation
Trust
London
UK

Dr Sivakumar Sathasivam PhD
MRCP(UK)
Consultant Neurologist
The Walton Centre for Neurology and
Neurosurgery NHS Trust
Liverpool
UK

Dr Hilary Tyne MB ChB (Hons)
FRCP MD
Consultant Neurologist
Salford Royal Hospital
Salford
UK

Dr Udo C Wieshmann MD PhD FRCP
The Walton Centre for Neurology and
Neurosurgery NHS Trust
Liverpool
UK

Dr Martin Wilson FRCP DM
Consultant Neurologist and
Clinical Director of Neurology
The Walton Centre for Neurology
and Neurosurgery NHS Trust
Liverpool
UK

Acknowledgements

The third edition of Medical Masterclass has been produced by a team. The names of those who have written and edited are clearly indicated, and along with all these contributors I gratefully acknowledge the contributions of those who wrote and edited the first and second editions. This third edition is based on their foundations, and some of their material has been retained. But my acknowledgements must not stop there, because the Medical Masterclass would not have been published without the efforts of many other people. Naming names is risky, but I must name Claire Daley, who has worked as editor of the third edition with a wonderful combination of quietness and efficiency, and with an attention to detail that has made me feel triumphant if I have ever spotted a misplaced comma in a proof.

Dr John Firth DM FRCP
Medical Masterclass Editor-in-Chief

Cover image courtesy of: Zephyr / Science Photo Library

Published by:
Royal College of Physicians of London
11 St Andrews Place
Regent's Park
London NW1 4LE
United Kingdom

Typeset by Manila Typesetting Company, Makati City, Philippines

Printed by The Lavenham Press Limited, Suffolk

First edition published 2001
Reprinted 2004
Second edition published 2008
Updated and reprinted 2010
Third edition published 2018

ISBN: 978-1-86016-662-4 (this book)
eISBN: 978-1-86016-663-1 (this book)
ISBN: 978-1-86016-670-9 (set)
eISBN: 978-1-86016-671-6 (set)

Royal College of Physicians of London
11 St Andrews Place
Regent's Park
London NW1 4LE
United Kingdom
Tel: +44 (0)20 3075 1379
Email: medical.masterclass@rcplondon.ac.uk
Web: www.rcplondon.ac.uk/medicalmasterclass

Preface

This third edition of Medical Masterclass is produced and published by the Royal College of Physicians of London. It comprises 12 books and an online question bank. Its aim is to interest and help doctors in their first few years of training, to enable them to improve their medical knowledge and skills, and to pass postgraduate medical examinations, most particularly the MRCP(UK): Part 1, Part 2 and PACES (the practical assessment of clinical examination skills that is the final part of the exam).

The 12 textbooks are divided as follows: two cover the scientific background to medicine; one is devoted to general clinical skills, including medicine for older people, palliative care and specific guidance on exam technique for PACES; one deals with acute medicine; and the other eight cover the range of medical specialties.

The medical specialties are dealt with in eight sections:

> Case histories – you are presented with letters of referral that are commonly received in each specialty and led through the ways in which the patients' histories should be explored, and what investigations and/or treatments should follow, as in Station 2 of PACES.

> Physical examination scenarios – these emphasise solid and reliable clinical method, logical analysis of physical signs and sensible clinical reasoning ('having found this, what would you want to do next?'), as in Stations 1 and 3 of PACES.

> Communication and ethical scenarios – you are presented with difficult issues that can arise in each specialty. What should you actually say in response to the 'frequently asked (but nonetheless tricky) questions', as required in Station 4 of PACES?

> Brief clinical consultations – how should you take a focused history and perform a focused examination of a patient who has a medical problem when there isn't much time? This section explains how to do this while working as a medical registrar on take, or in Station 5 of PACES.

> Acute presentations – what are your priorities if you are the doctor seeing a patient in the emergency department or the medical admissions unit? The material in this section is relevant to all parts of the MRCP(UK) exam.

> Diseases and treatments – concise structured notes that are of particular relevance to the Part 1 and Part 2 exams.

> Investigations and practical procedures – short and concise notes.

> Self-assessment questions – in the form used in the Part 1 and Part 2 exams.

The online question bank, which is continually updated, enables you to take mock Part 1 and Part 2 exams, or to be selective in the questions that you tackle (if you want to do 10 questions on cardiology, or any other specialty, then you can do so). You can see how your scores compare with those of others who have attempted the same questions, which helps you to know where to focus your learning.

I hope that you enjoy using the Medical Masterclass to learn more about medicine. I know that medicine is tough at the moment, with hospital services under unprecedented pressure and the medical registrar bearing more than their fair share of the burden. But careers are a long game, and being a physician is a wonderful occupation. It is sometimes intellectually and/or emotionally very challenging, but with these challenges come great rewards, and few things give more substantial satisfaction than being a doctor who provides good care for a patient. The Medical Masterclass should help you do to that, as well as to pass the MRCP(UK) exam along the way.

Dr John Firth DM FRCP
Medical Masterclass Editor-in-Chief

Key features

We have created a range of icon boxes that sit among the text of the various Medical Masterclass books. They are there to help you identify key information and to make learning easier and more enjoyable. Here is a brief explanation:

This icon is used to highlight points of particular importance.

Key point

A patient with a normal physical examination, a normal ECG and a normal echocardiogram is at very low risk of significant arrhythmia.

This icon is used to indicate common or important drug interactions, pitfalls of practical procedures, or when to take symptoms or signs particularly seriously.

Hazard

Acute lymphoblastic leukaemia may present in an identical manner to infectious mononucleosis.

Case examples / case histories are used to demonstrate why and how an understanding of the scientific background to medicine helps in the practice of clinical medicine.

Case history

A man with a renal transplant is immunosuppressed with ciclosporin, azathioprine and prednisolone. He develops recurrent gout and is started on allopurinol.

Neurology

Authors

**Dr A Larner, Dr R Menon, Dr S Sathasivam, Dr H Tyne,
Dr U Wieshmann and Dr M Wilson**

Editor

Dr S Sathasivam

Editor-in-Chief

Dr JD Firth

The neurology section of the second edition of Medical Masterclass was written by
Dr LJ Coward, Dr FJ Rugg-Gunn, Dr S Sathasivam, Dr C Turner and Dr NS Ward (editor).
This third edition of Medical Masterclass contains entirely new material, but many sections
from the second edition have been retained and updated, and we gratefully acknowledge the
contribution of these authors.

Neurology: Section 1

1 PACES stations and acute scenarios

1.1 History taking

1.1.1 Episodic headache

Dear Doctor,
Re: Mrs Lucy Carter, aged 29 years

I would be grateful for your opinion regarding this woman who suffers frequent severe headaches. She is a teacher with no significant past medical history, but has had to take an unacceptable amount of time off work since going back after maternity leave 4 months ago because of the pains. I have prescribed her regular codeine phosphate, which she finds is of some benefit. Examination is normal, including blood pressure (BP).

Yours sincerely,

Introduction

The diagnosis of an episodic headache, as with facial pain (see Section 1.1.2), can virtually always be made on the history alone. It is certainly worth taking time over this: the commonest cause of an incorrect diagnosis is an incorrect history. It is important to note that the severity of pain is not an indicator of whether a headache is life threatening or not. Your approach to the patient presenting with headache should be to establish:

> Are the headaches benign?

> If so, then what is their cause?

In this patient there is a worry that the headaches are related to raised intracranial pressure secondary to a space-occupying lesion, hydrocephalus or idiopathic raised intracranial hypertension; or that they are caused by a systemic condition. However, it is much more likely that her headaches are benign. It is important to make the correct diagnosis in benign headaches to have the best chance of treating them effectively.

History of the presenting problem

The following are a list of points that it is useful to establish:

> How long has the patient had these headaches? Long-standing headaches (present for over 1 year) are almost always benign, so establish when the headaches truly began and not just when they got worse. In this case, did the headaches start during her pregnancy or after delivery?

> How often do they occur and for how long? Determine whether she is describing episodic discrete headaches or exacerbations with a constant background, which may also be described as recurrent – ask specifically about the period in between headaches (Fig 1).

> Where does she get the pain? Is it bilateral, strictly unilateral, alternating unilateral, frontal, temporal or occipital? The use of a finger or hand to indicate the position will give some clue as to the quality of the pain (Fig 2).

> What is the pain like? Is it throbbing (migraine); a deep, boring, intense

unilateral pain (cluster headache); or band-like tightness/pressure around the head (tension-type headache)? The pain of a raised intracranial pressure headache is non-specific (causes of raised intracranial pressure include a space-occupying lesion, intracranial bleed, Arnold–Chiari malformation and cerebral venous sinus thrombosis).

> What does she do with herself during an attack? Most patients with severe headache prefer to remain still, but agitation during an attack is characteristic of cluster headache.

> Are there any precipitating or aggravating factors? Light, noise, smell, movement and stress aggravate most headaches and so are not helpful in differentiating one type of headache from another. Exacerbation by coughing, sneezing or straining is also relatively non-specific. Alcohol can precipitate migraine and cluster headache (during a bout) but may alleviate tension-type headaches.

> Are there any associated features? 'Classical migraine' may be associated with visual phenomena such as seeing dazzling zigzag lines (fortification spectra). Many patients who experience this feel intensely nauseated. Additional features such as weakness, paraesthesiae, aphasia, diplopia and visual loss are often worrying but can all happen as part of migraine aura. Establish how closely these symptoms are

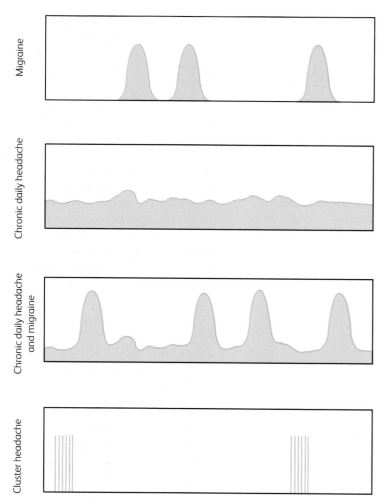

Fig 1 Periodicity of pain in different headache syndromes.

associated with the headache. Any residual deficit should be taken seriously and investigated further. The diagnosis of giant cell arteritis should be considered in anyone over the age of 50 years with severe headache: visual symptoms, jaw claudication, proximal muscle pain (polymyalgia rheumatica) and constitutional symptoms would all support this diagnosis.

> What medication is she on now? Either it is not working and needs to be changed, or it is contributing significantly to the headache and so should be stopped. The codeine that has been prescribed to this lady is unlikely to be helping her and may be precipitating the headaches.

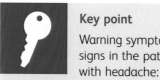

Key point

Warning symptoms or signs in the patient with headache:

> headaches of subacute onset with steady progression over days or weeks

> a recent change in pattern or character of an established headache

> association with fever or other systemic features

> association with focal neurological signs, papilloedema, personality change or seizures could indicate a space-occupying lesion as the underlying cause

> new onset of headache in people older than 50 years.

Other relevant history

Ask about the following:

> A previous history of depression, anxiety or neck trauma will be relevant if considering tension-type headache.

> Current or previous use of tetracyclines, corticosteroids or vitamin A derivatives may be associated with idiopathic intracranial hypertension.

> Pregnancy, an underlying autoimmune disorder (eg antiphospholipid syndrome), history of deep venous thrombosis (DVT) or pulmonary embolism, family history of DVT, use of the oral contraceptive pill (especially the combined pill) and underlying malignancy can be associated with cerebral venous sinus thrombosis.

> Recent weight gain or pregnancy in a woman of childbearing age (such as in this case) can precipitate idiopathic intracranial hypertension.

> Previous head injury, subarachnoid haemorrhage or meningitis may predispose to communicating hydrocephalus.

Plan for investigation and management

You should begin by explaining that under normal circumstances you need to confirm that her neurological examination is normal.

Investigation

Consider the following:

> Blood tests – erythrocyte sedimentation rate and C-reactive protein are important tests to carry out if giant cell arteritis is suspected (see Section 1.1.2), otherwise blood tests are rarely helpful unless systemic disease is suspected.

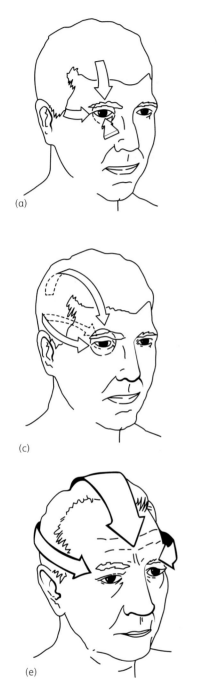

(a)

(b)

(c)

(d)

(e)

Fig 2 Site of pain in different headache diagnoses. **(a)** Classical migraine. Pain is centred in and around the eye, and the forehead on one or other side; and usually extends to involve the whole half-head. **(b)** Orbital onset migraine. The pain tends to start in and around the orbit and may extend across to the opposite eye and to the adjacent facial, frontal and temporal areas, but the main pain remains in the orbit itself. **(c)** Occipital onset migraine. The pain may start as a tightness in the occipital area, rather like tension headache, but will typically extend forward around the temporal area or over the top of the head. The ultimate location of the headache is in and around the eye. **(d)** Cluster headache. The pain is located in the eye and nostril. It is strictly unilateral and rarely changes sides. Lacrimation, nasal blockage and discharge (autonomic features) are common. **(e)** Tension headache. The pain has a quality like a tight band around the head, coming forwards to the forehead.

> Brain imaging – it is often difficult to decide whether or not a patient with headache needs a brain scan. The yield will be very low and not infrequently an incidental finding will cause some difficulty. There is also an increasing awareness of the exposure to radiation associated with computerised tomography (CT) scanning (equivalent to approximately 100–150 chest X-rays). However, if a clear diagnosis cannot be made and there are uncertainties as to whether the headache is benign, then it may be appropriate to perform a scan to exclude a space-occupying lesion or hydrocephalus. Imaging may demonstrate slit-like ventricles in a patient with idiopathic intracranial hypertension, but may also be completely normal.

> Lumbar puncture – a diagnosis of idiopathic intracranial hypertension is confirmed by measuring an elevated opening pressure on lumbar puncture (>25 cm H_2O) after normal brain imaging has been obtained.

Management

Management depends on the particular cause:

> migraine, cluster headache and tension-type headache with exacerbations – see Section 2.6

> Idiopathic intracranial hypertension:
  > dietary advice to lose weight
  > repeat lumbar punctures
  > acetazolamide 750–1,000 mg daily
  > deterioration in vision is likely to need optic nerve sheath fenestration
  > progressively worsening headaches with neurological symptoms may require shunt insertion (lumboperitoneal shunt).

Further discussion

In a young woman of childbearing age who has recently been pregnant or gained weight, idiopathic intracranial hypertension must be considered. Patients characteristically present with a gradual onset headache associated with features of raised intracranial pressure. They may also complain of visual obscurations (transient bilateral visual loss occurring with changes in posture) and occasionally tinnitus. The headache itself has no specific features.

Hazard

Idiopathic intracranial hypertension is no longer called 'benign' because of the danger of progressive visual loss associated with papilloedema. Sight must be monitored by regular formal visual field testing and intraocular pressure measurement, not simply by testing of acuity.

1.1.2 Facial pain

Letter of referral to neurology outpatient clinic

Dear Doctor,

Re: Mrs Edna Smith, aged 60 years

Many thanks for seeing this woman who complains of having a 'chronic' pain in the right side of her face for the last 6 weeks. The pain comes and goes and is not relieved by simple analgesia.

She has no significant past medical history apart from mild chronic obstructive pulmonary disease due to smoking (now 5–10 cigarettes/day). Physical examination and routine blood tests are normal.

I would be grateful for your help in diagnosis and management.

Yours sincerely,

Table 1	Causes of facial pain
Type of facial pain	**Causes**
Intermittent	Trigeminal neuralgia Cluster headache Giant cell arteritis Costen's syndrome
Constant	Postherpetic neuralgia Atypical facial pain Tolosa–Hunt syndrome

Introduction

The clinical history is the most important tool in reaching a diagnosis for the cause of facial pain (Table 1). Physical examination and investigations will often be normal. There are several causes of intermittent facial pain, but although the symptoms can be distressing it is usually possible to improve matters if the correct diagnosis is made. Constant facial pain is less common and often harder to treat than intermittent pain.

History of the presenting problem

First, it is important to characterise the pain. Then you must identify the presence of any associated features that may give clues to the underlying diagnosis. Ask the patient to describe the pain as fully as possible and then, if not already volunteered, enquire specifically:

> Where do you feel the pain? (See Fig 3.)

> Is it intermittent or constant? (See Table 1.)

> How long have you had it for?

> Does anything make the pain better or worse?

As you obtain the answers to these questions, consider the diagnoses shown below.

Trigeminal neuralgia

A unilateral, lancinating sharp pain that lasts for seconds, affecting the lower jaw and upper lip and set off by touch, chewing or talking (see Section 2.6).

Postherpetic neuralgia

The constant unilateral burning sensation (with occasional lancinating pains) comes on after 10% of instances of herpes zoster ophthalmicus. This usually affects the upper face, especially the eyebrow.

Cluster headache

An episodic deep boring pain situated on or around one eye (see Section 2.6).

Giant cell arteritis

A diagnosis that should be considered in any patient over 60 years of age with recent onset headache or facial pain. It may cause diffuse unilateral or bilateral headache, although the patient may concentrate on the symptom of temporal tenderness.

Costen's syndrome

Severe pain over the temporomandibular joint when eating.

Atypical facial pain

Described as a continuous unbearable pain – usually maxillary – and either unilateral or bilateral. This is a diagnosis of exclusion and is not to be made before other possibilities have been exhausted.

Tolosa–Hunt syndrome

An idiopathic granulomatous process in the anterior portion of the cavernous sinus or at the superior orbital fissure. Causes intra- and retro-orbital pain that may simulate cluster headache. Involvement of the third, fourth and sixth cranial nerves leads to variable ophthalmoplegia.

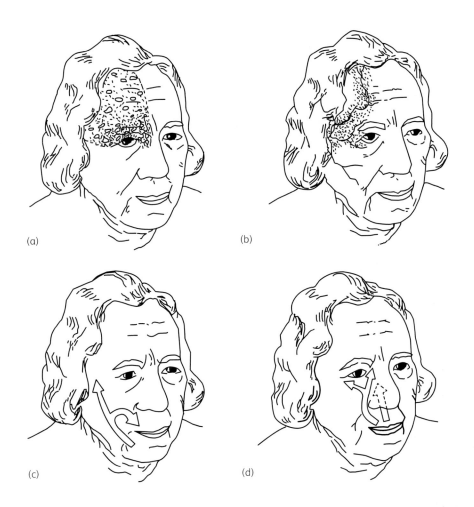

(a)   (b)

(c)   (d)

Fig 3 Site of facial pain in different diagnoses. **(a)** Postherpetic neuralgia. The whole area of the first division of the fifth nerve may have been involved, but typically the most persistent and unpleasant pain is in the eye itself and the eyebrow. **(b)** Cranial arteritis. Although involvement of the superficial temporal artery has always been stressed, any artery in the head can be involved. There is a tendency for the pain to be worse nocturnally, but still present 24 hours a day and associated with systemic symptoms (weight loss and general ill health). In most instances the patient's erythrocyte sedimentation rate (ESR) and C-reactive protein (CRP) will be markedly elevated. **(c)** Trigeminal neuralgia. The commonest pattern is pain radiating from the lower jaw, particularly the canine tooth, up to a position deep in front of the ear. The less common variant **(d)** involves pain starting in the incisors or canines of the upper jaw, and radiating up to and around the eye or – at its worst – up inside the nose.

Other relevant history

Are there any associated features? Consider the following points:

> Has there been any visual disturbance? This, together with jaw claudication, is an important clue to the diagnosis of giant cell arteritis, as is the presence of constitutional symptoms.

> Has an eye gone red? Primary angle closure glaucoma often causes an intermittently painful red eye, but it may cause non-specific headaches. In milder, less acute cases coloured haloes seen around lights may be the main diagnostic clue.

> Is there painful ophthalmoplegia? This would suggest ophthalmoplegic

migraine (less likely to occur *de novo* at this age) or Tolosa–Hunt syndrome.

> Has there been a rash or any spots? Postherpetic neuralgia will have been preceded by herpes zoster ophthalmicus.

> Cluster headache has a number of associated features (see Section 2.6).

> Has there been discharge or bleeding from the nose? These would suggest a sinus problem in this context.

> If facial pain is associated with signs or symptoms suggestive of cerebral ischaemia then look very closely for an ipsilateral Horner's syndrome, as there may have been a carotid artery dissection.

> Paget's disease affecting the skull base may result in symptoms similar to trigeminal neuralgia.

> Atypical facial pain is said to be associated with depressive symptoms, but this may be a feature of any chronic pain syndrome.

Plan for investigation and management

You should explain to the patient that you would normally examine her face, throat, head and neck to confirm that there are no abnormalities as stated in the letter from her general practitioner (GP).

Investigations

These will be dictated by the likely diagnosis. In a woman of this age, the most important diagnosis to exclude is giant cell arteritis, but the most likely diagnosis is trigeminal neuralgia. In general, if a confident clinical diagnosis cannot be made, the following tests or advice should be obtained:

> Inflammatory markers (CRP and ESR) – it is best to check these yourself since they may not be part of the GP's 'routine blood tests'. If they are normal, then the diagnosis of giant cell arteritis can be excluded with almost complete certainty.

> Temporal artery biopsy – if giant cell arteritis is suspected.

> CT scan of head – to rule out structural causes of pain, particularly in the cavernous sinus.

> Ophthalmological opinion – especially if there is a red eye or ophthalmoplegia.

> Ears, nose and throat opinion.

Management

Management depends on the diagnosis:

> Trigeminal neuralgia – see Section 2.6.

> Postherpetic neuralgia – amitriptyline provides relief in 50% of cases; other useful drugs include gabapentin and pregabalin. Topical capsaicin cream may help. A transcutaneous electrical nerve stimulation (TENS) machine relieves pain in some patients.

> Giant cell arteritis – the response to steroids is characteristic and often dramatic.

> Cluster headache – see Section 2.6.

> Atypical facial pain – there may be a limited response to amitriptyline, the dose of which may need to be titrated up according to response.

> Costen's syndrome – surgical correction of bite may be required.

> Tolosa–Hunt syndrome – usually responds to treatment with steroids.

Most cases of facial pain can be appropriately managed as an outpatient. Patients should be reviewed with the results of investigations as they become available and GPs must be informed of any new treatment that is to be prescribed, particularly high-dose steroids, so that regular monitoring for potential side effects can be arranged.

Hazard

Action must be taken on the same day in patients with suspected giant cell arteritis. The results of inflammatory markers should be checked and, if raised, steroids started immediately. If a temporal artery biopsy is planned, it should not delay the initiation of steroids but should be arranged within 3 weeks of starting treatment to have the best chance of detecting any inflammation. A negative biopsy does not exclude the diagnosis since the inflammation can occur as 'skip lesions' with normal tissue in between.

1.1.3 Funny turns/blackouts

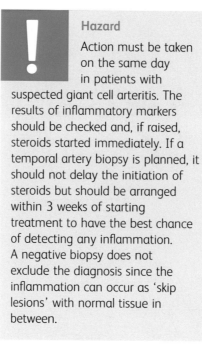

Letter of referral to general medical outpatient clinic

Dear Doctor,

Re: Mr Thomas Barnett, aged 76 years

Thank you for seeing this retired schoolteacher with a 6-month history of recurrent episodes of impaired consciousness. These seem to come on at any time and do not have any obvious distinguishing features, such that I am unable to tell whether they are cardiac or neurological in origin, or indeed are caused by something else.

He has mild hypertension, for which he has taken bendroflumethiazide 2.5 mg od for some years, but has no other past medical history of note.

I would be grateful for your help with diagnosis and management.

Yours sincerely,

Introduction

'Funny turn' is a vague term that can be used to describe a multitude of different symptoms ranging from light-headedness to a loss of consciousness. Making the diagnosis depends critically on the history. This can be difficult to obtain since the patient may have a poor recollection of events, and ideally a witness account of at least one attack needs to be obtained (although this is clearly not possible in the PACES examination!). The key points to establish are whether or not the patient is experiencing vertigo, and whether there has been a loss of consciousness. The differential diagnosis will vary accordingly (see Table 2).

History of the presenting problem

Is the patient describing vertigo?
It can sometimes be difficult to be certain. Ask about the following:

> A sensation of rotation of self or environment by definition is vertigo. However, many patients will not be this explicit and will describe to-and-fro or up-and-down movement of the body or head, or that the wall/floor moves, or that they veer to one side during symptoms 'as if being pulled down by a magnet'. These symptoms, which merge into the very non-specific complaint of 'unsteadiness', are difficult to sort out. Further probing is required.

> Are the symptoms aggravated by moving, closing the eyes or riding in a car? Is he disinclined to walk during an attack? All suggest that the symptom should be regarded as vertigo.

> The duration of attacks is crucial: benign positional vertigo (BPV) lasts only minutes, whereas the vertigo of Ménière's disease can last for hours.

Table 2 Common or important causes of recurrent 'funny turns'		
Symptom	Common causes	Other causes
Vertigo	Ménière's disease BPV Cerebellopontine angle lesion	Vertebrobasilar TIA (rare) Drugs, eg aminoglycosides
Giddy/dizzy/unsteady	Anxiety Drugs (various) Multiple deficits of sensory input	Cervical spondylosis TIA Anaemia or polycythaemia Hypoglycaemia
Presyncope or syncope	Postural hypotension Cardiac arrhythmia Vasovagal Ventricular outflow obstruction, eg aortic stenosis or hypertrophic obstructive cardiomyopathy Specific precipitant, eg carotid sinus syncope	Specific precipitant, eg cough or micturition syncope Myocardial ischaemia
Transient loss of awareness/consciousness	Epilepsy Causes of syncope Non-epileptic (psychogenic) attacks	Transient global amnesia

BPV, benign positional vertigo; TIA, transient ischaemic attack.

> The role of posture in the generation of vertiginous symptoms is often over-played: most cases of vertigo will be worse on movement. If movement of the neck, eg twisting to look when reversing the car, precipitates vertigo then vertebrobasilar ischaemia is possible. However, this is an exceedingly rare cause of vertigo and should be considered only if other symptoms suggesting brain ischaemia also occur.

Key point

A peripheral vestibular disorder is strongly suggested by a history of the symptoms being provoked by rolling over in bed.

It is not uncommon for the patient to be unable to describe their symptoms in any more detail than light-headedness, giddiness, dizziness or intermittent unsteadiness. In these cases the wide differential diagnoses listed in Table 2 need to be considered.

Is the patient describing presyncope? Does he describe early visual symptoms, muffled sounds, feelings of hot or cold, or feeling lightheaded? These features would be suggestive of a transient fall in cerebral blood flow. Symptoms on standing suggest postural hypotension, and those associated with effort, chest pain, shortness of breath or palpitations are more likely to have a cardiac cause. Was it preceded by coughing vigorously or by micturition, suggesting a specific syncopal syndrome?

New onset of vasovagal presyncope or syncope would not be expected to occur in a patient aged 76 years, but when such episodes do occur they are typically when a patient has been standing up in hot and stuffy rooms, have quite a long prodrome of 'feeling faint' and culminate in a dizzy feeling where noises seem to become loud before the patient collapses. Consciousness is restored almost as soon as the patient falls to the ground or is encouraged to lie down by someone who recognises what is happening. In those susceptible, vasovagal syncope can also be induced by painful or unpleasant stimuli. Vasovagal syncope is frequently accompanied by brief myoclonic limb movements, which are commonly misinterpreted as epileptic.

Was there loss of consciousness in these attacks (syncope)?
If syncope has occurred, was it preceded by presyncopal symptoms that could give a clue to the diagnosis? A witness account of pallor followed by flushing would be very suggestive of a Stokes–Adams attack (due to the intermittent development of complete heart block), but this does not occur in all patients.

Could the cause be epilepsy?

Hazard

The presence of jerking limbs and incontinence does not prove epilepsy as the primary cause. Anoxic fits can occur following prolonged cerebral anoxia, such as when an individual is propped up after passing out. A helpful differentiating factor can be the length of time taken to come round after an episode, which may be prolonged in a postictal state and short after an anoxic event.

If the patient was awake but unresponsive during an attack, ask specifically about any warnings that they or any witness may have noticed. Features such as lip smacking, fiddling with clothes or stereotyped movements would be suggestive of a complex partial seizure.

Are there any additional features in the history to help?
Consider the following points:

> A history of tinnitus and deafness in the context of episodic vertigo points towards Ménière's disease or even a cerebellopontine angle lesion (acoustic neuroma), particularly if ataxia and/or facial weakness is also present.

> Do other neurological symptoms occur? In their absence, transient ischaemic attacks (TIAs) of either the anterior or posterior circulation are unlikely.

> If the patient mentions feeling unsteady, then ask about how they find walking – particularly over uneven ground – or if they have tripped on paving stones; also ask about numbness in the feet and hands. Those with peripheral neuropathy may be susceptible to bouts of unsteadiness – especially when other sensory modalities such as vision are simultaneously impaired, eg getting out of bed at night in the dark.

> Does he have any biological features of depression? It is not uncommon for depression to present with somatic symptoms.

> Do not forget alcohol. Many are familiar with the 'funny turns' that can be precipitated by drinking!

Could the cause of a funny turn be transient global amnesia?
Did the patient have an episode of amnesia and confusion lasting for several hours? If so consider the diagnosis of transient global amnesia, in which self-identity is preserved. The degree of retrograde amnesia shrinks significantly after the attack. The significance of recognising this not uncommon condition is that it is benign, recurs only very infrequently and does not require investigation.

Other relevant history
Has the patient ever suffered from stroke, myocardial infarction, angina, heart valve disease, cardiac dysrhythmia or epilepsy? A full history of current and recently prescribed drugs is clearly important – especially those likely to cause or exacerbate postural hypotension, eg diuretics (as in this case) and antihypertensives. Ask about risk factors for atheromatous vascular disease: smoking, hypertension, diabetes mellitus, family history of stroke, ischaemic heart disease and hyperlipidaemia.

Plan for investigation and management
Investigations
In many cases a diagnosis can be made on the basis of the history, when selected confirmatory investigations may be required. When no clear diagnosis can be made, then consider the following:

> Are the 'funny turns' a marker of ill health? Check the patient's full blood count (FBC), electrolytes, renal and liver function tests, glucose, inflammatory markers and chest X-ray. In some cases other tests, eg thyroid function or vitamin B_{12} levels, may be indicated.

> Are the episodes cardiac? Check resting 12-lead electrocardiogram (ECG), 24-hour ambulatory ECG and the echocardiogram (if there is clinical suspicion of valvular or other structural abnormality). In the patient with frequent, troublesome and potentially life-threatening syncope, repeated monitoring or even inpatient observation may be required.

> Are the episodes neurological? Any patient with focal neurological features or new onset seizures must have a CT scan of the brain. A magnetic resonance imaging (MRI) scan of the brain and internal auditory meati is indicated if an acoustic neuroma is suspected. An electroencephalogram is usually unhelpful and is unnecessary unless a seizure disorder is strongly suspected.

> If there is vertigo, then specialist otological referral should be considered.

Management
Management will depend on the precise diagnosis, but note in particular the following:

> Vestibular retraining may be useful for those with BPV.

> Vestibular suppressants can help in other forms of vertigo.

> Cardiac arrhythmias may require permanent pacemakers and/or drug therapy, and structural cardiac lesions – eg aortic stenosis – may warrant surgery.

> A clear history of seizures warrants treatment with antiepileptic medications, but these should not be given as a 'therapeutic trial'.

In many patients, particularly older patients, it is likely that several factors will be identified without any one of them being clearly responsible for the 'funny turns'. It is always difficult to know how far to pursue investigation, the severity of symptoms and the patient's wishes being important considerations. In any case of 'funny turns, cause unknown' it is important to adopt a sensible approach to symptomatic treatment, eg giving advice regarding postural symptoms, provision of a stick to provide extra sensory input and control of hypertension, diabetes, etc.

Further discussion

There are specific guidelines issued by the UK Driver and Vehicle Licensing Agency (DVLA) regarding driving restrictions for patients who have episodes of loss of awareness. A clear history of a vasovagal episode carries no restrictions, whereas an attack with seizure markers results in a 1-year driving licence suspension. Episodes with no aetiological basis are stratified according to their perceived chance of recurrence and range from a 4-week to 6-month suspension. Further details are available from the DVLA website (www.dvla.gov.uk).

1.1.4 Memory problems

Dear Doctor,
Re: Mr Jack Shaw, aged 60 years

I'd be grateful if you could review this 60-year-old retired schoolteacher who has had episodes of forgetfulness for the past 2 months. His mother, who he cared for, died 6 months ago from probable Alzheimer's disease. Please could you advise me as to whether you feel his memory problems are the early stages of dementia as he is especially concerned about this.

His past medical history is pretty unremarkable. He was diagnosed as having hypertension about 5 years ago and has been on amlodipine and bisoprolol since then, with blood pressure (BP) 140/78 mmHg when last checked.

Yours sincerely,

Introduction

Impairment of cognitive function, affecting the content but not the level of consciousness, may signify dementia if there is memory impairment and decline in social and occupational function, or mild cognitive impairment if activities of daily living are relatively preserved despite memory deficit.

In all memory complaints, it is essential to obtain collateral history from a relative, friend or carer who knows the patient well since a 'forgetful' patient's history may be unreliable (this will not be possible in PACES, although details may be given in the letter of referral). Attending the clinic alone despite memory complaints ('attended alone sign') has been shown to be a robust indicator of the absence of cognitive impairment.

There are many neurological causes of cognitive impairment and dementia (Table 3), very few of which are reversible or potentially reversible, although it is obviously important to rule these out.

Key point

The most common and important condition to distinguish from dementia is depression ('pseudodementia') since this is eminently treatable.

History of the presenting problem

What are the characteristics of the memory impairment?

Ask initially for the patient's own account: 'Give me some examples of the problems you've been having with your memory'; 'How does your memory let you down?' If the patient turns to the accompanying relative/friend/carer ('head turning sign'), this is suggestive (but not diagnostic) of the presence of cognitive impairment.

If relevant details do not emerge spontaneously, then ask the following questions:

> Was the onset of memory difficulties associated with a precipitating cause, such as a head injury (eg traumatic brain injury, subdural haematoma)?

> Was the onset of cognitive impairment chronic (as in Alzheimer's disease (AD), subcortical ischaemic vascular dementia), or subacute (as in Creutzfeldt–Jakob disease (CJD))?

> Has the course of cognitive impairment been gradually progressive (neurodegenerative disorders) or stepwise (as in multi-infarct vascular dementia)?

> Is there fluctuating cognitive impairment affecting both memory and higher cortical functions (eg visuospatial abilities), suggesting dementia with Lewy bodies?

> Does the patient seem slowed down, with impaired attention/concentration and loss of motivation? These features are more suggestive of so-called 'subcortical' dementia (Section 3.1) in which, as the name implies, there is less cortical dysfunction (amnesia, agnosia, aphasia) and more disturbance of structures such as the basal ganglia and basal forebrain. Subcortical features are more frequent in progressive supranuclear palsy, Huntington's disease, and subcortical ischaemic vascular dementia and less frequent in AD.

> Is there prominent behavioural change, with disinhibition, loss of social skills (eg table manners), emotional blunting, neglect of personal hygiene, change in dietary habits (predilection for sweet foods) and language dysfunction (paucity of output, or loss of meaning)? These features are seen in the frontotemporal lobar degenerations (FTLD).

Table 3 Differential diagnosis of cognitive impairment and dementia

Common	Uncommon
AD/MCI Vascular cognitive impairment/vascular dementia: multi-infarct, SIVD Mixed dementia (AD and vascular disease) Parkinson's disease dementia and DLB Alcohol-related dementia Traumatic brain injury	FTLD, including frontotemporal dementia with motor neurone disease Prion diseases (eg Creutzfeldt–Jakob disease) Huntington's disease Other parkinsonian disorders: progressive supranuclear palsy, corticobasal degeneration, idiopathic normal pressure hydrocephalus Neurosyphilis Brain tumour HIV-associated neurocognitive disorder Drug toxicity Hypothyroidism Chronic subdural haematoma Vitamin B_{12} deficiency

AD, Alzheimer's disease; DLB, dementia with Lewy bodies; FTLD, frontotemporal lobar degenerations; MCI, mild cognitive impairment; SIVD, subcortical ischaemic vascular dementia.

Associated features

Consider the following:

> Is there associated headache with features suggesting raised intracranial pressure (eg worse on recumbency, stooping, coughing, sneezing; early morning wakening)? Tumour is rarely a cause of cognitive decline but must not be missed.

> Are there any neuropsychiatric symptoms (eg depression, apathy, irritability) or motor abnormalities (eg extrapyramidal features)? These are more common in subcortical than cortical dementias.

> Are there formed visual hallucinations (eg children, animals; Section 1.1.8) or the sleep disturbances suggestive of rapid eye movement (REM) sleep behaviour disorder ('dream enactment'), with or without associated motor features of parkinsonism? These are suggestive of dementia with Lewy bodies (DLB).

> Is there prominent and early gait disturbance with urinary incontinence, which might suggest idiopathic normal pressure hydrocephalus?

Other relevant history

Ask about the following:

> Are there vascular risk factors (smoking, hypertension, hypercholesterolaemia, diabetes), previous cerebrovascular events (strokes) or signs of heart disease (eg atrial fibrillation)?

> Could there be hypothyroidism?

> Is there a family history of dementia, particularly younger onset dementia? Although rare, genetic causes of dementia are increasingly defined, eg in Alzheimer's disease (AD) (APP, presenilin 1, presenilin 2), frontotemporal lobar degenerations (FTLD) (tau, progranulin, C9orf72), prion disease (PrP gene), Huntington's disease. A positive family history may also explain why a patient is concerned about the possibility of dementia even if there is no clinical evidence to support the diagnosis.

> A detailed drug history is essential, especially for agents with anticholinergic activity, but drugs tend to cause confusion rather than dementia.

> Sexual history: neurosyphilis is now extremely rare in the developed world, and acquired immune deficiency syndrome (AIDS) dementia likewise, although the prevalence of HIV-associated neurocognitive disorder is increasing with improved survival in HIV disease. If suspected, questioning should adopt a tactful approach, eg 'Some infections of the brain can rarely cause this sort of problem – the sort of infections that can be spread by sexual contact. What sexual contacts have you had in the past?'

> Alcohol history: explain why you need the information before embarking on direct questions that some might find intrusive and objectionable, eg 'Sometimes alcohol can cause problems like this. Are you a heavy drinker now? Have you ever been a heavy drinker in the past?'

> Could this be depression ('pseudodementia'), perhaps precipitated in this patient's case by the death of his mother? How is his mood? Does he enjoy anything? Has he lost interest in things he used to do? Is he tearful at times? What time does he wake in the mornings? Has he felt depressed or thought of his death/suicide since the death of his mother?

Plan for investigation and management

Investigations

Any clinical clue to the conditions listed in Table 3 should be followed, but controversy surrounds what constitutes a cost-effective series of investigations because of different estimates of the incidence of reversible dementias. Many physicians would consider the following.

Blood tests

Check FBC; electrolytes; renal, liver and thyroid function tests; inflammatory markers (erythrocyte sedimentation rate or C-reactive protein); serum vitamin B_{12} level; and syphilis serology.

Hazard

Genetic testing raises complex ethical issues. Consequences of genetic testing must be carefully considered as significant harm can result from inadequate counselling (see Section 1.3.2).

Structural neuroimaging

CT and MRI have conventionally been used to rule out structural and rarely treatable causes of dementia such as tumours, normal pressure hydrocephalus or chronic subdural haematoma. Patterns of cerebral atrophy, particularly if quantifiable in serial volumetric MRI scans, may help differentiate cases of AD (temporoparietal atrophy) from frontotemporal dementia (frontal and temporal atrophy).

Functional neuroimaging

Single-photon emission CT (SPECT) typically shows temporoparietal hypoperfusion in AD, and frontal hypoperfusion in frontotemporal dementia. Positron emission tomography (PET), particularly with amyloid ligands (eg Pittsburgh compound B (PiB),

florbetapir) is now recommended in preference to SPECT for diagnosis of AD as this detects a disease biomarker; however, such scanning facilities are not currently widely available.

Cerebrospinal fluid

Examination of cerebrospinal fluid (CSF) (Section 3.2) is usually reserved for patients with atypical clinical features such as systemic symptoms, rapid progression or unusual signs. The CSF cell count, protein and glucose are typically normal in patients with AD. If neurosyphilis is suspected, CSF treponemal serology should be performed, as this is specific but not very sensitive (unlike serum testing). Empirical treatment should be commenced if there is diagnostic doubt.

14-3-3 protein may be raised in the CSF in any condition where there is rapid neuronal loss and gliosis, and has proved sensitive for the diagnosis of sporadic CJD. CSF protein biomarkers of AD are increasingly used, namely Aβ1-42 (low) and total-tau and phospho-tau (both raised).

Electroencephalogram

This is not particularly useful because of the overlap in electroencephalography (EEG) patterns in different forms of dementia. In AD there is loss of alpha activity and increase in diffuse slow waves. In sporadic CJD periodic sharp wave complexes may become apparent with time; they are not seen in variant CJD (Section 2.10.1).

Management

Management will depend on precise diagnosis. For AD, see Section 2.4.1. Patients and those connected to them should be seen after their investigations for explanation and the provision of information, and where possible for a trial of treatment.

Key point

If a depressive element is suspected to be contributing to some or all of the clinical picture of memory complaint, then a trial of antidepressants, usually for 6 months, is warranted followed by clinical reassessment.

Further discussion

It is very common for patients with depressive pseudodementia to have a high degree of insight into their memory disturbance, whereas in cases of AD (after the initial stages) patients often have very little awareness of their memory problems (cognitive anosognosia) and are often not distressed by their difficulties. A knowledgeable relative or friend is therefore essential for accurate history taking, and in PACES you would emphasise that you wished to talk to a relative/close friend to supplement your history from the patient.

1.1.5 Chorea

Letter of referral to a neurology outpatient clinic

Dear Doctor,

Re: Mrs Ethel Lane, aged 72 years

I would be grateful for your urgent review of this woman who is known to you with Parkinson's disease. She has started to develop writhing and jerky spontaneous movements over the past few weeks, which have become very disabling and tiring. I have been gradually increasing her parkinsonian medications since you commenced them 5 years ago. Please could you advise as to the cause of these movements and their management.

Yours sincerely,

Introduction

Chorea is a continuous or intermittent flow of irregular, jerky and sometimes explosive movements that move from one part of the body to another. Each movement is brief and often appears as a fragment of what might have been a normal movement. Causes of chorea are shown in Table 4, the commonest cause being in the context of chronic levodopa treatment in Parkinson's disease – clearly the presumptive diagnosis in this case – or as a part of Huntington's disease (HD).

History of the presenting problem

Which parts of the body are affected?

Chorea often affects movement and speech, and can be extremely disabling for some patients. A useful trick in routine practice (but not in PACES) to bring out any minor degree of chorea is to give the patient a repetitive task to perform or ask them to walk.

When did the condition begin?

Patients who present with chorea as young adults often have a different cause from older patients, although there is significant overlap. A young adult with chorea should raise suspicions of HD, Wilson's disease and other rare genetic disorders. Young adults are also more likely to present with post-Sydenham's chorea, especially in women who are pregnant or taking the oral contraceptive pill.

Antiphospholipid syndrome, systemic lupus erythematosus (SLE) and thyrotoxicosis are also commoner in young adults.

Older patients with chorea often have a history of at least 2 years' treatment with levodopa, usually for Parkinson's disease – as in this case.

How fast was the onset?

If the onset is acute, then the commonest cause of chorea in older patients is in association with a stroke in the basal ganglia, which often affects the contralateral side of the body. When the stroke involves the contralateral subthalamic nucleus, patients develop severe chorea or 'hemiballismus'.

Key point

Late onset chorea is a controversial diagnosis where no cause of chorea can be found in older patients. But many of these patients probably have chorea that is drug-induced or in association with basal ganglia strokes, and some have been found to have late onset HD.

Other relevant history

The most important aspects of the history to elucidate in a patient with chorea are:

> a full drug history

> family history

> vascular risk factors.

Relatives of the patient may be helpful in clarifying these events. Note HD can present in the young as severe parkinsonism rather than chorea; this is the Westphal variant.

Plan for investigation and management

Investigation

> Blood tests – these should include FBC (particularly noting the haematocrit); fresh blood film for acanthocytes (look in three samples for cells with many thorn-like projections from the surface membrane in an extremely rare condition called amyotrophic chorea-acanthocytosis); clotting (prolonged activated partial thromboplastin time in lupus anticoagulant); and erythrocyte sedimentation rate.

> Urea and electrolytes, glucose, liver function test, thyroid function test, copper, caeruloplasmin, antinuclear antibody, anticardiolipin antibodies and antistreptolysin O titres.

> Imaging – CT scans may demonstrate multiple infarcts in older patients or atrophy of the caudate nucleus in those with HD. MRI is more sensitive at detecting subcortical infarcts and caudate nucleus atrophy in HD.

> Genetic tests – HD (see Section 1.3.1).

Table 4 Causes of chorea	
Common	**Uncommon**
Levodopa-induced dyskinesias HD Basal ganglia strokes	SLE / primary antiphospholipid syndrome Carbon monoxide poisoning Pregnancy Sydenham's chorea (post-streptococcal) Genetic (neuroacanthocytosis, Wilson's disease and benign hereditary chorea) Hyperthyroidism Polycythaemia rubra vera Drugs, especially neuroleptics and oral contraceptives Cerebral palsy Late onset chorea

HD, Huntington's disease; SLE, Systemic lupus erythematosus.

Management

Any underlying disorder, eg Wilson's disease, should be treated. Some forms of chorea are self-limiting, eg Sydenham's and post-stroke. Some patients with HD do not find their chorea troublesome. If the patient becomes significantly symptomatic then pharmacological therapies to reduce chorea are available, including tetrabenazine (although this can cause depression) and neuroleptics, eg risperidone, sulpiride and olanzapine. Patients with Parkinson's disease should have a thorough drug and 'on/off' history taken. Some patients can convert part of their levodopa therapy to smaller doses in conjunction with a dopamine agonist. In older patients who are sensitive to the neuropsychiatric side effects of agonists, total levodopa dose reduction is often required, resulting in poor mobility. Deep brain stimulation is also used in selected patients with fluctuations and dyskinesia. Neuroleptics should be avoided in Parkinson's disease and are not used in the management of dyskinesia in Parkinson's disease.

Hazard

Genetic causes of chorea

The pattern of inheritance may help, although the family history, especially in patients with HD, may be missing or incomplete because of a high incidence of early mortality in affected relatives.

Further discussion

Genetic testing for HD is now readily available in genetic reference laboratories. This needs to be undertaken sensitively, with the help of trained geneticists and with full informed consent. Pre-symptomatic testing is a difficult issue and many patients at risk of developing HD choose not to be tested (see Section 1.3.1).

1.1.6 Muscle weakness and pain

Letter of referral to neurology outpatient clinic

Dear Doctor,
Re: Mr Mark Perrin, aged 25 years

I would be grateful if you could see this man who complains of pain in his muscles and weakness on exercise that has been getting worse for the last few months and is now preventing him from playing football.

He has no significant past medical history, except for mild asthma for which he occasionally uses a salbutamol inhaler.

I cannot find anything abnormal on neurological examination. Is there anything going on?

Yours sincerely,

Introduction

The list of causes of muscle pain is extensive, but pain or muscle cramps occurring on exercise limits the differential diagnosis (Table 5).

Key point

Examination may be normal between attacks in cases of McArdle's disease or carnitine palmitoyltransferase (CPT) deficiency, although some cases develop a myopathy following recurrent episodes.

History of the presenting problem

In a young, otherwise fit, man the important differential is between a disorder of lipid or carbohydrate metabolism. These conditions are described in Section 2.2, which will explain the significance of the questions shown below.

Is this a disorder of energy production? Find out:

> How much exercise is possible before the onset of pain?

> Is a 'second wind' phenomenon experienced?

> Are there associated painful muscle cramps?

> Have there been episodes of dark urine (indicating rhabdomyolysis)?

> Is there a family history? Autosomal recessive inheritance is seen in CPT deficiency and McArdle's disease; maternal inheritance in mitochondrial disorders.

Table 5	Causes of muscle pain on exercise
Cause	**Diagnoses**
Metabolic	CPT deficiency and other disorders of fatty acid metabolism
	McArdle's disease and other disorders of glycogen metabolism Mitochondrial myopathy
Other	Hypothyroidism
Ischaemia	Lumbar canal stenosis[1]
	Claudication[1]

1 Muscular pain restricted to the legs, excepting rare cases of arm claudication.
CPT, Carnitine palmitoyltransferase.

Is this hypothyroidism?

Ask about weight gain, lethargy, cold intolerance and other symptoms of hypothyroidism.

Is this mechanical (lumbar canal stenosis)?

Find out if the symptoms are:

> confined to the legs

> improved by bending over.

Lumbar canal stenosis would be unusual in a young man. It is usually caused by progressive hypertrophy of the facet joints and disc degeneration leading to narrowing of the lumbar canal. Lumbar claudication (pain and heaviness of the legs, often proximal) is experienced on standing or walking. Flexion improves the diameter of the canal and therefore the symptoms, hence patients often report no problems with cycling, in which the lumbar spine is often flexed.

Is this muscle ischaemia?

Unlikely in a young man, but in other cases check if the patient is an arteriopath with multiple vascular risk factors.

Other relevant history

Was the patient sporty as a child/teenager? If so, this suggests an 'acquired' illness rather than a metabolic myopathy, which is a lifelong condition.

Plan for investigation and management

You should explain to the patient that under normal circumstances you would examine him to confirm that there are no abnormalities, as stated in the letter from the GP. If the condition is acute or subacute, the patient may need to be admitted for investigations. If it is a chronic condition, then outpatient investigations followed by a review in clinic is appropriate.

Blood tests

Check FBC; erythrocyte sedimentation rate / C-reactive protein (if raised suggests an inflammatory cause); electrolytes, renal, liver and bone function (routine screen); thyroid function; and creatine kinase.

Other tests

An electromyelogram may show spontaneous activity or myopathic features; a muscle biopsy is most likely to reveal a specific diagnosis; an MRI can show patterns of wasting, which may assist in diagnosis.

For a fuller discussion see Section 2.2. Lumbar canal stenosis is diagnosed by imaging (MRI) and treated by surgical decompression.

Further discussion

It is important to counsel patients with metabolic myopathy about the need to avoid situations that are likely to precipitate myoglobinuria, which may lead to acute renal failure. Patients with disorders of carbohydrate metabolism should be advised to slow down exercise if they begin to recognise the first onset of symptoms of muscle pain and weakness, and then only resume it in small increments. By contrast, patients with disorders of lipid metabolism are prone to more severe attacks of myoglobinuria, which usually develop after prolonged exercise and are worse in a fasting state, and they should be advised to avoid any situation that provokes muscle pain or cramps.

1.1.7 Sleep disorders

Letter of referral to neurology outpatient clinic

Dear Doctor,

Re: Mr Frank Richards, aged 60 years

Thank you for seeing this self-employed businessman with excessive daytime sleepiness, which is now interfering with his work and social life. Most recently he fell asleep while driving and is understandably concerned.

He has a past history of ischaemic heart disease, with a myocardial infarction 5 years ago followed by coronary artery grafting. But he is now free of cardiac symptoms. His regular medications consist of bisoprolol, enalapril, atorvastatin and aspirin. He is obese (weight 113 kg, BMI 35.7).

Yours sincerely,

Introduction

'This patient complains of daytime sleepiness' is not an infrequent referral, but the narcoleptic syndrome is much less common and even if the patient tells you that they have 'narcolepsy', other causes should be considered (see below and Table 6).

Key point

Differential diagnosis of excessive daytime sleepiness:

> insomnia (insufficient sleep)

> non-restorative sleep

> narcolepsy.

Table 6	Causes of insomnia
Cause	**Diagnosis**
Wrong environment	Noisy Too light/cold/hot Disturbed by partner Antisocial conditions – shift work, etc
Psychophysiological	Anxiety/depression Bipolar affective disorders
Endocrine	Thyrotoxicosis
Physical	Pain Nocturia Restless legs syndrome Parkinson's disease
Drugs	Alcohol Coffee Prescription: steroids, beta-blockers, phenytoin, bronchodilators, diuretics, stimulants
Hereditary	Fatal familial insomnia

History of the presenting problem

A sleep history is required: what time does the patient go to bed; when do they wake up in the morning; how often do they wake during the night; and what do they do when they do so? Exactly what does their 'excessive daytime sleepiness' mean? How often do they actually fall asleep and have they ever fallen asleep when they were trying to stay awake, eg when driving, as in this man's case? The answers to these questions will help to place the problem into one of two categories:

> Insomnia – Table 6 lists the most common causes for an inability to get sufficient sleep; further questioning should be designed to address these issues.

> Non-restorative sleep – where the patient appears to spend a sufficient time asleep but does not awake refreshed. The main causes of this are shown in Table 7.

Could the patient have any of the conditions listed in Tables 6 or 7, or narcolepsy? Further history should be directed to looking for evidence of the following conditions in particular.

Obstructive sleep apnoea

Does the patient have a morning headache? Patients with obstructive sleep apnoea retain carbon dioxide, resulting in headache. The observations of a partner are essential: these will not be directly available in PACES but may be recorded in the referral letter. The important issues being:

> Does he snore loudly?

> Does he sometimes appear to stop breathing?

> Does he resume breathing with a large gasp?

Central sleep apnoea

There will usually be a history of a brainstem event or of other symptoms to suggest more widespread neurodegenerative disease.

Parasomnias

These are a group of disorders that usually start in childhood and can be linked to particular stages of sleep. They can either be disorders of movement, including hypnic jerks, periodic movements of sleep, sleep paralysis and sleepwalking; disorders of autonomic function with symptoms of sympathetic overdrive; or more complex abnormalities such as sleep terrors.

Key point

Parasomnias are rare in an adult population and can only be diagnosed by a witness account.

Table 7	Causes of non-restorative sleep	
Aetiology		**Causes**
Obstructive sleep apnoea		Associated with obesity
Central		Brainstem lesions Degenerative brain conditions
Mixed		Seen in myotonic dystrophy

Narcoleptic syndrome

This is classically defined as the triad of narcolepsy, cataplexy and hypnogogic hallucinations (and other parasomnias, especially sleep paralysis) although not all patients will have all the symptoms.

> Narcolepsy – when daytime sleep attacks are often without warning, at times of emotion and after a carbohydrate load. Typically patients feel refreshed after each episode of sleep.

> Cataplexy – these are episodes of partial (often face or jaw) or complete loss of muscle tone that result in the patient falling to the ground. They are often triggered by strong emotional stimuli, usually laughter.

> Hypnogogic hallucinations – presleep dreams associated with sleep onset rapid eye movement (REM) activity. In sleep paralysis, which is not restricted to the narcoleptic syndrome, the patient feels completely paralysed at sleep onset (less commonly on waking), and this feeling is often associated with terror, anxiety and fear. Recovery is spontaneous.

Other relevant history

This is important in the case of central sleep apnoea. Adults with parasomnias may have been sleepwalkers or tooth-grinders as children.

The family history may be relevant in some rare diseases. Familial fatal insomnia is an hereditary disease caused by an Asp Asn mutation at codon 178 of the human prion protein gene in the presence of a methionine at codon 129. The same mutation at codon 178 but with a valine at codon 129 results in a familial Creutzfeldt–Jakob disease. Fatal familial insomnia is a rapidly fatal disease characterised by insomnia and dysautonomia, and also more

widespread neurological involvement including pyramidal, cerebellar and cognitive signs.

Plan for investigation and management

The approach to investigations and management will be determined by findings in the history. It may be that nothing more than simple advice is required.

Insomnia

It is often sufficient to improve sleep hygiene, whether that means sleeping with ear plugs, lining the curtains or not drinking coffee after 6pm. Psychiatric and physical disorders that are felt to be contributing must be addressed.

Sleep apnoea

Patients who might have sleep apnoea should be referred to a respiratory specialist with an interest in sleep disorders for further investigation and/or treatment. The initial test will be to monitor arterial oxygen tension overnight using a pulse oximeter, looking for characteristic drops in oxygen saturations at frequent intervals. Treatment involves weight loss and non-invasive ventilatory support at night.

Narcoleptic syndrome

This diagnosis should be confirmed with a multiple sleep latency test, which is performed in a specialist sleep centre. During this test, five episodes of sleep are permitted during the day; a rapid onset of sleep and REM sleep within 15 minutes of the onset in the absence of sleep deprivation are both features indicative of narcolepsy. The excessive sleepiness of narcolepsy can be treated with modafinil or dexamphetamine. The cataplexy, sleep paralysis and hypnagogic/

hypnopompic hallucinations respond to REM-suppressing antidepressants, such as venlafaxine or other selective serotonin reuptake inhibitors. More recently, sodium oxybate has been approved for use in narcolepsy, and is effective for both daytime sleepiness and cataplexy.

Further discussion

The Epworth Sleepiness Scale provides a quantitative measure of the patient's general level of sleepiness (Fig 4). Patients rate the chance that they would fall asleep during different routine daytime situations during the past week. Answers to the questions are rated from 0 to 3, with 0 meaning that they would never fall asleep in a given situation, and 3 representing a high chance. A score of 10 or more suggests the need for further evaluation.

More than 85% of patients having narcolepsy with cataplexy have the human leukocyte antigen (HLA) allele DQB1 0602, often in combination with HLA DRB1 1501, while only around 40% of the patients having narcolepsy without cataplexy have HLA DQB1 0602 suggesting increased heterogeneity in narcolepsy without cataplexy. Although the association of HLA DQB1 with narcolepsy is more specific, its usefulness as a screening or diagnostic test is limited by the fact that it has a high prevalence (as high as 12–38%) in the general population.

A loss of the hypothalamic neuropeptide hypocretin (also called orexin) causes narcolepsy with cataplexy; an autoimmune mechanism may be responsible for this loss. Approximately 90% of patients of narcolepsy with cataplexy have low cerebrospinal hypocretin levels while only 10–20% of patients classified as having narcolepsy without cataplexy show low cerebrospinal hypocretin levels.

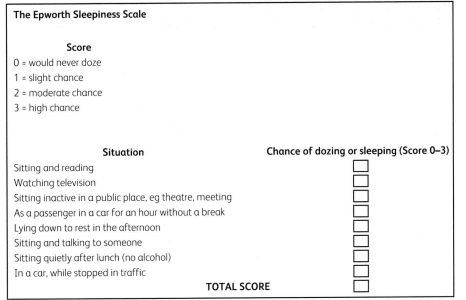

The Epworth Sleepiness Scale	
Score	
0 = would never doze	
1 = slight chance	
2 = moderate chance	
3 = high chance	
Situation	**Chance of dozing or sleeping (Score 0–3)**
Sitting and reading	☐
Watching television	☐
Sitting inactive in a public place, eg theatre, meeting	☐
As a passenger in a car for an hour without a break	☐
Lying down to rest in the afternoon	☐
Sitting and talking to someone	☐
Sitting quietly after lunch (no alcohol)	☐
In a car, while stopped in traffic	☐
TOTAL SCORE	☐

Fig 4 The Epworth Sleepiness Scale.

It is thought that simply a less severe injury to the orexin neurons occurs resulting in a small reduction in hypocretin levels in patients of narcolepsy without cataplexy.

1.1.8 Visual hallucinations

Dear Doctor,

Re: Mrs Christina Churchill, aged 63 years

I would be grateful for your opinion regarding this woman who has begun to experience visual hallucinations over the last 2 months. She has a history of depression in the past and takes amitriptyline 100 mg on, which she has done for many years, but is otherwise well. Physical examination is unremarkable.

Yours sincerely,

Introduction

There are many causes of visual hallucinations, which can usefully be classified as described in Table 8. Some cases present in the context of identifiable pre-existing disease (eg psychoses, dementia with Lewy bodies, Parkinson's disease dementia, migraine) but in those occurring *de novo* you must decide which patients are likely to have an intracranial structural lesion.

History of the presenting problem

Keeping in mind the working classification shown in Table 8, establish the features of the hallucination:

> Does the patient think it is real or not?

> What form does it take: simple (colours, shapes) or complex (people, animals)?

> Does it affect the whole visual field or just a hemifield?

> Is it affected by closing or moving the eye(s)?

> How long does it last?

> If the patient has experienced more than one, are they always the same?

> Are any other senses involved?

A full drug history is essential, including prescribed and non-prescribed drugs, as is a careful history of alcohol consumption.

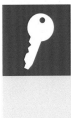

Key point

Medication for Parkinson's disease is particularly likely to induce visual hallucinations.

Other relevant history

Is the patient known to have a history of any of the following:

> stroke

> Parkinson's disease

> dementia

> psychiatric disease

> visual disturbance

> epilepsy

> alcohol abuse

> drug abuse?

Plan for investigation and management

Begin by explaining that under normal circumstances you need to confirm that the patient's neurological examination is normal.

Investigations

Key point

Any patient with complex visual hallucinations in the absence of a known neurological disease (Parkinson's disease, dementia, delirium tremens or acute confusional state) should have a brain scan.

Table 8 Working classification of visual hallucinations	
Type of hallucination	**Associated conditions**
Perceived by the patient as real	Psychiatric disorders Acute confusional states (delirium) Delirium tremens Parkinson's disease, associated with dopaminergic drugs and dementia Dementia with Lewy bodies Creutzfeldt–Jakob disease Some epileptic phenomena Drugs
Recognised as unreal by the patient (pseudohallucinations)	Purely visual: > Visual hallucinations secondary to eye disease, occurring in the whole visual field and disappearing with eye closure. Causes include cataracts, macular degeneration, glaucoma, choroidal neovascularisation > Hemianopic hallucinations indicate occipital lobe lesions (infarct, haemorrhage or tumour) causing unilateral (usually complex) visual hallucinations, which disappear with saccadic eye movements
	May involve hallucinations in other sensory modalities: > Associated with epileptic aura or seizures, stereotyped and usually short lived (<30 seconds), may be simple or complex occurring in a hemifield and not affected by saccadic eye movements. May be perceived as real by some patients > Associated with migraine aura: usually simple images, lines, fortification spectra and flashing lights > Peduncular hallucinosis: a rare syndrome of often complex visual hallucinations, sleep disturbance and agitation, that is secondary to a lesion in the midbrain or thalamus > Drugs

In addition, simple visual hallucinations that are stereotyped may well be ictal and patients with these should also have a brain scan.

The following investigations may also be appropriate:

> 'Screening tests' – FBC, electrolytes, renal and liver function tests (including gamma-glutamyl transpeptidase), glucose, inflammatory markers and chest X-ray.

> Electroencephalogram only if frequent suspected ictal events.

Management
This will obviously depend on the aetiological diagnosis:

> Epileptic visual hallucinations usually respond to antiepileptic medications.

> Occipital lobe lesions: the hallucinations are often self-limiting and the outcome will depend on the nature of the lesion, eg stroke or tumour.

> Parkinson's disease: if anticholinergic medications are being used (eg for tremor) these should be reduced and stopped; if hallucinations persist, dopaminergic medications should be reduced (dopamine agonists before levodopa preparations). With levodopa agents, there is a risk of worsening motor features of disease and therefore a risk:benefit calculation needs to be considered and discussed with the patients, eg if the patient is not unduly disturbed by the hallucinations there may be no indication to reduce therapy.

> Delirium tremens: this is an unlikely diagnosis in a patient who is not acutely unwell.

Further discussion
How might clinical examination help distinguish the cause of the hallucinations?

> Visual system: the presence of severely impaired visual acuity may be the cause. Visual field defects (see Section 1.2.11) will be extremely useful in alerting you to the presence of a space-occupying lesion and its likely location.

> Other neurological signs: evidence of Parkinson's disease, or particularly brainstem signs ('peduncular hallucinosis'), will also direct towards a particular cause.

1.2 Clinical examinations

1.2.1 Numb toes and foot drop

 Instruction
This 50-year-old man complains of numbness and tingling in his toes. He also says that he trips up frequently when walking. Please examine his legs.

General features

Although it might appear that these symptoms are most likely the result of peripheral nerve pathology, do not immediately rule out the possibility of central nervous system or combined (peripheral and central nervous system) pathology. In addition, the symptoms may be part of a more generalised disorder. Is the patient systemically well? Are there indications of any of the conditions discussed in Section 2.1? Look in particular for:

> Cachexia – which may suggest malignancy or alcoholism.

> Evidence of alcoholism/chronic liver disease.

> Vasculitic rash – probably indicating systemic vasculitis in this context.

> Signs of hypothyroidism – which can produce mild neuropathy.

> Postural hypotension (evidence of this is not likely to be available in PACES, but it is an issue that could be mentioned in discussion) – which is likely to indicate an autonomic component.

Neurological examination
Is this a peripheral or central nervous system disorder?
Look for the following patterns as you examine the legs.

Peripheral nervous system
Typical findings are:

> distal weakness

> absent ankle reflexes (+ knee reflexes)

> stocking distribution sensory loss

> wasting (if the problem is severe).

If there is a loss of sensation to temperature, but preservation of proprioception, power and reflexes, then consider a small-fibre neuropathy (see Section 2.1).

Central nervous system
Typical findings are:

> spastic tone

> weakness both proximally and distally, but predominantly in leg flexors

> brisk reflexes

> extensor plantars

> possible sensory level on abdomen or higher.

The arms may also provide useful information:

> Distal blunting to pin-prick with absent reflexes indicates a peripheral neuropathy.

> Loss of dexterity, absent biceps and supinator reflexes, and brisk triceps reflexes (inverted supinator / biceps reflex pattern) suggests a lesion at C5/6 leading to cervical cord compression below this level, as well as compression of the C6 root.

Are the signs symmetrical?
In this case, asymmetry in the context of an upper motor neurone syndrome would represent a Brown-Séquard syndrome, with loss of proprioception ipsilateral to the weak leg, and loss of pain and temperature sensation contralateral to the weak leg. Asymmetric lower motor neurone findings suggest mononeuritis multiplex or entrapment neuropathies (for a discussion on peripheral nerve lesions, see Section 1.2.2).

Further discussion
Hereditary motor and sensory neuropathy
This is common in PACES. Note the following:

> It is divided into type I (demyelinating), type II (axonal), type III (Dejerine–Sottas) and some other subtypes.

> Previously called Charcot–Marie–Tooth disease and peroneal muscular atrophy.

> Inverted champagne bottle legs (and similar process in arms/hands).

> Sensory abnormalities are much less prominent than motor ones.

> Lateral popliteal nerves are sometimes palpable.

Subacute degeneration of the spinal cord

> Vitamin B_{12} deficiency may cause a peripheral neuropathy, but can also result in additional corticospinal tract and dorsal column degeneration, which leads to combined upper and lower motor neurone features.

> Either the peripheral nervous system or spinal cord may be affected first in the early stages, but objective sensory abnormalities usually result from posterior column involvement and less often from peripheral neuropathy.

> Early in the course impaired joint position and vibration sense predominate.

> Typically the legs are affected before the arms.

> At presentation, 50% of patients have absent ankle jerks but are hyperreflexic at the knees; their plantars may be flexor initially, but eventually become extensor.

The clinical picture can be variable, but remember that this is a treatable condition and must not be missed.

1.2.2 Weakness in one leg

Instruction

This 46-year-old woman complains of weakness in her right leg. Please examine her legs.

General features

Is it painful for the patient to move about? In the presence of coexistent back and leg pain, a radiculopathy or plexopathy/sciatic nerve lesion should be suspected (Figs 5 and 6). More distal symptoms in the absence of back pain would indicate a more peripheral nerve lesion, eg common peroneal nerve palsy.

Neurological examination

The back
Check for:

> local tenderness – consider vertebral collapse or fracture

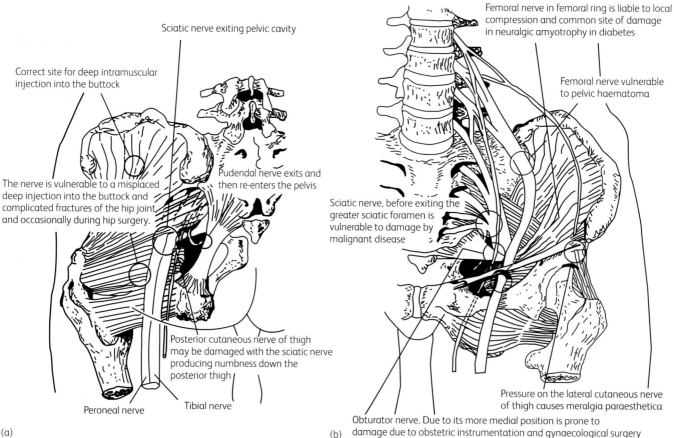

Sciatic nerve exiting pelvic cavity

Correct site for deep intramuscular injection into the buttock

The nerve is vulnerable to a misplaced deep injection into the buttock and complicated fractures of the hip joint and occasionally during hip surgery.

Pudendal nerve exits and then re-enters the pelvis

Posterior cutaneous nerve of thigh may be damaged with the sciatic nerve producing numbness down the posterior thigh

Peroneal nerve

Tibial nerve

(a)

Femoral nerve in femoral ring is liable to local compression and common site of damage in neuralgic amyotrophy in diabetes

Femoral nerve vulnerable to pelvic haematoma

Sciatic nerve, before exiting the greater sciatic foramen is vulnerable to damage by malignant disease

Pressure on the lateral cutaneous nerve of thigh causes meralgia paraesthetica

Obturator nerve. Due to its more medial position is prone to damage due to obstetric instrumentation and gynaecological surgery

(b)

Fig 5 Posterior **(a)** and anterior **(b)** nerve supply to the leg.

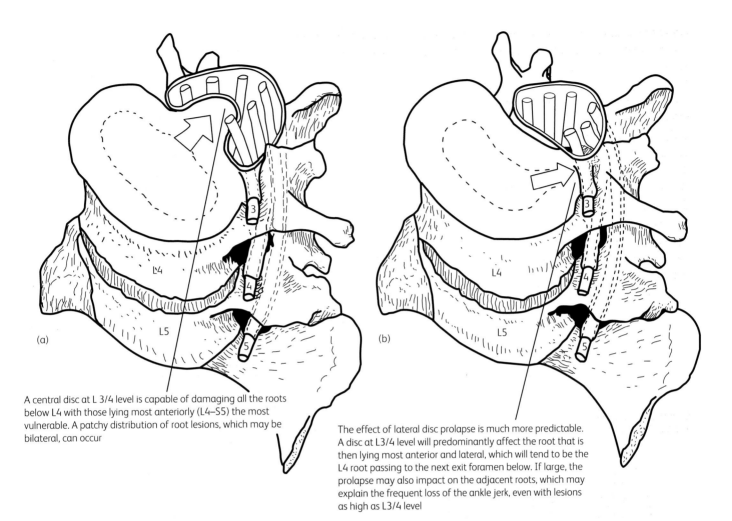

(a)

A central disc at L 3/4 level is capable of damaging all the roots below L4 with those lying most anteriorly (L4–S5) the most vulnerable. A patchy distribution of root lesions, which may be bilateral, can occur

(b)

The effect of lateral disc prolapse is much more predictable. A disc at L3/4 level will predominantly affect the root that is then lying most anterior and lateral, which will tend to be the L4 root passing to the next exit foramen below. If large, the prolapse may also impact on the adjacent roots, which may explain the frequent loss of the ankle jerk, even with lesions as high as L3/4 level

Fig 6 Anatomy of a central **(a)** and lateral **(b)** disc protrusion.

> paraspinal muscular spasm (in response to pain)

> restricted movement

> radiation of pain (Table 9).

Straight leg raising
Unilateral restriction may signify sciatic tension, but may also be limited by pain in the absence of nerve or root compression.

Legs
Check carefully for the following:

> Is there any wasting or fasciculation?

Table 9	Pain radiation in radicular lesions
Nerve	**Pain radiation**
L2 and L3	Pain radiates to anterior thigh
L4	Pain radiates through the knee and down the medial side of the calf to the medial malleolus
L5	Pain radiates through the buttock, down the posterolateral aspect of the thigh, through the lateral aspect of the calf and across the dorsum of the foot to the big toe
S1	Pain radiates through the inner buttock to the posterior aspect of the thigh, then through the posterolateral aspect of the calf to the lateral border of the foot

> Is there any weakness? If so, what is the distribution? Specifically check for lesions of the following roots:

> L2 weakness of hip flexion and thigh adduction

> L3 weakness of thigh adduction and knee extension

> L4 weakness of knee extension and ankle inversion

> L5 weakness of ankle dorsiflexion, inversion and eversion and dorsiflexion of the big toe

> S1 weakness of plantar flexion, eversion and knee flexion.

> Reflexes – are they normal? Hyporeflexia or areflexia is only seen with lesions of the following roots:

> L3 and L 4 – knee jerk

> S1 – ankle jerk.

> Sensation – sensory abnormalities in a well-defined distribution will help with localisation (Fig 7).

Look for evidence of the following peripheral nerve lesions
Common peroneal (or fibular) nerve palsy:

> causes foot drop with loss of ankle and toe dorsiflexion, and ankle eversion

> causes numbness over the lateral aspect of the lower leg and dorsum of the foot

> is usually due to pressure over the fibular head.

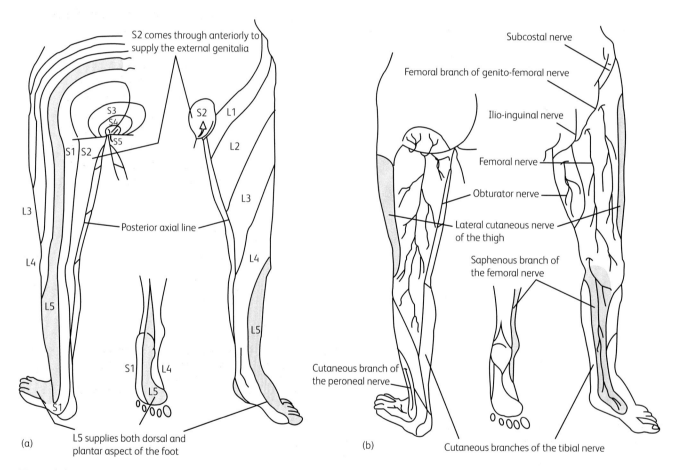

Fig 7 (a) Cutaneous nerve root supply of the leg (note the sensory areas spiral round the leg as shown). **(b)** Cutaneous nerve supply of the leg (the sensory areas are vertically distributed).

Key point
Differentiation between a common peroneal nerve lesion and an L5 root lesion is a common clinical dilemma: a common peroneal nerve lesion will cause weakness of ankle dorsiflexion and eversion, but will not affect inversion.

Posterior tibial nerve palsy (tarsal tunnel syndrome):

> may result in wasting in the intrinsic muscles of the foot, leading to weakness of toe flexion

> causes a burning sensation in the toes and sole of the foot, with reduced sensation on the sole

> usually results in entrapment behind and below the medial malleolus.

Femoral nerve lesion:

> causes wasting and weakness of knee extensors

> results in a depressed or absent knee jerk

> causes sensory loss in the anterior thigh and medial part of knee

> may be compressed by a psoas abscess or haematoma, or damaged by fractures of the pelvis, traction during surgery or thrombotic lesions of the vasa nervorum, eg in diabetes mellitus.

Sciatic nerve lesion:

> as the sciatic nerve splits to form the common peroneal nerve and posterior tibial nerve, damage to the sciatic nerve encompasses both of the above

> causes weakness in all muscles below the knee, as well as knee flexors

> causes sensory loss over the lateral border of the lower leg and entire foot, except the medial malleolus which is supplied by the saphenous nerve.

Key point
Because muscle groups receive innervation from more than one root, weakness may be minimal in someone with a single root lesion. Thus, in the case of severe weakness, eg complete foot drop, a peripheral nerve lesion or multilevel radiculopathy must be implicated. Furthermore, weakness that fails to conform to a simple pattern may be due to a lumbosacral plexus lesion.

Hazard
A common clinical mistake is to expect loss of the ankle jerk with foot drop. If this is the case it suggests involvement of both L5 and S1.

Further discussion
What are the causes of back and unilateral leg pain?
There are many causes of back pain. Radiation to a leg implies involvement of nerve root or lumbosacral plexus and limits the differential diagnosis (Table 10). L5 and S1 are the most commonly affected nerves in degenerative disease; L4 is involved occasionally, but L2 and L3 rarely – and if they are, the diagnosis is not likely to be simple degeneration.

Table 10 Causes of back and leg pain

Site of lesion	Diagnoses
Radiculopathy	Disc disease Degenerative spinal disease Infective spinal disease (pyogenic abscess and tuberculosis) Malignant spinal disease (secondary tumour and myeloma) Intrinsic, eg secondary tumour and myeloma Extrinsic, eg extramedullary, nerve sheath tumour and meningeal infiltration
Plexopathy/sciatic nerve lesion	Pelvic retroperitoneal mass Tumour Haematoma Abscess Hip fracture Misplaced deep muscular injection

Table 11	Causes of spastic paraparesis	
Common	**Uncommon**
Multiple sclerosis Cerebral palsy Spinal injury Cord compression, eg cervical spondylosis, tumours, abscess and vertebral fracture/dislocation	Genetic conditions, eg hereditary spastic paraplegia, Friedreich's ataxia and spinocerebellar ataxias Vitamin B_{12} and E deficiencies Vascular malformations Syphilis/HIV/human T-cell lymphotropic virus-1 Syringomyelia Anterior spinal artery occlusion Motor neurone disease

1.2.3 Spastic legs

Instruction

This man complains of stiffness and heaviness in his legs and has difficulty walking. Please examine his legs.

General features

Stiffness or heaviness is more suggestive of upper rather than motor neurone weakness, ie spastic paraparesis rather than peripheral neuropathy. The causes of a spastic paraparesis are listed in Table 11. Patients with weak legs will often have walking aids or wheelchairs next to the bed. There is often coincidental sphincter involvement so a catheter bag may be present.

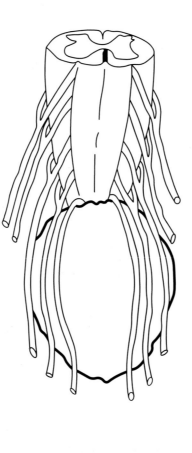
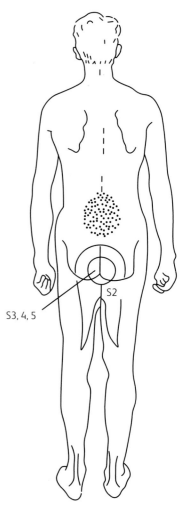

Fig 8 Conus lesion of the spinal cord. A lesion of the conus will affect the sacral roots from the inside outwards, hence the perianal and perineal areas are involved first, with progressive numbness and often surprisingly little pain.

Take note of the patient's speech during introductions: if it is slurred, then the patient may have multiple sclerosis, cerebral palsy, one of the rare genetic conditions or motor neurone disease. While you are shaking the patient's hand, also have a look to see if there is wasting (motor neurone disease) or ataxia (multiple sclerosis or genetic conditions) in the hands. Look for signs of surgical or traumatic injury along the whole of the spine.

Neurological examination

Motor

Tone will be increased in the leg muscles, particularly in the extensors. This results in an increase in tone on rapid flexion at the knee (a 'spastic catch'). There may be clonus at the ankles, which is best tested with the knee flexed. Power will be reduced in a 'pyramidal pattern', ie extensors less affected than flexors in the legs – indeed the extensors may be strong. Deep tendon reflexes will be brisk. If the weakness is severe then coordination will be difficult to assess. Plantar responses will be extensor, unless there is concurrent peripheral neuropathy (eg subacute combined degeneration of the cord).

 Key point

Vitamin B_{12} deficiency may cause a peripheral neuropathy, but may also result in additional corticospinal tract and dorsal column degeneration, leading to combined upper and lower motor neurone features. The clinical picture can be variable, but remember that this is a treatable condition and must not be missed.

Sensory

There may be a 'sensory level' if the sensory tracts are also involved, but they may also be spared (eg motor neurone disease).

 Hazard

Although demonstrating a sensory level points to the spinal cord, it is notoriously inaccurate at localising the level of the pathology. You should therefore use all possible clinical signs to help you. For example, a patient with a sensory level at the umbilicus (T10) who also has brisk arm reflexes is likely to have a lesion in the cervical cord above C5, rather than at T10. The significance of this is that it is the cervical cord that requires imaging, not the thoracic cord. It is generally much better to start imaging at the top (cervical) and work down, rather than the other way round (Fig 9).

Gait

In routine clinical practice and in PACES always ask the patient to walk, giving them whatever assistance is necessary (the examiner will stop you if there isn't time and they want to start asking questions). The patient may walk with a spastic gait which, if severe, becomes 'scissoring', ie legs crossing over each other as the patient walks.

Further discussion

An acute onset or an acute deterioration on the background of a chronic progressive story is a medical emergency and should prompt urgent imaging of the spine. A more slowly progressive onset can be investigated less urgently.

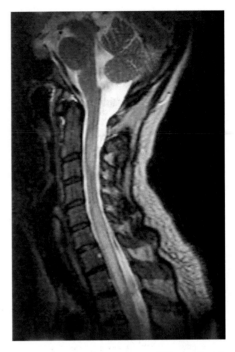

Fig 9 Increased signal on a T2-weighted sagittal MRI of the cervical cord, which is indicative of an intrinsic lesion and probably inflammatory.

Remember that bilateral cortical lesions affecting the leg areas of both primary motor cortices can cause a spastic paraplegia: this is classically associated with a parasagittal meningioma.

1.2.4 Gait disturbance

 Instruction

This woman has unsteadiness and difficulty in walking. Please examine her gait and proceed with your neurological examination to establish the diagnosis.

General features

The common causes of gait disturbance are given together with their main characteristics in Table 12.

Table 12 Commonly encountered abnormal gaits

Diagnosis	Main characteristic
Parkinson's disease	Shuffling/stooped
Cerebellar ataxia	Wide based
Peripheral neuropathy	High stepping
Diffuse cerebrovascular disease	*Marche à petit pas*
Proximal myopathy	Waddling
Pyramidal tract involvement – unilateral	Circumduction
Pyramidal tract involvement – bilateral	Scissor gait

General observation on introduction to the patient may yield some clues to the diagnosis:

> Parkinson's disease is suggested by the patient looking hypomimic (paucity of facial expression), infrequently blinking and having difficulty with holding saliva in the mouth due to a poor swallow frequency. Careful observation of the hands may reveal an asymmetrical 3–6 Hz resting 'pill-rolling' tremor.

> The patient with cerebellar ataxia may infrequently have a head tremor or 'titubation' and an intention tremor in the arms on shaking hands; they may also have a slurring dysarthria.

> The patient with peripheral neuropathy may have wasting in the hands and be wearing bilateral splints or ankle–foot orthoses.

> Diffuse cerebrovascular disease is often associated with a dementia when severe enough to cause gait impairment and the patient may have a pseudobulbar palsy with dysarthria.

Neurological examination

The patient should be asked to walk a distance of at least 10 metres as normally as possible. Make sure that you walk alongside the patient as you test their gait if they appear to be very imbalanced. Based on this inspection the most probable diagnosis should be made and then corroborating signs sought on examination.

Is it Parkinson's disease?
Look specifically for these features, remembering that many of them may be asymmetrical:

> Gait is typically short stepped, shuffling and festinant, with reduced or absent arm swing. In early disease, a slight reduction in arm swing on one side may be the only abnormality. Freezing of gait occurs later in the disease. The patient will often have problems initiating walking, but once they have started they then have difficulty stopping.

> Posture is flexed, stooped and when severe is referred to as 'simian'.

> Hypomimia, ie paucity of facial expression with 'mask-like' facies and a reduced blink rate.

> The rest tremor of the hands is classically pill-rolling and most marked at rest. It is best seen with the hands resting, palms facing inwards on the lap or over the edge of an armchair. The tremor may be intermittent and if not seen can be elicited by mental distraction, such as counting back from 20, or it often comes on with walking. It is typically asymmetrical. Tremor seen in the legs is highly suggestive of Parkinson's disease. Tremor may also occur in the chin, neck and tongue.

> Bradykinesia, ie slowness and fatigability of rapid movements. Ask the patient to open and close each hand as widely and as rapidly as possible, or to tap the thumb of one hand with each finger of the same hand in rapid succession with the widest amplitude possible. If they are not obviously slow, then continue this exercise at least 10 times to demonstrate decrement in rate and amplitude. An extra-pyramidal syndrome cannot be diagnosed without this feature.

> Extra-pyramidal rigidity with 'cogwheeling', ie the combination of rigidity and tremor, is best demonstrated by a slow and gentle rotation of the wrist.

> Ask the patient to write a phrase such as 'Mary had a little lamb' several times, looking for the development of micrographia. Ask the patient to draw a spiral, which may demonstrate tremor as well as micrographia.

> Note that the glabellar tap (which involves tapping the glabella and observing whether the patient blinks) is a non-specific test that is not clinically useful, although it used to be said that failure of this response due to fatigue (ie blinking to stop with repeated taps) indicated Parkinson's disease, especially in younger patients.

Drug-induced parkinsonism may appear clinically identical, although it tends to be more symmetrical. Wilson's disease may present with parkinsonism and is associated with Kaiser–Fleisher rings (which are usually only visible with a slit lamp).

Is it cerebellar disease?

The following are features of cerebellar disease:

> titubation (head tremor) – is uncommon

> dysarthria (scanning speech)

> nystagmus (horizontal and jerky) and jerky pursuit eye movements

> limb ataxia – upper limb (failure of rapid alternating movements, intention tremor and dysmetria with past pointing) and lower limb (heel–shin ataxia, wide-based gait and unable to perform heel–toe walking).

Is it peripheral neuropathy?

See Section 2.1.1 for further detail on peripheral neuropathy. The neuropathy may be a polyneuropathy, which will lead to symmetrical signs in a 'glove-and-stocking' distribution, or less commonly is due to bilateral mononeuropathies affecting the common peroneal or sciatic nerves, which are more likely to be asymmetrical. The patient's gait is often 'high-stepping' as a consequence of both bilateral foot drop and sensory loss. The main findings are:

> wasting distally in the legs, feet and hands

> possible fasciculations if there is axonal loss

> atrophic changes in the skin (oedematous, purple, hairless and pigmented) due to loss of autonomic and sensory fibres

> ulcers associated with pressure points (heel, between toes and sacrum)

> reduced tone, although this is often difficult to differentiate from normal

> distal weakness (foot drop and hand weakness)

> reduced or absent reflexes

> glove-and-stocking sensory loss.

Is it diffuse cerebrovascular disease?

Patients with either bilateral large vessel frontal infarcts or subcortical ischaemic leucoencephalopathy may have a 'frontal apraxic' gait, which characteristically leads to a *marche à petit pas* appearance and is commonly mistaken for the gait of Parkinson's disease. In *marche à petit pas*, the steps are small, broad-based, 'stuck to the floor' and shuffling. Turning requires several steps and there may (in contrast to Parkinson's disease) be excessive arm swing. The stance is upright with the centre of gravity being normal, as opposed to shifted forwards as in Parkinson's disease. There is often poor gait initiation, but this is also seen in Parkinson's disease.

In the patient with diffuse cerebrovascular disease there are often symmetrical extra-pyramidal signs that are more severe in the legs than the arms or face. *Marche à petit pas* is therefore sometimes termed 'lower-body parkinsonism'. There is no resting tremor and the bradykinesia is symmetrical. The rigidity seen with frontal lobe disease (sometimes called *Gegenhalten*) is often due to poor attention and not due to a true increase in tone. Other diseases that can cause a frontal apraxic gait include hydrocephalus and subdural haematomas: these should be considered in any patient, especially if their gait disorder is isolated.

Is it myopathic?

Look for the following features:

> The patient may have 'myopathic facies' with wasting of temporalis and muscles of mastication.

> Waddling gait – failure to stabilise the pelvis caused by predominant involvement of pelvic girdle and proximal leg muscles.

> Wasting of affected muscle groups.

> Usually more prominent proximal weakness – distal myopathies are rare apart from myotonic dystrophy.

> Reflexes are preserved until there is severe muscle wasting.

> No sensory signs.

Is it a spastic gait?

In unilateral upper motor neurone syndromes, the gait is stiff with circumduction and toe dragging of the affected leg. When bilateral upper motor neurone lesions occur both legs are stiff and patients develop a scissoring gait (see Section 1.2.3). The common signs are:

> Spastic tone, pyramidal weakness, brisk reflexes and extensor plantar responses – these are all upper motor neurone signs.

> There may be a sensory level when there is spinal cord disease.

Hazard

In routine clinical practice, do not forget to look beyond the neurological system for important diagnostic clues.

> Does the patient look as though they have lost weight? Is there lymphadenopathy? Are there masses in the breast, or on abdominal and rectal examination? Is the chest examination normal? If metastatic disease is suspected, which may apply to some cases of cerebellar, neuropathic, spastic or myopathic gait disturbance, then a full systemic examination should be performed.

> If vascular disease is suspected then a full cardiovascular assessment is required, including heart rhythm, murmurs, bruits and evidence of hypercholesterolaemia and chronic smoking.

Further discussion

The differentiation of frontal gait apraxia and idiopathic Parkinson's disease can sometimes be difficult, especially in older patients where the two diseases may coexist. Patients who have Parkinson's disease and have been treated for it can sometimes be difficult to assess blindly without the history, but the presence of only extra-pyramidal signs and the predominance of the upper limbs and face being affected should make the diagnosis of idiopathic Parkinson's disease clearer.

1.2.5 Cerebellar syndrome

Instruction

This woman presents with a 2-month history of progressive imbalance and slurred speech. Please examine her gait/cranial nerves/arms (instruction could be to focus on any one of these).

General features

Multiple sclerosis, common in routine clinical practice and in PACES, would be high on the list of differential diagnoses. It is quite likely that her imbalance is due to cerebellar involvement, but you should also consider a spastic paraparesis (see Section 1.2.3). The common causes of a cerebellar syndrome are given in Table 13. The patient with cerebellar ataxia may have a head tremor or 'titubation' and an intention tremor in the arms when shaking hands. They may also have a slurring dysarthria and use walking aids or a wheelchair.

Table 13	Causes of a cerebellar syndrome	
Common	**Uncommon**
Multiple sclerosis	Genetic syndromes including spinocerebellar ataxias, Friedreich's ataxia, ataxia telangiectasia
Drugs: alcohol, phenytoin and carbamazepine	Prion disease
Neoplasms	Infections, eg tuberculosis and meningitis
Infarction/haemorrhage	Arnold–Chiari malformation
Paraneoplastic syndrome	Vitamin B_{12} and E deficiencies

Neurological examination

Gait ataxia

If you have not yet observed the gait, ask the patient to walk a distance of at least 10 metres as normally as possible. Make sure that you walk alongside the patient as you test their gait if they appear to be very imbalanced. A broad-based (to improve stability) ataxic gait is characteristic of cerebellar disease, but in mild cases the unsteadiness may be apparent only when walking heel-to-toe (tandem walking). In a unilateral cerebellar hemisphere lesion, there is unsteadiness towards the side of the lesion. In truncal ataxia there is difficulty sitting or standing without support. For discussion of other gait abnormalities see Section 1.2.4.

Subsequent examination should focus on the cerebellar system and then go on to examine other features to delineate the cause.

Key point

In midline or generalised cerebellar disease, an abnormal gait is likely to be the most prominent physical sign and coordination of the arms may appear normal.

Incoordination of movement

Cerebellar dysfunction causes impairment of the process of controlling movements once they have been initiated. This gives rise to ataxia (incoordination) with the following signs:

> Intention tremor – there is no tremor at rest, but when the patient moves a limb an oscillating tremor develops that increases in amplitude as the limb moves towards the target.

> Dysdiadochokinesia – this is the inability to carry out rapid alternating movements with regularity.

> Dysmetria – this is the inability to control smooth and accurate targeted movements. The movements are jerky with overshooting of the target, as manifested in the finger–nose and heel–shin tests.

Ataxic dysarthric speech

Speech can be slow, slurred and scanning in quality. In scanning speech, there is loss of variation of intonation and the words may be broken up into syllables. Ask the patient to say words with several consonants such as 'baby hippopotamus' and 'British constitution'.

Abnormal eye movements

> 'Jerky' pursuits – pursuit movements are slow, with catch-up saccadic movements on attempting to maintain fixation on the moving target.

> Dysmetria of saccades – on attempting to fixate on a target, the eyes overshoot and oscillate several times before fixation is achieved.

> Nystagmus – this is maximal on gaze towards the side of the lesion and is jerky, ie it has a slow and a fast phase. Nystagmus results from damage of the vestibular connections of the cerebellum.

Titubation

Nodding tremor of the head may occur, mainly in the anterior–posterior (nodding) plane.

Altered posture

A unilateral cerebellar lesion may cause the head (and when the lesion is recent and severe, also the body) to tilt towards the side of the lesion.

Hypotonia

Hypotonia is a relatively minor feature of cerebellar disease, resulting from depression of alpha and gamma motor neurone activity. Hypotonia can sometimes be demonstrated clinically by decreased resistance to passive movement (eg extension of a limb), by 'pendular' reflexes or by the rebound phenomenon. This occurs when the patient's outstretched arms are pressed down for a few seconds and then abruptly released by the examiner. The arms may rebound upwards and continue to oscillate for longer than expected.

Other features

Once it has been determined that the patient has a cerebellar syndrome, neurological and general examinations should be conducted to try and delineate the cause.

> If the patient has multiple sclerosis then they may have a spastic tetra/paraparesis, other brainstem signs (eg internuclear ophthalmoplegia) or evidence of sphincter dysfunction (eg a suprapubic or transurethral catheter).

> If they have had a cerebellar stroke, then there may be other features of a lateral medullary syndrome (ipsilateral Horner's syndrome, ipsilateral facial and contralateral limb spinothalamic loss, ipsilateral palatal weakness and contralateral hemiparesis). The ataxia in such cases is ipsilateral and the patient may have evidence of other cardiovascular risk factors, eg a coronary artery bypass graft scar, atrial fibrillation or diabetes mellitus. A cerebellar haemorrhage can have catastrophic consequences and lead to rapid deterioration in the patient's level of consciousness due to brainstem compression: they may have a surgical scar over the occiput where decompression has been performed and this should be looked for at the end of the examination.

> Cerebellar tumours usually present slowly but can present in a stroke-like manner. The patient may be pale and thin. The commonest tumours to metastasise to the cerebellum are from the lung and breast, and in routine clinical practice these systems need to be examined.

> Patients with chronic alcohol abuse often develop a chronic cerebellar syndrome that characteristically affects the lower limbs and gait more than the eyes and upper limbs. In such patients there may be signs of chronic liver disease and portal hypertension.

> Rare genetic syndromes may prominently affect the cerebellum and other neurological systems may be involved, eg spastic paraparesis and peripheral polyneuropathy in Friedreich's ataxia.

Further discussion

There are many rare causes of a cerebellar syndrome, but common ones such as alcohol and anticonvulsants must not be forgotten and should be mentioned before the rarer causes in giving a differential diagnosis. The examiners may ask you to discuss the molecular mechanism of the spinocerebellar and Friedreich's ataxias, which are part of a group of rare genetic disorders called the 'triplet repeat diseases' because they are associated with an expanded number of trinucleotide repeats in disease states. If you are led into this line of questioning then it is a good sign: the examiners think you have done well!

1.2.6 Weak arm/hand

Instruction

This 60-year-old woman has pain in her right arm and hand. Please examine her arms.

General features

It is unlikely in the context of PACES, but is the patient cachectic or clubbed? Is there lymphadenopathy? Any of these features would suggest malignancy. Check carefully for breast masses and also for any abnormal chest signs, particularly at the lung apex where a Pancoast tumour might be found (indicated by wasting of the intrinsic hand muscles and Horner's syndrome). Are both radial pulses equally palpable, and is the blood pressure (BP) the same in both arms? A positive Adson's test (decrease in the radial pulse when the patient turns her head to the affected side and breathes in deeply) may indicate subclavian artery compression, eg by a cervical rib, but the test may also be positive in normal subjects. Is there a characteristic skin rash of herpes zoster?

Musculoskeletal

> Observe how the woman moves her neck and shoulder, eg when removing her clothing before being examined. If movement of the neck is painful, then this will be held rigid: if the shoulder is painful then the normal scapulohumeral rhythm of movement, whereby the arm moves in the shoulder joint before the scapula moves, will be reversed.

> Feel for local tenderness of muscles of the back of the scalp, neck and shoulder, and also for tenderness of the shoulder joint itself.

Neurological examination

Root/radicular lesion

Look for signs of nerve root lesions as shown in Table 14, the most common roots to be affected being C5–C7. Look also for the following:

> An inverted brachioradialis jerk, which occurs when finger flexion is the only response to an attempt to elicit the normal biceps or supinator jerk. This may indicate

Nerve root	Weakness	Hyporeflexia	Sensory changes
C5	Deltoid Infraspinatus Supraspinatus	Biceps Brachioradialis Biceps	Shoulder tip Outer part of upper arm
C6	Biceps Brachioradialis Wrist flexors	Brachioradialis	Lateral aspect of forearm, thumb and index finger
C7	Triceps Wrist extensors	Triceps	Middle finger
C8	Intrinsic muscles of hand	Triceps Finger	Little and ring fingers
T1	Intrinsic muscles of hand	None	Medial aspect of forearm

Table 14 Signs in affected cervical nerve roots

a spinal cord lesion at C5–C6, resulting in lower motor neurone signs at the level of the lesion (ie loss of C5–C6 reflexes) and upper motor neurone signs below the lesion (ie brisk C7 (triceps) and C8 (finger flexion) reflexes; and pyramidal signs in the legs).

> If there is dissociated sensory loss (loss of pain and temperature with intact proprioception) in a cape-like distribution (ie suspended sensory level, see Fig 10) and lower motor neurone weakness, it is likely that there is an intrinsic cord lesion such as a syrinx. Other signs may include Horner's syndrome (if the lesion extends to the T1 segment) and pyramidal weakness below the level of the lesion.

Key point

If the T1 nerve root is affected, Horner's syndrome may be present because of damage to the adjacent sympathetic plexus.

Peripheral nerve lesion

Look for evidence of the following peripheral nerve lesions (see also Section 2.1).

Median nerve lesion:

> Signs and symptoms of carpal tunnel syndrome (see Section 2.1).

> If only the anterior interosseous branch of the median nerve is damaged, the patient will be unable to perform the ring sign (pinch grip) resulting in the thumb and index fingers assuming an extended position. Also there is pronation weakness when the elbow is in a flexed position (the latter is due to weakness of pronator quadratus). The ring sign involves flexion of the distal phalanges of the thumb (flexor pollicis longus) and index finger (flexor digitorum profundus); there are no sensory changes (pure motor branch).

> In an elbow lesion (pronator teres syndrome), apart from a weakness of thumb abduction there is a weakness of flexion of the distal phalanges of the thumb and the adjacent two fingers (anterior interosseous branch function); sensory changes are as in carpal tunnel syndrome plus there is decreased sensation over the thenar region extending up to the wrist.

Ulnar nerve lesion:

> Most commonly damaged at the elbow.

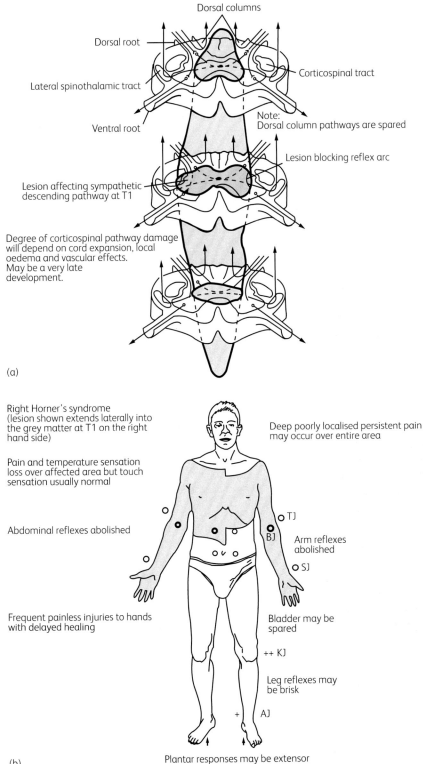

(a)

Dorsal columns

Dorsal root

Corticospinal tract

Lateral spinothalamic tract

Ventral root

Note:
Dorsal column pathways are spared

Lesion blocking reflex arc

Lesion affecting sympathetic descending pathway at T1

Degree of corticospinal pathway damage will depend on cord expansion, local oedema and vascular effects. May be a very late development.

(b)

Right Horner's syndrome (lesion shown extends laterally into the grey matter at T1 on the right hand side)

Deep poorly localised persistent pain may occur over entire area

Pain and temperature sensation loss over affected area but touch sensation usually normal

Abdominal reflexes abolished

TJ

BJ

Arm reflexes abolished

SJ

Frequent painless injuries to hands with delayed healing

Bladder may be spared

++ KJ

Leg reflexes may be brisk

+ AJ

Plantar responses may be extensor

Fig 10 Lesion in central cord at C5–T6 level. **(a)** Anatomical diagram. Note that the decussating spinothalamic pathways are blocked across the length of the central lesion. This may be slightly asymmetrical as shown, extending from C3 to T9 on the right and C4 and T8 on the left. Spinothalamic sensation below this level would be unaffected. **(b)** The clinical picture. AJ, ankle jerk; BJ, biceps jerk; KJ, knee jerk; SJ, supinator jerk; TJ, triceps jerk.

> Wasting of first dorsal interosseous appears first, but later there may be involvement of the other dorsal interossei and hypothenar eminence.

> Difficulty abducting and adducting outstretched fingers.

> Froment's sign – distal thumb flexion (adductor pollicis weakness) when a patient is asked to pinch a sheet of paper between the thumb and second metacarpal.

> Sensory loss over the little finger and the medial half of the ring finger.

> If the deep palmar branch (purely motor) is compressed in Guyon's canal (which runs between the pisiform and hook of the hamate) there will be wasting and weakness of the interossei, especially the first dorsal and adductor pollicis; hypothenar muscles are usually spared.

Radial nerve lesion:

> Most commonly damaged at the spiral groove of the humerus.

> Major feature is weakness of wrist and finger extensors (wrist drop).

> Weakness of forearm flexion with forearm midway between pronation and supination (due to brachioradialis involvement).

> Sparing of triceps occurs if the lesion is at or distal to spiral groove.

> Sensory loss over dorsum of hand between the lateral two digits.

> If only the posterior interosseous branch of the radial nerve is involved there is wrist extension, but with radial deviation because the extensor carpi radialis muscle is spared; brachioradialis and triceps normal; and there are no sensory changes (pure motor branch).

Axillary nerve lesion:

> wasting of deltoid

> weakness of shoulder flexion, abduction and extension

> sensory loss over lateral deltoid.

Key point

Generalised axonal peripheral neuropathies will affect the legs before the arms and are generally symmetrical. Inflammatory or demyelinating neuropathies may pick off individual nerve fibres and so could affect an arm first.

Hazard

Myopathies that affect distal before proximal muscles are rare. However, one form of inflammatory muscle disorder should be considered – inclusion body myositis (see Section 2.2). In this there is typically disproportionate and marked weakness in the wrist and finger flexors relative to the corresponding extensors (so would cause difficulty carrying a briefcase), and disproportionate weakness of knee extensors compared with hip flexors.

Further discussion

What are the neurological causes of pain in the arm?
See Table 15.

Neuralgic amyotrophy (brachial neuritis)
This is characterised by acute onset of excruciating unilateral (although it may be bilateral) arm (usually shoulder) pain, followed by shoulder and parascapular muscle weakness several days later; the pain is so severe that it is often confused with the pain of a myocardial infarction. Presentation and nerve involvement can be variable. Sensory changes are minimal. There may be subsequent rapid wasting of arm muscles.

Site of lesion	Diagnoses
Cerebral	Thalamic lesion and extrapyramidal disorder
Spinal cord	Syringomyelia and tumour
Nerve root	Disc prolapse, vertebral collapse, trauma and postherpetic
Brachial plexus	Pancoast's syndrome and brachial plexopathy, eg neuralgic amyotrophy, cervical rib, subclavian artery aneurysm and trauma
Peripheral nerve	Entrapment neuropathies, paraneoplastic, vasculitis and diabetes
Muscle	See Section 2.2

Table 15 Neurological causes of arm pain

Phrenic nerve involvement can result in significant breathlessness. Precipitating factors include recent trauma, severe exercise, surgery, infection or vaccination. It may rarely be hereditary. The prognosis is good, with a spontaneous recovery rate of over 90%.

1.2.7 Proximal muscle weakness

Instruction

This man has muscle weakness which has progressively got worse over the last 6 months. Please examine his limbs.

General features

Look for signs that may give diagnostic clues for the causes of proximal muscle weakness (Table 16), in particular:

> skin, eg purpura of steroid treatment, and much less likely malar rash in systemic lupus erythematosus (SLE), Gottron's papules and heliotrope rash in dermatomyositis

> skeletal, eg joint swelling in SLE and rheumatoid arthritis

> endocrine, eg cushingoid appearance in glucocorticoid excess and tremor in hyperthyroidism.

Consider 'could this man have myotonic dystrophy?', which is very much commoner in PACES than in routine clinical practice: look for myopathic

Cause	Diagnoses
Drugs	Alcohol, corticosteroids and statins
Endocrine	Adrenal insufficiency, Cushing's disease, hyperthyroidism, hypothyroidism and acromegaly
Inflammatory	Dermatomyositis and polymyositis
Rheumatological	SLE, rheumatoid arthritis and polymyalgia rheumatica
Metabolic	Glycogen and lipid storage diseases, and mitochondrial disease
Genetic	Limb girdle muscular dystrophies, facioscapulohumeral dystrophy and Duchenne/Becker muscular dystrophy

Table 16 Causes of proximal myopathy

SLE, systemic lupus erythematosus.

facies (drooping eyes/mouth and a sad/lifeless expression), ptosis, frontal balding and wasting of facial/neck/shoulder girdle muscles.

In routine clinical practice also check the following factors:

> cardiovascular, eg cardiomyopathy in alcohol, amyloidosis, glycogen storage diseases, inflammatory myopathies and muscular dystrophies

> gastrointestinal, eg hepatomegaly in metabolic storage diseases and amyloidosis.

Neurological examination

Look particularly for muscle wasting, and also for the presence of pseudohypertrophy of the calf muscles, most typically seen in Duchenne muscular dystrophy or Becker muscular dystrophy.

It is very important to determine the distribution of the weakness, eg bilateral, proximal or distal, or more focal. If the patient has difficulty rising from a squatting position (hip muscles) or combing his hair (shoulder girdle), then the weakness is proximal; if the patient has difficulty standing on his toes (gastrocnemius/soleus) or doing fine movement with the hands (intrinsic hand muscles), then the muscle weakness is distal.

If myotonic dystrophy is a possibility, try to elicit myotonia by asking the patient to grip your fingers as hard as they can, relax, and then repeat the grip/relaxation cycle a few times (offer two fingers, but not more or you may get hurt if the patient is strong!).

Hazard

Myopathy does not cause sensory signs. Do not diagnose a purely myopathic condition if sensory signs are present.

Key point

Do not forget to check whether there is also wasting and weakness in sternomastoid muscles (eg myotonic dystrophy) and facial muscles (some forms of muscular dystrophy or myotonic dystrophy).

Hazard

Is the weakness fatiguable? Think of myasthenia gravis! Do not forget to check for extraocular muscle weakness by examining eye movements.

Further discussion

What are the causes of proximal muscle weakness?
See Table 16.

What are the causes of predominantly distal muscle weakness?
Myotonic dystrophy, inclusion body myositis and genetic distal myopathies (the latter are rare).
See Section 2.2.

1.2.8 Muscle wasting

Instruction

This man has muscle wasting in his right arm and hand. Please examine his cranial nerves and his arms.

General features

Lesions that affect the ulnar nerve, T1 trunk or cord of the brachial plexus, T1 nerve roots, or the equivalent group of anterior horn cells can all cause wasting of the small hand muscles.

However, you need to establish whether the muscle wasting is limited to the hand or involves other regions as well, eg muscles in the shoulders or thighs, as the latter would indicate a more diffuse disease process, eg motor neurone disease (MND) (see Section 2.1.3).

Neurological examination

Cranial nerve examination

> Are there any upper motor neurone signs indicating a pseudobulbar palsy, eg a brisk jaw jerk, spastic tongue or emotional lability? This would indicate disease involvement of the corticobulbar pathways above the brainstem, eg in MND.

> Are there any lower motor neurone signs indicating a bulbar palsy, eg poor elevation of the soft palate or tongue weakness and atrophy? This would indicate the involvement of the motor nuclei of the cranial nerves IX–XII of the brainstem.

> If the T1 nerve root is involved (eg in a Pancoast tumour), Horner's syndrome may be present.

Limb examination

> Are there any upper motor neurone signs (spastic tone, brisk reflexes or extensor plantar responses)? These would be found in spinal cord lesions, eg cervical myelopathy above the level of C5, or diffuse disease processes, eg MND.

> Are there any lower motor neurone signs (wasting, fasciculations hypotonia or hyporeflexia)? These would be found in MND, chronic inflammatory demyelinating polyneuropathy (CIDP), multifocal motor neuropathy (MMN) or spinal cord compression at the levels of C5–T1 (indicating local anterior horn cell or radicular involvement).

> Sensory examination – in MND and MMN there is no sensory involvement. In cervical spondylosis, radicular findings often do not conform to textbook dermatomal descriptions. In CIDP there is often impairment of joint position and vibration sense, and less commonly of pain and temperature sensation.

Key point

MND and cervical myelopathy can sometimes be difficult to differentiate. The involvement of corticobulbar pathways, as suggested by the presence of a pseudobulbar palsy, would indicate the former as it puts the disease process above the spinal cord.

Hazard

It is crucial to differentiate MND from other potentially treatable conditions such as cervical spondylosis and MMN because of the better prognosis in the latter two conditions.

Further discussion

What are common mimics of motor neurone disease?
See Table 17.

Hazard

Wasting and weakness restricted to the small muscles of the hand (T1 lesion) should be considered the result of a Pancoast tumour until proven otherwise. Obtain a smoking history, look for nicotine staining and arrange a chest X-ray immediately.

Table 17   Mimics of motor neurone disease (MND)

Condition	Investigation(s)
Cervical/lumbar spondylotic myelopathy	MRI
Brainstem lesions, eg syrinx and stroke	MRI
MMN	Nerve conduction studies and anti-GM1 ganglioside antibody
Kennedy's disease (X-linked spinobulbar muscular atrophy)	Androgen receptor gene mutation
Myasthenia gravis	Single-fibre electromyelogram and anti-acetylcholine receptor antibody
CIDP	Nerve conduction studies and high protein in cerebrospinal fluid
Polymyositis or inclusion body myositis	Serum creatine kinase, electromyography and muscle biopsy
Thyrotoxicosis	Thyroid function tests
Paraproteinaemias	Serum protein electrophoresis

CIDP, chronic inflammatory demyelinating polyneuropathy; MMN, multifocal motor neuropathy.

1.2.9 Hemiplegia

Instruction

This man has weakness in his left arm and leg. Please examine his arms and legs.

General features

The most likely diagnosis is stroke, so look for evidence of vascular risk factors/disease, eg xanthelasma, corneal arcus, nicotine stains, scars on the chest or legs indicating surgery for ischaemic heart disease, scars in the neck indicating previous carotid surgery, the presence of a pacemaker, and bruising of the skin from use of antiplatelet agents or anticoagulants especially in older patients.

When introducing yourself to the patient take particular notice of how well he moves his limbs. Does he appear to have a visuospatial deficit suggesting right parietal cortical involvement? You should also note the presence of speech and language problems. Aphasia is unlikely in a right-handed subject, but you do not yet know if he is right or left handed. It is important to know if it is his dominant or non-dominant hand that is affected.

Neurological examination

The neurological examination should be broken down into motor, sensory, visual and cognitive elements.

Motor signs

The key features to look for are:

> Wasting – this may be present on the affected side due to disuse over time.

> Tone – usually increased on the affected side (may be normal or even reduced in the acute setting).

> Power – typically power is reduced in a pyramidal distribution (upper limb extensors weaker than flexors and lower limb flexors weaker than extensors, hence the arm tends to be held in flexion with a hyperextended leg).

> Reflexes – these are increased on the affected side.

> Plantar response – extensor (upgoing) on the affected side.

Key point

Do not forget to examine the power of the facial muscles. If weakness is present on the opposite side to the limb weakness, this would suggest a brainstem stroke. If the weakness is on the same side, the damage is most likely in the middle cerebral artery territory.

Sensory signs
Sensory signs are likely to be in the same distribution as the motor signs. Sensory loss has a negative impact on functional recovery, so it is important to assess it. Do not forget to assess proprioception as impairment in this modality will cause specific difficulties with rehabilitation.

Visual signs
The presence of a homonymous hemianopia has value in localising the lesion site. In acute stroke, there can be conjugate eye deviation ipsilateral to the side of the stroke.

Cognitive signs
Determine whether the patient has any deficit in either of these domains.

> Language function – briefly assess expressive and comprehension components (see Section 3.1).

> Visuospatial function – briefly look for visual and/or sensory inattention and/or extinction.

Once again, these features will have localising value to either the dominant (language) or non-dominant (visuospatial) hemisphere, and they suggest cortical involvement in the damage. Note that cortical signs can be present when only the white matter adjacent to the intact cortex is damaged, as this can effectively disconnect the cortical area from afferent and efferent connections. It is crucial to know about the presence of 'cognitive' signs when considering rehabilitation strategies.

Further discussion
In a patient with hemiplegic stroke the important questions are:

> Where is the lesion?

> What is the pathology?

> What is the mechanism?

Where is the lesion?
Hemiplegia may be caused by a lesion affecting the cerebral cortex in the arterial territory of the anterior or middle cerebral artery, the deep white matter or the brainstem. The Oxfordshire Community Stroke Project (OCSP) study classification is useful to help determine the anatomical site of the lesion (Table 18).

What is the pathology?
Stroke is much the commonest cause of hemiparesis, but there are various stroke mimics that need to be considered, such as a space-occupying lesion, seizure, migraine (hemiplegic migraine), hypoglycaemia, hyponatraemia and conversion disorder.

It is important to make the distinction between an ischaemic and a haemorrhagic stroke, but this cannot be reliably done by the bedside and neuroimaging is required to be certain.

What is the mechanism?
The classification of stroke is broadly into ischaemic and haemorrhagic.

Hazard

It is not possible to distinguish an ischaemic from a haemorrhagic stroke on the basis of the history and examination alone. Neuroimaging (usually with CT in the first instance) is the only reliable method of doing so.

Ischaemic stroke can be caused by thromboembolism from the heart (cardioembolic), extracranial atherosclerotic disease, small vessel disease (intracranial atherosclerotic disease) or can be cryptogenic. The presence of atrial fibrillation or carotid bruits is helpful in indicating the likely source of embolus, which has implications for optimal secondary preventative strategies.

Intracerebral haemorrhage are caused by:

1 Primary intracerebral bleed (80–85%):

> hypertension

> cerebral amyloid angiopathy.

2 Secondary intracerebral bleed (15–20%):

> oral anticoagulants

> underlying bleeding disorder

> tumour (primary or secondary)

> ruptured aneurysms and vascular malformations (eg arteriovenous malformations, cavernomas)

> cerebral venous sinus thrombosis

> cerebral vasculitis

> eclampsia.

3 Rare causes include:

> trauma

> reversible cerebral vasoconstriction syndrome.

Table 18 The Oxfordshire Community Stroke (OCS) Study sub-classification system

OCS classification	Site of infarction	A combination of
Total anterior circulation syndrome (TACS)	Implies large cortical stroke in middle cerebral artery, or middle and anterior cerebral artery territories	New higher cerebral dysfunction (eg dysphasia, dyscalculia and visuospatial disorder) *and* Homonymous visual field defect *and* Motor and/or sensory deficit involving at least two out of three areas of the face, arm or leg on the side opposite the lesion
Partial anterior circulation syndrome (PACS)	Implies smaller cortical stroke in the middle or anterior cerebral artery territories	Patients with two out of three components of TACS, *or* New higher cerebral dysfunction alone *or* A motor/sensory deficit more restricted than those classified as LACS (eg isolated hand movement)
Lacunar syndrome (LACS)	Implies a subcortical stroke due to small vessel disease	Pure motor stroke Pure sensory stroke Combined sensorimotor stroke Ataxic hemiparesis Dysarthria and clumsy hand Note that evidence of higher cortical involvement or disturbance of consciousness excludes a lacunar syndrome
Posterior circulation syndrome (POCS)		Ipsilateral cranial nerve palsy with contralateral motor/sensory deficit Bilateral motor and/or sensory deficit Disorder of conjugate eye movement Cerebellar dysfunction without ipsilateral pyramidal involvement (which if present is more likely to be ataxic hemiparesis – see LACS) Isolated homonymous visual field defect

1.2.10 Tremor

Instruction

This woman has a 12-month history of tremor. Please examine her neurologically to determine the cause.

General features

The common causes of a tremor are listed and discussed in Section 1.4.3. The main differential diagnosis is between essential tremor (ET) and the tremor of idiopathic Parkinson's disease.

Neurological examination

Is it Parkinson's disease?

Look specifically for these features, remembering that many of them may be asymmetrical:

> Hypomimia, ie paucity of facial expression with 'mask-like' facies and a reduced blink rate.

> The tremor, when present, is classically pill-rolling and most marked at rest, although in severe cases it will often be seen with posture and action. Rest tremor of the hands is best seen with the hands resting, palms facing inwards on the lap or over the edge of an armchair. The tremor may be intermittent and if it is not seen it can be elicited by mental taxation (eg asking the patient to count backwards from 100 by subtracting three each time, while saying the numbers out loud as they do so – this is known as 'serial threes') or it often comes on with walking.

> Bradykinesia, ie slowness and fatigability of rapid movements. Ask the patient to open and close each hand as widely and as rapidly as possible, or to tap the thumb with each finger of the same hand in rapid succession with the widest amplitude possible. If not obviously slow, continue

at least 10 times to demonstrate decrement in rate and amplitude. An extrapyramidal syndrome cannot be diagnosed without this feature.

> Extrapyramidal rigidity with 'cogwheeling', which feels like the combination of rigidity and tremor. This is best demonstrated by a slow and gentle rotation of the wrist.

Key point

Tremor seen in the lower limbs is highly suggestive of Parkinson's disease.

> Ask the patient to write a phrase such as 'Mary had a little lamb' several times until micrographia develops or you are sure it is absent (eg after two lines of writing).

> Ask the patient to draw a spiral, which may demonstrate tremor as well as micrographia.

> Note that the glabellar tap (which involves tapping the glabella and observing whether the patient blinks) is a non-specific test that is not clinically useful.

> Drug-induced parkinsonism may look identical to idiopathic Parkinson's disease, although it tends to be more symmetrical. Wilson's disease may present with parkinsonism and is associated with Kaiser–Fleisher rings (which are usually only visible with a slit lamp).

If time and the examiners allow it, ask the patient to walk if the following are present.

> Their posture is stooped, severe cases of which are referred to as 'simian'.

> Their gait is typically short stepped, shuffling and festinant, with reduced or absent arm swing. In early disease, a slight reduction in arm swing on one side may be the only abnormality. Freezing of gait occurs later in the disease.

Is it benign essential tremor?

This can look quite similar to the tremor of Parkinson's disease, but notice the absence of other signs of parkinsonism:

> Examination may be normal except for the tremor of outstretched arms, which may be worsened as the patient changes posture, eg to hold the palms of their hands downwards under their nose or to do the finger–nose test.

> If possible, ask the patient to hold a cup and saucer, or a glass of water, which often exacerbates tremor.

> The key difference in distinguishing ET from the tremor of Parkinson's disease is that ET occurs mostly

with posture and action and not at rest; whereas the tremor of Parkinson's disease is mostly at rest, although there is often a postural component.

> The tremor of ET interferes with activities, whereas some patients with Parkinson's disease do not notice their tremor initially or find it socially embarrassing because it is worst when they are not active.

Is it cerebellar disease?

The tremor of cerebellar disease is called an 'intention' tremor because it occurs with action, although when severe it can also occur at rest. The tremor is often severely functionally disabling and can render a patient virtually incapable of walking or using their arms. There will be other signs of cerebellar disease as outlined in Section 1.4.3.

Further discussion

The examiners may ask how you would proceed to differentiate the tremor types by investigation and their management. If there is still doubt after clinical examination then brain imaging can rule out other rarer diseases of the basal ganglia; and a fluoro-L-dopa or fluorodeoxyglucose positron emission tomography scan can sometimes be very helpful in demonstrating the characteristic asymmetrical reduction in signal in the basal ganglia seen in Parkinson's disease. Beta-blockers, anticholinergics and some anticonvulsants may help tremors, but often they only have a relatively modest effect. The use of anticholinergics in older patients needs to be undertaken with caution because they can produce neuropsychiatric deterioration, eg hallucinations and confusion.

1.2.11 Visual field defect

Instruction

This man has been noted by his optometrist to have restricted visual fields. Please examine his eyes.

General features

Is the patient thin and pale with 'waxy' skin (suggesting panhypopituitarism) or are there features of acromegaly? Are there signs of a previous stroke (facial asymmetry, upper limb held flexed and internally rotated and a lower limb extended with a circumducting gait)? Are there any aids for those with visual impairment present (white stick, magnifying glass or Braille books) beside the bed?

Examination of vision

Key point

In determining the site of the lesion, it is important to decide whether the visual field defect affects one or both eyes.

Monocular field defects

Visual field defects affecting one eye only are due to lesions in the visual pathway anterior to the optic chiasm, either within the eye or in the optic nerve (Fig 11a).

> A central or paracentral scotoma (loss of the visual field within or adjacent to the central area of vision) usually indicates damage to the macular photoreceptors (eg macular degeneration) or macular nerve fibres at or within the optic nerve (eg optic neuritis) (Table 19). It is important to look for associated features such

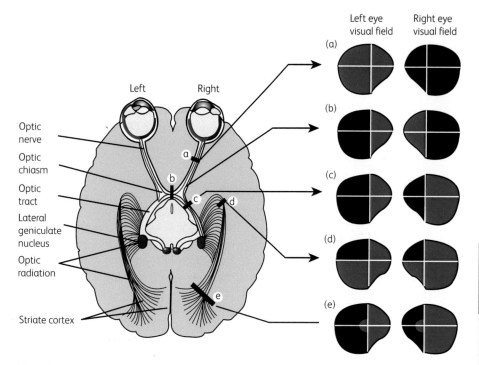

Left eye visual field   Right eye visual field

(a)

(b)

(c)

(d)

(e)

Fig 11 Patterns of visual field loss depend on the site of the lesion.

as reduced visual acuity, colour desaturation and a relative afferent pupillary defect. Is there papilloedema suggesting a local compressive lesion, such as optic nerve glioma?

> A dumb-bell shaped scotoma that covers both the central visual field and the blind spot is termed a caecocentral scotoma, which strongly implies optic nerve pathology.

> It is occasionally difficult to distinguish between an enlarged blind spot and a paracentral scotoma. Fundoscopy will reveal an abnormality of the optic disc (eg drusen or papilloedema) in the case of an enlarged blind spot.

> Horizontal/altitudinal field defects extend to the periphery but do not cross the horizontal midline. They most commonly occur in anterior ischaemic optic neuropathy due to vascular disease or giant cell (temporal) arteritis.

> A monocular segmental defect, for example a quadrantanopia in one eye only, may be due to retinal disease, such as ischaemia from a retinal artery branch occlusion or retinal detachment. Careful fundoscopy of the dilated eye is usually diagnostic.

Binocular field defects

Field defects affecting both eyes may be due to bilateral ocular pathology (eg glaucoma or macular degeneration) or bilateral optic nerve pathology (eg due to toxins or multiple sclerosis). More frequently, however, binocular field loss is due to chiasmal or retrochiasmal lesions.

> Does the field defect respect the vertical midline? If so, the lesion is either chiasmal (bitemporal hemianopia) or retrochiasmal

(homonymous hemianopia). Chiasmal lesions will eventually progress to involve the other visual field if left untreated.

> If the field defect crosses the vertical midline in each eye, the lesion must be anterior to the optic chiasm, indicating either ocular or optic nerve pathology.

> Bitemporal hemianopias (Fig 11b) are seen in lesions affecting the optic chiasm.

Key point

Typically pituitary lesions expand upwards into the optic chiasm resulting in a predominantly superior bitemporal hemianopia. Hypothalamic lesions expand downwards resulting in a bitemporal hemianopia that is most dense inferiorly.

> Lesions within the optic tract, optic radiation or striate (occipital) cortex cause homonymous visual field defects. These are typically hemianopic (Fig 11c), although quadrantanopias (Fig 11d) are seen in focal lesions within the temporal lobe (superior quadrants affected) or parietal lobe (inferior quadrants affected). The field defects tend to become more congruous, ie more similar in each eye, the more posterior the lesion.

> Macular-sparing homonymous field defects implicate the striate cortex (Fig 11e), which is commonly affected in a posterior circulation ischaemic event. The occipital pole, which is important in resolving the macular visual field, may additionally receive some blood supply from the middle cerebral artery.

Other examination

Once the characteristics of the visual field have been elucidated, it may be important to extend the clinical examination outside the visual system:

> If a pituitary lesion is suspected, look for features of acromegaly or panhypopituitarism.

> Other signs of multiple sclerosis should be sought in a young patient with signs of optic neuropathy: reduced visual acuity, a central scotoma, reduced colour appreciation and a relative afferent pupillary defect (Section 1.2.12). Look for ataxia and spastic paraparesis, etc.

> Check the vascular status in a patient with a homonymous hemianopic visual field defect. Look for signs of coexistent hemiparesis or hemisensory loss. Are there any cortical parietal signs such as alexia, acalculia or apraxia?

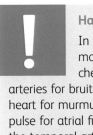

Hazard

In patients with monocular visual loss, check the carotid arteries for bruits, auscultate the heart for murmurs and feel the pulse for atrial fibrillation. Palpate the temporal arteries looking for tenderness suggesting giant cell arteritis. Check the inflammatory markers, particularly in any patient over the age of 50 years.

Further discussion

What are the possible causes of optic neuropathy?
See Table 19.

1.2.12 Unequal pupils

Instruction

This woman has an abnormality of her eyes. Please examine them.

Table 19	Causes of optic neuropathy
Type of lesion	**Example**
Genetic	LHON, Friedreich's ataxia
Compressive	Optic nerve glioma, sphenoidal wing meningioma or dysthyroid eye disease
Vascular	Ischaemia: due to arterial or venous compromise
Inflammatory	Sarcoidosis[1]
Demyelinating	Multiple sclerosis,[1] neuromyelitis optica,[1] ADEM
Infections	Syphilis,[1] tuberculosis[1]
Toxic	Tobacco–alcohol amblyopia, heavy metals
Nutritional	Vitamin B_{12} and folate deficiency
Iatrogenic	Drugs: chloramphenicol, isoniazid, ethambutol
Other	Paraneoplastic

1 Also a cause of optic neuritis.
LHON, Leber's hereditary optic neuropathy; ADEM, acute demyelinating encephalomyelitis.

Note that this case might also be found in Station 5: Eye examination.

General features

The causes of unequal pupils (anisocoria) are listed in Table 20. There is a clear clinical distinction to be made between patients who are noticed to have anisocoria but are asymptomatic, and those in whom the unequal pupils are part of a well-defined symptomatic disorder, eg brainstem stroke. Patients in PACES will virtually always fall into the former category. In a normal pupil miosis is caused by stimulation of the parasympathetic efferent fibres in the oculomotor nerve, whereas mydriasis is caused by activation of the sympathetic fibres from the superior cervical ganglion.

Key point

Simple or physiological anisocoria (<0.6 mm) is seen in about 20% of normal people.

Table 20	Common causes of miosis and mydriasis		
Abnormality	**Unilateral**		**Bilateral**
Miosis	Horner's syndrome Iritis Pilocarpine		Argyll Robertson pupils Pontine bleed
Mydriasis	Holmes–Adie syndrome Oculomotor nerve palsy Midbrain lesion Atropine Unilateral afferent pupillary defect		Bilateral afferent pupillary defect, eg bilateral optic atrophy

Eye examination

Which is the abnormal pupil? If the pupils respond to direct light, proceed to inspect them in bright and dim light:

> If anisocoria is greater in bright light than dim (ie is less marked in the dark), then the iris sphincter on the side of the lesion is defective. This indicates that there is a local iris problem or a parasympathetic defect such as oculomotor nerve palsy, ie the problem is on the side of the large pupil.

> If anisocoria is greater in dim light than bright (ie is more marked in the dark), then the iris dilator muscle on the side of the smaller pupil is defective. This indicates simple anisocoria or Horner's syndrome, ie the problem is on the side of the small pupil.

Having decided which is the abnormal pupil, then look for those of the following specific features that are relevant:

> ptosis

> irregularity of pupil

> inflammation of the iris

> light–near dissociation: the pupil does not react to light but does to accommodation. This is tested by asking the patient to look at something in the distance and then to focus on your finger held reasonably close to their nose (Table 21).

> afferent pupillary defect: the pupil will not react to light because of optic atrophy or severely diminished visual acuity from another cause. The swinging light test is used: on shining a light directly into the normal pupil, the normal pupil will constrict and so will the affected pupil through the consensual response to light. On quickly moving the light to shine directly on the affected pupil, the affected pupil will dilate because it has an impaired direct response to light.

> ophthalmoparesis

> optic atrophy.

When examining this woman, consider the conditions listed in Table 20, but particularly the following.

Horner's syndrome

Horner's syndrome consists of miosis, ipsilateral partial ptosis and sometimes anhidrosis. Although part of the syndrome, enophthalmos is not a useful sign. It results from impairment of ocular sympathetic innervation. If anhidrosis affects an entire half of the body and face, then the lesion is in the central nervous system; if it affects only the face and neck, then the lesion is in the preganglionic fibres; and if sweating is unaffected, the lesion is above the carotid artery bifurcation (see Section 1.2.13 and Fig 14). In the patient with Horner's syndrome, look for wasting of the muscles of the ipsilateral hand. This indicates a T1 lesion and flags the possibility of a Pancoast tumour.

Argyll Robertson pupils

This is almost always bilateral and consists of small irregular pupils that show light–near dissociation (ie poorly reactive to light, with better constriction to accommodation; Table 21).

Holmes–Adie syndrome

There is usually unilateral pupillary dilatation with poor constriction to light and accommodation, occurring in association with depressed deep tendon reflexes. This commonly affects young women. The pupil may become small over time. Results from a peripheral lesion of the parasympathetic autonomic nervous system.

Further discussion

Would you like to ask this woman some questions?

Your initial question would naturally be to ask the woman if she was aware of the problem with her pupil(s) or had any other problems with her eye(s) or brain. Regarding ocular/visual symptoms, check the following, the answers to which may be 'no':

> Is there any pain or redness, which might indicate iritis or acute angle closure glaucoma?

> Does she have any diplopia, suggesting oculomotor palsy in this context?

> Does she suffer from headache? Both migraine and cluster headache can cause episodic Horner's syndrome, which may become permanent.

> Does she suffer from photophobia when moving from dark to light? This is caused by a fixed dilated pupil failing to protect the retina in bright light.

> Is there a history of poor night vision in a patient with small, poorly reactive pupils?

If she says that she has no ocular/visual symptoms, then it would be appropriate to make brief enquiry about any general medical problems and follow any leads that this produces. Note new chest symptoms, particularly if she is a smoker (Pancoast tumour); also check for vascular risk factors and take a drug history, which must include the use of eye drops.

Table 21	Causes of light–near dissociation	
Pupil size	**Diagnoses**
Small pupils	Argyll Robertson pupils Long-standing Holmes–Adie pupils Diabetic neuropathy
Large pupils	Bilateral afferent pupillary defects Holmes–Adie pupils/tonic pupils Pretectal lesions (eg Parinaud's syndrome)

What would your approach to investigations and management be? This depends on the findings of history and examination. Remember the following:

> Any patient with bilateral tonic pupils, poorly reactive or irregular pupils, or pupils with light–near dissociation should have a Venereal Disease Research Laboratory test.

> Perform a chest X-ray in cases of Horner's syndrome (especially if preganglionic) (Fig 12).

> Imaging of the carotid artery is required in postganglionic Horner's syndrome.

> Imaging of the head is only required if other neurological features are present.

Hazard

Think of Pancoast tumour! Look for unilateral wasting of small hand muscles. Get a chest X-ray.

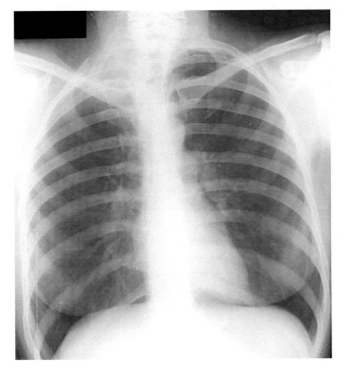

Fig 12 Right Pancoast tumour.

1.2.13 Ptosis

Instruction

This woman has an abnormality of her eyes. Please examine them.

Ptosis is abnormal lowering of the upper eyelid and is due to a problem with the levator palpebrae superioris muscle or its nerve supply (via the third, oculomotor, cranial nerve) or involvement of the sympathetic supply of the smooth muscle fibres of the superior tarsal muscle (Table 22). In assessing this patient, remember that many of the causes of ptosis would not be asymptomatic; those that might present without symptoms include congenital ptosis, disinsertion of levator, myasthenia gravis or Horner's syndrome.

General features

Look for the following:

> Are there any scars on the neck or chest wall which may be a result of previous surgery (eg carotid endarterectomy) or trauma?

> Is there any evidence of malignancy?

> Is there any wasting of the small muscles of the hand? This indicates involvement of the C8/T1 nerve roots, which may be affected, along with the sympathetic supply to the eyelid, by lesions in the neck.

Eye examination

The upper eyelid normally covers 1–2 mm of the cornea, and the lower lid just reaches the level of the cornea. Are the pupils normal? Are ocular movements normal? Are the irises different colours (heterochromia iridis), indicating either a congenital Horner's syndrome or Horner's syndrome occurring before the age of 2 years?

Look for the following patterns:

> Miosis, anhidrosis and enophthalmos with partial ptosis in Horner's syndrome. The pupillary asymmetry is more pronounced in low-light conditions.

> Complete ptosis and abnormal eye position and movement in third (oculomotor) nerve palsy, with a normal or dilated pupil.

> Partial ptosis with a sixth cranial nerve palsy and numbness in the distribution of the first or second division of the trigeminal nerve suggests a cavernous sinus or post-orbital lesion.

> Fatigability of the ptosis on looking up persistently, which would suggest myasthenia gravis; this may appear unilateral at onset.

> A loss of upper eyelid skin crease is suggestive of levator disinsertion.

Key point

Levator disinsertion
Disinsertion of the aponeurosis of levator palpebrae superioris from the tarsal plate is a common cause of unilateral ptosis in older patients, and is also associated with trauma. The important clinical sign is that the crease normally found on the upper eyelid is lost. There are no accompanying disorders of the pupil or external ocular movements. It is important to realise that these patients may complain of increasing ptosis at the end of the day, and may even report subjective (without objective) improvement after a Tensilon test. Therefore, differentiation from myasthenia gravis should be on different grounds (other neurological signs, positive response to an ice pack test, or the presence of anti-acetylcholine receptor antibodies). Surgical reinsertion can be offered for symptomatic cases.

It may be important to proceed with examining the remaining cranial nerves and the limbs, particularly if Horner's syndrome is present. For example, a brainstem lesion may present with a central Horner's syndrome, hemisensory loss, dysarthria, dysphagia, ataxia, vertigo and nystagmus. An assessment of limb fatiguability should also be made if myasthenia gravis is suspected.

Further discussion

What are the causes of ptosis?
See Table 22.

What are the causes of a Horner's syndrome?
See Figs 13 and 14.

What is the localising significance of anhidrosis?

Depending on the level of the lesion, impaired flushing and sweating may be found ipsilaterally. Anhidrosis affects the ipsilateral side of the body with central lesions. Lesions affecting

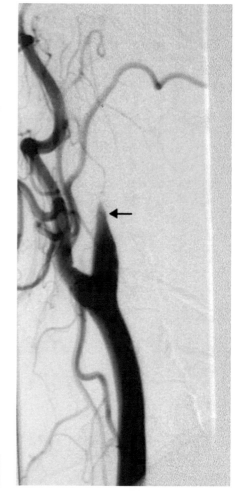

Fig 13 Carotid artery dissection, a possible cause of Horner's syndrome. Arrow shows abrupt termination of flow in the internal carotid artery.

second-order neurons, which exit the spinal cord at the level of T1, pass in close proximity to the pulmonary apex before synapsing in the superior cervical ganglion, and may cause anhidrosis of the ipsilateral face. With postganglionic lesions, anhidrosis is either absent or limited to an area above the ipsilateral brow.

Hazard

Think of Pancoast tumour in any patient with Horner's syndrome and look for associated wasting of the intrinsic hand muscles, which is consistent with a T1 root lesion.

Table 22   Causes of ptosis

	Type of disorder	Example
Unilateral	Neuromuscular	Third (oculomotor) nerve palsy
		Horner's syndrome
		Levator palpebrae muscle paralysis
	Local anatomical	Levator aponeurosis dehiscence or disinsertion
		Inflammation (eg chalazion) or infiltration (eg amyloidosis) of eyelids or conjunctiva Lost contact lens
	Ischaemic	Hemispheric stroke (rare)
	Congenital	Congenital cranial dysinnervation disorder
Bilateral	Neuromuscular	Myasthenia gravis
		Myotonic dystrophy
		Chronic progressive external ophthalmoplegia
		Ocular dystrophy
		Oculopharyngeal dystrophy
		Guillain–Barré syndrome
	Congenital	Congenital cranial dysinnervation disorder

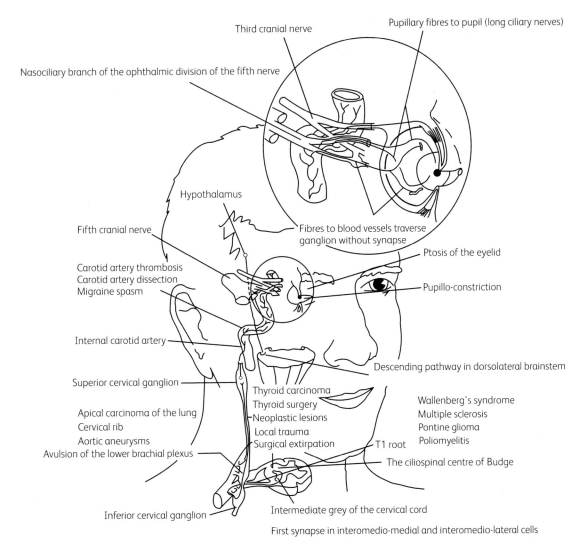

Third cranial nerve

Pupillary fibres to pupil (long ciliary nerves)

Nasociliary branch of the ophthalmic division of the fifth nerve

Hypothalamus

Fibres to blood vessels traverse ganglion without synapse

Fifth cranial nerve

Ptosis of the eyelid

Carotid artery thrombosis
Carotid artery dissection
Migraine spasm

Pupillo-constriction

Internal carotid artery

Superior cervical ganglion

Descending pathway in dorsolateral brainstem

Thyroid carcinoma
Thyroid surgery
Neoplastic lesions
Local trauma
Surgical extirpation

Wallenberg's syndrome
Multiple sclerosis
Pontine glioma
Poliomyelitis

Apical carcinoma of the lung
Cervical rib
Aortic aneurysms
Avulsion of the lower brachial plexus

T1 root

The ciliospinal centre of Budge

Inferior cervical ganglion

Intermediate grey of the cervical cord

First synapse in interomedio-medial and interomedio-lateral cells

Fig 14 Horner's syndrome.

1.2.14 Abnormal ocular movements

Instruction
This woman has worsening diplopia. Please examine her eyes.

Diplopia is caused by misalignment of the visual axes. You need to establish whether this is an isolated local problem, or whether it is due to neurological disease (Table 23).

General features

Is there a head tilt? The head tilts in the direction of action of the weak muscle. For example, in a left fourth cranial nerve palsy, the head tilts towards the right to compensate for the loss of intorsion of the left eye.

Are there any signs of thyroid disease?

Does the patient have a pacemaker, which in conjunction with an external ophthalmoplegia would suggest a diagnosis of the rare mitochondrial disorder Kearns–Sayre syndrome?

Eye examination

On inspection, look for:

> Proptosis – suggesting an orbital lesion (unilateral) or thyroid eye disease (bilateral).

> Ptosis and a dilated pupil – indicating a third cranial nerve palsy (Fig 15).

> Partial ptosis and a small pupil – indicating Horner's syndrome, which may be associated with ophthalmoplegia (see Section 1.2.13)

Does covering either eye relieve the diplopia? If not, the two images are coming from the same eye, which is relatively unusual. This can be due to refractive error (in which case asking the patient to look through a pinhole will relieve the symptoms) or a retinal problem (which will be evident on fundoscopy).

Table 23   Cuuses of diplopia

Eyes involved	Causes	Diagnoses
Binocular	Physiological	At extremes of vision
	Pathological	Neuromuscular: Any cause of third, fourth or sixth nerve palsy, eg multiple sclerosis
		Myasthenia gravis
		Brainstem ischaemic event (not isolated diplopia)
		Miller Fisher variant of Guillain–Barré syndrome
		Cavernous sinus thrombosis
		Chronic progressive external ophthalmoplegia
		Mitochondrial diseases, eg Kearns–Sayre syndrome

		Local anatomical:
		    Orbital infiltration, eg metastases
		    Dysthyroid eye disease

Monocular	Psychogenic	
	Pathological	Astigmatism
		Cataract
		Retinal pathology, ie detachment
		Foreign body in aqueous or vitreous media
		Poor optical equipment, eg defective contact lenses

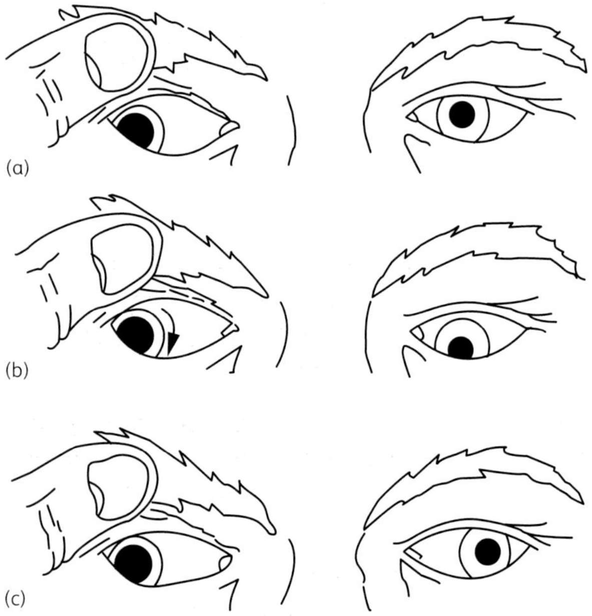

(a)

(b)

(c)

> **Key point**
>
> **Analysis of diplopia**
> In which direction is the diplopia worse?
> This occurs on looking in the direction in which the weak muscle has its purest action (Fig 16).
>
> Are the images separated horizontally or vertically? Horizontal separation is likely to indicate sixth nerve palsy (Figs 17 and 18). The common cause of isolated vertical diplopia is superior oblique palsy, in which the patient may describe a difficulty looking down – often notable when reading or walking down stairs.

Fig 15 Right third nerve palsy. **(a)** The patient is at rest when the eyelid is lifted by the examiner, the eye is looking down and out and the pupil is fixed and dilated. **(b)** On attempted down-gaze the affected eye ball will be seen to rotate inwards, best demonstrated by watching a conjunctival vessel during the attempt. **(c)** Attempted gaze to the left. The right eye remains stationary while the left lateral achieves full abduction.

The most important aspect is to check eye movements and at the point of maximum separation of an image, cover one eye.

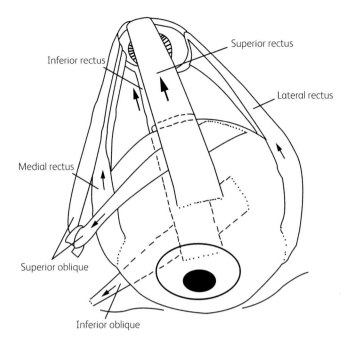

Fig 16 The eyeball and eye movements. The left eyeball is shown from above, the optic nerve is shown cut off so that the inferior rectus muscle can be seen. Note that due to the angulation of the orbit, the superior and inferior rectus muscles have their main elevating and depressing effect when the eyeball is looking laterally, whereas the oblique muscles (superior and inferior) that depress and elevate the eyeball (respectively) are maximally effective when the eye is looking medially. The medial and lateral recti simply pull the eyeball inwards and outwards.

Loss of the lateral image indicates that the covered eye is the abnormal one; careful consideration of Figs 15–18 should then enable you to decide which muscle or nerve is causing the problem.

Always deliberately consider the question 'Is there internuclear ophthalmoplegia' (nystagmus in abducting eye and failure of adduction of the affected side), which would suggest multiple sclerosis (Fig 18)?

A complete neurological examination is required to look for clues to differentiate the possible causes of diplopia given in Table 24, eg reduced visual acuity, optic atrophy or cerebellar signs in multiple sclerosis; or fatigability in myasthenia gravis.

Further discussion

What are the causes of a third cranial nerve palsy?
See Table 24 and Fig 18.

Hazard

Cavernous sinus syndrome

This may result in ophthalmoplegia, pain, proptosis, Horner's syndrome (resulting in a mid-sized pupil caused by the combination with a third nerve palsy, ie both sympathetic and parasympathetic paresis) and prominent scleral vessels. Intracavernous carotid artery aneurysm, mass lesions or thrombophlebitis may be causes; the latter is sometimes due to mucormycosis in the case of immunocompromised or diabetic patients.

What if the diplopia is worse in the evenings?
Consider myasthenia gravis.

1.2.15 Facial weakness

Instruction

This woman has a problem with her face. Please examine her cranial nerves.

Key point

The differential diagnosis depends on whether the facial weakness is due to a central or peripheral (upper motor neurone versus lower motor neurone) lesion. This is assessed by testing the muscles of the forehead, which are generally affected in a lower motor neurone lesion but not with a central lesion (Fig 19). Note, however, that some lower motor neurone lesions may spare the forehead, eg focal lesions within the lower parotid gland.

General features

> Does the patient have a stick, frame or other walking aid, suggesting the presence of limb weakness or ataxia?

> Does the patient wear a hearing aid, which clearly suggests the possibility of an eighth nerve lesion in this context?

> Is there a generalised rash, such as erythema nodosum, suggesting an inflammatory or infective cause? (This is unlikely in PACES.)

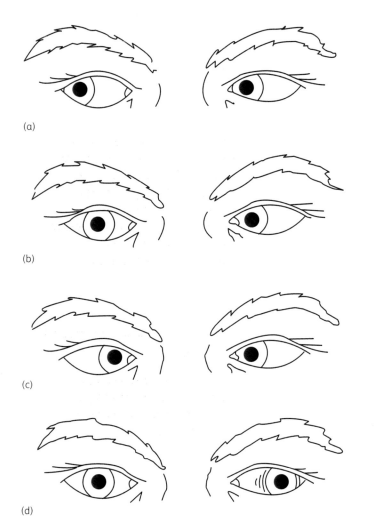

(a)

(b)

(c)

(d)

Fig 17 Eye movements in internuclear ophthalmoplegia and sixth nerve palsy. **(a)** Normal on right gaze – both eyes move normally and single vision is retained with no nystagmus. **(b)** Sixth nerve palsy (produced by a lesion at position B on Fig 18) at rest – the left eye is slightly medially deviated giving a disconcerting diplopia best prevented by closing the eye or tilting the head round to the left, such that the normal right eye abducts to line up its ocular axis with the abnormal left eye. **(c)** Sixth nerve palsy on attempted left lateral gaze – the right eye achieves full adduction and the left eye remains static, producing widely separated images. **(d)** Internuclear ophthalmoplegia (produced by a lesion at position A on Fig 18) prevents the activation of the right medial rectus muscle on attempted left lateral gaze. On attempted lateral gaze the left eye abducts nearly completely but shows nystagmus. The right eye makes little or no movement medially, but due to minimal displacement no nystagmus occurs.

Neurological examination

If unilateral facial weakness is due to a lower motor neurone lesion, it is important to look for a number of other abnormalities to aid localisation:

> Is there involvement of the fifth, sixth and eighth cranial nerves, with ipsilateral ataxia suggesting a lesion at the cerebellopontine angle? Large acoustic neuromas at this site may also expand to involve the ninth, tenth and eleventh cranial nerves, although this is uncommon.

> Is the sixth cranial nerve affected, either in isolation or with contralateral upper motor neurone limb signs suggesting a pontine lesion, such as a glioma?

> Are an extensive number of cranial nerves affected ipsilaterally? This may be seen in an infiltrative neoplastic process such as a meningioma en plaque.

> Multiple cranial nerve palsies may also be due to a leptomeningeal process, eg sarcoidosis or malignant meningitis.

> Is there hyperacusis, implying a lesion proximal to the branch to stapedius muscle? This is seen in approximately one-third of patients with Bell's palsy.

 Hazard

Facial nerve palsy The head and neck must be carefully inspected for masses, eg parotid tumours, and scars, particularly just behind the ear (surgical removal of cerebellopontine angle tumours).

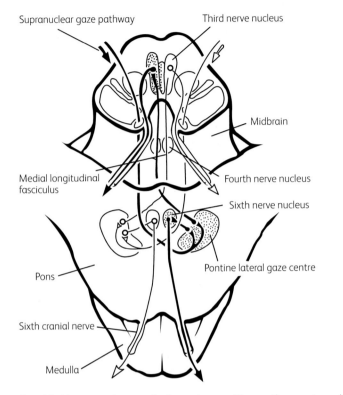

Fig 18 Nerve pathways for lateral gaze. The pathways to achieve left lateral gaze are shown in thicker lines and stippled areas.

Further discussion

What is the course of the facial nerve? See Fig 20.

What are the causes of an upper motor neurone facial weakness? This may be due to any process above the level of the facial nerve nucleus in the pons. Remember that cerebral hemispheric lesions such as stroke, tumour or demyelination result in contralateral upper motor neurone signs affecting the face and limbs.

What are the causes of bilateral facial palsy? The differential diagnosis for bilateral facial palsy includes:

> Myasthenia gravis – look for fatiguable weakness, complex ophthalmoplegia and lack of sensory signs.

Table 24	Causes of third cranial nerve palsy
Location	**Diagnoses**
Central (brainstem)	Infarction
	Haemorrhage
	Tumour
	Abscess
Subarachnoid space	Aneurysm
	Infectious meningitis: bacterial, fungal/parasitic and viral
	Carcinomatous/lymphomatous/leukaemic infiltration and granulomatous inflammation (sarcoidosis, lymphomatoid granulomatosis and Wegener's granulomatosis)
Cavernous sinus	Tumour: pituitary adenoma, meningioma, craniopharyngioma and metastatic carcinoma
	Giant intracavernous aneurysm
	Carotid artery–cavernous sinus fistula
	Cavernous sinus thrombosis
	Ischaemia from microvascular disease in vasa nervosa
	Inflammatory: Tolosa–Hunt syndrome (idiopathic or granulomatous inflammation)
Orbit	Inflammatory: orbital inflammatory pseudotumour, orbital myositis
	Endocrine (thyroid orbitopathy)
	Tumour (eg haemangioma, lymphangioma and meningioma)

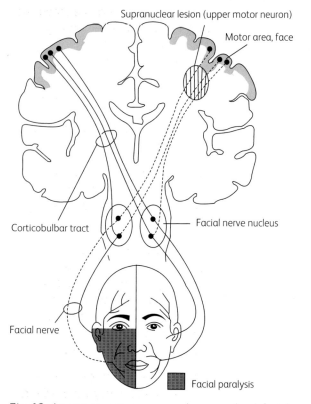

Supranuclear lesion (upper motor neuron)

Motor area, face

Corticobulbar tract

Facial nerve nucleus

Facial nerve

Facial paralysis

Fig 19 An upper motor neurone (supranuclear) facial nerve lesion causes weakness of only the lower half of the face (hatched area) because the upper part of the face receives bilateral upper motor neurone (supranuclear) input.

> Myotonic dystrophy – check for grip and percussion myotonia; wasting and weakness of temporalis; and masseter and sternocleidomastoid muscles.

> Facioscapulohumeral dystrophy – look for winging of the scapulae, bilateral foot drop and normal eye movements.

> In the acute setting, Guillain–Barré syndrome must also be considered.

What is the prognosis and treatment of idiopathic Bell's palsy?
Bell's palsy is a common idiopathic facial palsy, possibly caused by viral infection (particularly herpes simplex 1) and oedema of the seventh nerve within the facial canal. There is an increased incidence during pregnancy and in cases of diabetes mellitus. Maximal deficit occurs within 48 hours. Postauricular pain is experienced by about 50% of patients, typically shortly before facial paralysis occurs. Treatment with steroids and antiviral agents will improve the

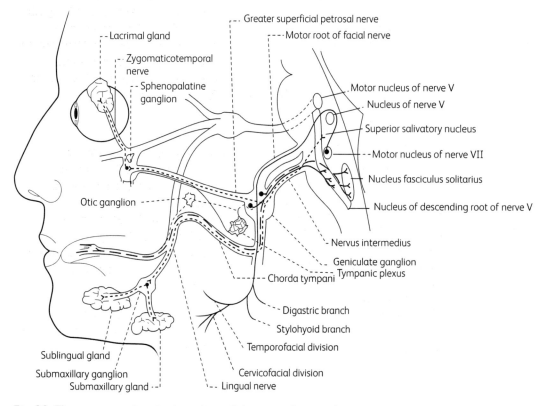

Greater superficial petrosal nerve

Lacrimal gland

Motor root of facial nerve

Zygomaticotemporal nerve

Sphenopalatine ganglion

Motor nucleus of nerve V

Nucleus of nerve V

Superior salivatory nucleus

Motor nucleus of nerve VII

Nucleus fasciculus solitarius

Otic ganglion

Nucleus of descending root of nerve V

Nervus intermedius

Geniculate ganglion

Chorda tympani

Tympanic plexus

Digastric branch

Stylohyoid branch

Temporofacial division

Sublingual gland

Cervicofacial division

Submaxillary ganglion

Submaxillary gland

Lingual nerve

Fig 20 The course and major branches of the seventh cranial nerve.

outcome if given within 3 days of symptom onset. Complete recovery is seen within 60 days in 75% of patients.

What if the patient presenting with facial palsy had a rash on their ear? In Ramsay–Hunt syndrome, herpes zoster vesicles may be seen in areas supplied by the sensory portion of the seventh nerve – tympanic membrane, external auditory canal, pinna, buccal mucosa and neck.

1.2.16 Lower cranial nerve assessment

Instruction

This woman has trouble swallowing fluids. Please examine her cranial nerves.

General features

The instruction suggests that any abnormality is most likely to be found in the lower cranial nerves, but from the foot of the bed:

> Look at the patient's nutritional status – is she cachectic, suggesting difficulty with swallowing solids as well as fluids?

> Look for generalised loss of muscle bulk, perhaps due to motor neurone disease.

> Is there any evidence of previous trauma or surgery, eg any scars in the neck?

> Is there anything to suggest a stroke, eg hemiparesis or speech disturbance? This could mean carotid artery dissection in the neck causing lower cranial nerve palsies by direct compression or ischaemia of the nerves.

> Look for signs of conditions associated with dysphagia, eg myasthenia gravis, myotonic dystrophy and polymyositis.

> Is there any respiratory compromise, indicating a condition with respiratory muscle involvement, eg myasthenia gravis or motor neurone disease?

> Important in routine clinical practice, but less likely in PACES, is to check if there are any swellings in the neck. A swelling may indicate a tumour, which can compress or infiltrate lower cranial nerves, or cervical lymphadenopathy associated with a malignancy elsewhere.

Neurological examination

The lower cranial nerves are: IX (glossopharyngeal), X (vagus), XI (spinal accessory) and XII (hypoglossal). Your examination should check the following:

> Voice (IX and X) – note the quality and sound of the patient's voice. Is it weak, hoarse or nasal?

> Swallowing (IX and X) – a drink should be available: note any difficulty or regurgitation of fluid.

> Gag reflex (IX and X) – observe the palate, which should rise symmetrically. If the cranial nerve is abnormal on one side, the palate will rise to the normal side. Also note elevation and symmetry of the uvula. Unilateral lesions usually result in deviation of the uvula away from the affected side.

> Trapezius and sternocleidomastoid (SCM; XI) – look for wasting, weakness and asymmetry. Peripheral lesions of cranial nerve XI produce ipsilateral SCM weakness and ipsilateral trapezius weakness. Central lesions produce ipsilateral SCM weakness and contralateral trapezius weakness, because of differing sources of cerebral innervation. This is a common clinical misunderstanding.

> Tongue (XII) – observe the tongue at rest in the mouth. Are there any fasciculations or wasting that may suggest motor neurone disease? Does the tongue deviate from the midline on protrusion? If there is a unilateral peripheral XII nerve lesion, the tongue will deviate towards the side of the lesion.

Although you have been asked to examine the cranial nerves, you should extend your examination as necessary, checking:

> Is there bulbar weakness, eg depressed gag reflex or a weak cough, as well as a wasted and fasciculating tongue? A brisk jaw jerk, spastic tongue and emotional lability suggest pseudobulbar palsy (Fig 21).

> In the limbs, upper motor neurone signs only (ie spasticity, hyperreflexia and extensor plantars) are seen in primary lateral sclerosis. Lower motor neurone signs only (ie flaccidity, atrophy, fasciculations and hyporeflexia) are seen in poliomyelitis and adult onset spinal muscular atrophies. Both upper and lower motor neurone signs are seen in motor neurone disease. See Section 2.1 for further discussion.

Further discussion

It is rare to have isolated lower cranial nerve lesions. More often several lower cranial nerves will be involved together – especially cranial nerves IX, X and XI, which leave the skull together through the jugular foramen. Localisation of any lesion will usually require MRI scanning of the head and neck.

The commonest causes of multiple lower cranial nerve lesions are shown in Table 25.

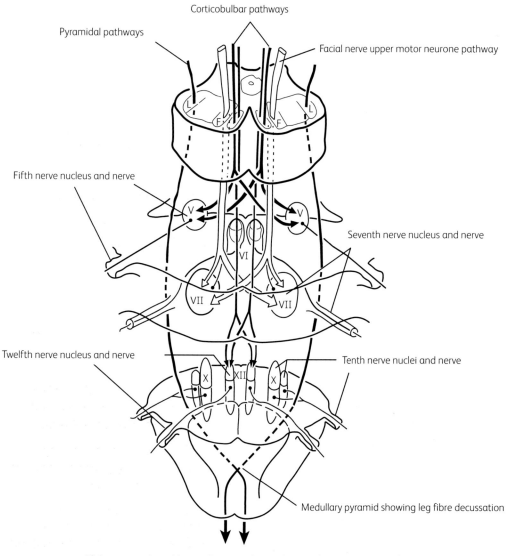

Corticobulbar pathways

Pyramidal pathways

Facial nerve upper motor neurone pathway

Fifth nerve nucleus and nerve

Seventh nerve nucleus and nerve

Twelfth nerve nucleus and nerve

Tenth nerve nuclei and nerve

Medullary pyramid showing leg fibre decussation

If there is a unilateral lesion of supranuclear pathway, subsequent supranuclear pathway lesion on the other side will produce sudden and complete paralysis of fifth, seventh, ninth, tenth, eleventh and twelfth cranial nerves

Fig 21 Anatomy of pseudobulbar palsy. The supranuclear pathways for the tenth nerve are not depicted, but are exactly like the fifth and twelfth nerves that are shown, with each supranuclear pathway contributing 50% to each right and each left nucleus. The facial nerve is different, with some 90% of fibres decussating; hence a lesion in the right supranuclear pathway will produce significant left facial weakness, whereas corresponding supranuclear lesions of the other motor cranial nerves will produce no abnormality (or at worst only transient abnormality).

Table 25 Causes of multiple lower cranial nerve lesions

Site	Eponym	Cranial nerves involved	Usual cause
Extramedullary lower cranial nerve syndromes			
Cerebellopontine angle		V, VII, VIII, sometimes IX	Acoustic neuromas and meningiomas
Jugular foramen	Vernet	IX, X and XI	Tumours, aneurysms, trauma and Paget's disease
Posterior laterocondylar space	Collet–Sicard	IX, X, XI and XII	Tumours of parotid gland and carotid body Carotid artery dissection Tuberculous adenitis
Posterior retroparotid space	Villaret	IX, X, XI and XII	As above plus granulomatous lesions, eg sarcoid
Within the nerve		IX, X, XI and XII	Invasion of tumours, eg squamous cell cancer Granulomatous lesions Infectious, eg HIV, Lyme disease, herpes zoster Post-infectious, eg Guillain–Barré syndrome
Intramedullary (brainstem) lower cranial nerve syndromes			
Tegmentum of medulla	Jackson	X and XII	Infarct or tumour
Lateral tegmentum of medulla	Wallenberg	Spinal V, IX, X and XI	Occlusion of vertebral or posterior inferior cerebellar artery

Key point

Swallowing is best assessed by asking the patient to take a small sip of water. If there is any difficulty with this, urgent speech and language therapy assessment is required. Having difficulty swallowing is a common occurrence after an acute stroke, but is of little localising value.

1.2.17 Speech disturbance

Instruction

This man is unable to communicate as well as he would like. Please examine his speech.

General features

The differential diagnosis of speech disturbance is determined by the type of disorder present: dysarthria, aphasia or dysphonia.

> Dysarthria is a disorder of articulation in which the content of the speech is unaffected, the underlying diagnosis almost always being determined by eliciting other physical signs (Table 26).

> Aphasia (or dysphasia; the former term is preferred to avoid confusion with dysphagia) is a disorder of language caused by a cortical lesion of the dominant cerebral hemisphere (Table 27).

> Dysphonia is a disorder of voice production but articulation and language content are normal (Table 28).

Key point

The most important step in making the correct diagnosis of speech disturbance is to characterise accurately the abnormality: is it dysarthria, aphasia or dysphonia?

General inspection should therefore look for clues that point to any of the causes indicated in Tables 26–28.

Look for evidence of neck surgery or swellings, indicating possible damage to the patient's vocal cords.

Is there anything to suggest a particular diagnosis associated with speech difficulties, eg myasthenia gravis, stroke or motor neurone disease?

Neurological examination

The type of speech defect is characterised by listening to the speech itself. Assessment of speech includes the following elements.

Phonation and articulation

When the patient talks, listen for dysphonia (a whispering, hoarse or otherwise abnormal voice) or disturbances of articulation that are characteristic of dysarthria. It may be possible to exaggerate dysarthria by asking the patient to repeat phrases such as 'biblical criticism' or 'West Register Street'. Repetition of particular

Table 26   Causes of dysarthria

Cause	Diagnosis
Cerebellar dysarthria	Any cause of a cerebellar syndrome
Bulbar palsy	Myopathy or myositis
	Myasthenia gravis
	Motor neurone disease
	Bulbar poliomyelitis
	Guillain–Barré syndrome
Pseudobulbar palsy	Small-vessel cerebral ischaemia
	Motor neurone disease
	Multiple sclerosis
Hypokinetic dysarthria	Extrapyramidal disease, especially Parkinson's disease
Hyperkinetic dysarthria	Chorea (eg Huntington's disease) or myoclonus
Isolated cranial nerve palsies	Cranial nerves V, VII, X and XII
Other	Hypothyroidism

Table 27   Causes of aphasia

Cause	Diagnosis
Stroke	Dominant (L>R) middle cerebral artery territory
Tumour	Dominant hemisphere
Trauma	
Cerebral abscess	
Herpes simplex encephalitis	
Degenerative central nervous system disease	Frontotemporal dementia (progressive non-fluent aphasia) more than Alzheimer's disease

letters can be used to assess individual parts of the articulatory process: lips ('pa'), tongue ('ta') and soft palate and posterior tongue ('ka'). Putting them all together rapidly ('pa-ta-ka') will uncover mildly dysarthric speech, but it is often difficult to characterise dysarthric speech purely on the basis of the way it sounds. It is frequently of mixed type, and the type(s) present can usually be deduced from the associated signs.

> Cerebellar speech is characterised as scanning or staccato, eg artillery pronounced 'art-til-ler-y', uneven and irregular output with improper stresses; may be associated with ataxic gait.

> Pseudobulbar or spastic dysarthria, caused by bilateral lesions in the upper motor neurone projections to the bulbar nuclei in the brainstem (see Section 1.2.16), is associated with dysphagia, small spastic tongue

and a brisk jaw jerk. There may also be signs of small vessel ischaemic brain damage such as *marche à petit pas*, brisk reflexes and extensor plantars.

> Bulbar dysarthria is due to a deficit in the bulbar cranial nerves (lower motor neurone type) or the bulbar muscles per se, hence there may be wasting and fasciculation of the tongue, proximal muscle weakness or fatiguability dependent on cause.

> Check carefully for isolated cranial nerve palsies.

Fluency

If phonation and articulation are normal, then consider whether the speech disturbance is an aphasia. If the speech is not fluent (ie hesitant or 'telegraphic', missing out words such as 'and'), then this may indicate a motor (anterior, 'expressive') aphasia such as occurs with lesions in Broca's area. If the speech sounds fluent but patients substitute alternative words for those they may have forgotten (paraphasias) or use nonsense words (neologisms), then this is compatible with a sensory (posterior, 'receptive') aphasia.

Comprehension

Early in the assessment it is wise to check that the patient understands what you are asking; indeed, it may be appropriate to do this right at the beginning if initial attempts at conversation with the patient are not rewarding. Comprehension is not an all-or-nothing skill, the level of comprehension being gauged by the complexity of the task that can be performed: one-, two- or three-step commands. You might approach

Table 28	Causes of dysphonia
Cause	**Diagnosis**
Paralysis of both vocal cords	Post-thyroidectomy Neck malignancy Guillain–Barré syndrome Brainstem stroke Multiple sclerosis Syringobulbia Poliomyelitis
Paralysis of one vocal cord / recurrent laryngeal nerve palsy	Post-thyroidectomy Carcinoma (bronchial, thyroid) Lymphoma Cervical node enlargement Aortic aneurysm Pulmonary tuberculosis Ortner syndrome (enlarged left atrium)
Neuromuscular respiratory failure	Guillain–Barré syndrome Myasthenia gravis Polymyositis
Other neurological disorders	Spasmodic dysphonia (may be isolated or associated with dystonia elsewhere) Essential tremor

testing as follows, starting with simple instructions and gradually increasing the complexity.

> 'I wonder if you are having some difficulty in understanding what I say?'

> 'I would like to test this …'

> 'Is that alright …?'

> 'Can you open your mouth, please – open your mouth?' If the patient does not do this, then open your own mouth and see if they copy you.

> 'Can you show me your left hand?'

> 'Can you put your right hand on top of your head?'

> 'Can you touch your left ear with your right hand, and put your left hand on your nose?'

Naming

The patient may not be able to name objects (anomia), but may be able to describe them (circumlocution; preserved semantics). This may indicate a lesion deep in the temporal lobe.

Repetition

Failure to repeat single words or phrases usually occurs as a result of a sensory aphasia. However, there may be severe impairment of repetition with preserved comprehension. This dichotomy is said to be the essential feature of conduction aphasia in which the lesion is localised to the left Sylvian fissure.

Reading

Test silently so as to test only visual comprehension, which is usually preserved in motor aphasia and impaired in sensory aphasia.

Writing

Use verbal and written requests to get the patient to write something. Poor writing with errors similar to speech is a feature of motor aphasia.

Further discussion

Management of speech disturbance depends on the underlying cause and ranges from ear, nose and throat (ENT) referral for some forms of dysphonia to neurosurgery for some space-occupying lesions causing aphasia.

What are the types of dysphasia?

Classification of language disorders has been based on various theoretical models, none of which show absolutely consistent correlation with anatomical lesions. Many consider it appropriate to think in terms of motor/anterior or sensory/posterior aphasia.

Motor/anterior dysphasia

Also sometimes known as 'expressive aphasia', this is characterised by the following.

> Speech is non-fluent or hesitant, ie 'agrammatic' or 'telegraphic' output, missing out words such as 'and'.

> Words or syllables are substituted.

> Writing is poor, with errors similar to speech.

> Naming may be impaired.

> Comprehension, repetition (except for some word or syllabic substitution) and reading are preserved.

Sensory/posterior dysphasia

Also sometimes known as 'receptive aphasia', this has the following characteristics:

> Fluent speech with normal rhythm. However, because of poor comprehension the patient is unable to monitor his or her speech output and so it may contain neologisms and paraphasias as well as substitutions (ultimately ending up as incomprehensible jargon, so-called 'jargon aphasia'). The patient also talks incessantly.

> Comprehension, repetition and reading are poor.

1.3 Communication skills and ethics

1.3.1 Genetic implications

Scenario

Role: you are a junior doctor in the neurology outpatient clinic.

Scenario: Mr David Johnson, aged 54 years, is referred to the neurology clinic because of behavioural change and increasing cognitive difficulties. His son, who attends with him, has also noticed that his father has become increasingly 'fidgety'. Mr Johnson has no significant past medical history, but an extended family history – given by the son – reveals that Mr Johnson's mother (the son's grandmother) died in middle age with dementia, but this is something that 'the family don't talk about'. It is difficult to be sure how much Mr Johnson understands, but he tells you that you should 'talk about anything you want with my son'. He has also said the same thing to his GP, who arranged for the son to attend the clinic with his father. The view of the neurological team is that the most likely diagnosis is Huntington's chorea, which could be confirmed by genetic testing.

Your task: to discuss the implications of genetic testing for Huntington's disease with Mr Johnson's son.

Key issues to explore

> The son's knowledge of the disease and the diagnostic testing that is available.

> 'If you have Huntington's disease, would you like to know?'

> Why test when the disease is incurable?

Key points to establish

> The fact that any test results will have widespread implications for other family members, including the son himself.

> That testing may or may not clarify matters, but if the results are negative the problem will not be cured and so further investigations may be needed.

> That there is no treatment for Huntington's disease.

> Although it is difficult to produce 'black and white' rules in an area where much is grey, most physicians with experience of Huntington's disease feel that it is inadvisable to test in the following circumstances: children under 18 years; for insurance purposes; if the patient is reluctant; and if the result automatically reveals someone else (ie a parent) to have the disease without their consent.

> After any test, follow-up will be required whatever the result.

Key points

Genetic testing
Issues to consider if this is to be used are:

> Depression may follow a positive or negative result ('survivor guilt').

> Suicide after a positive result has occurred, but this is no more common than for any other disease or chronic disability.

Appropriate responses to likely questions

Son: *I don't know about having the genetic test. Is there anybody else I can speak to about it?*

Doctor: yes – I can make a referral to the regional specialist clinical genetics service, where you and your father would be able to receive further counselling regarding the test.

Son: *can my father and I have the test done today?*

Doctor: because of all the things that the test might mean, I feel that it is important for you to have pre-test counselling. This is provided by the regional specialist clinical genetics service – I will refer your father and you to them.

Son: *what do you mean when you say 'all the things that the test might mean'?*

Doctor: Huntington's is a genetic disease, which means that it runs in the family. If your father has Huntington's – and we don't know that at the moment – but if he does, then there is a 50% chance that he will have passed it on to each of his children. I'm afraid that means there's a one-in-two chance that you will have it, and also a one-in-two chance that any of your brothers and sisters will have it.

Son: *if the test shows that someone's got Huntington's, can anything be done about it?*

Doctor: I'm afraid that there is no specific treatment for Huntington's. There are things that can be done to help the symptoms, for instance drugs can sometimes help the distressing movements, but there isn't any treatment that will deal with the underlying disease.

Son: *if I was tested and was positive, will I then know at which point the disease would start to cause me trouble?*

Doctor: no, the timing can be variable and the onset of the disease could only be established by examining you neurologically.

Son: *so, do we have to have the test done?*

Doctor: no, you don't. As you can see it's a difficult issue, which is why I think that talking to someone in the clinical genetics service is necessary rather than just racing into the test. Some people decide that they want to know, and some people decide that they don't – there isn't a 'right' and a 'wrong' answer to the question.

1.3.2 Explanation of the diagnosis of Alzheimer's disease

Scenario

Role: you are the neurology junior doctor working in a general neurology outpatient clinic.

Scenario: Mr Harry Wilson is a 69-year-old man who has come to clinic with his wife and one of his sons. He saw your colleague 2 months ago for investigation of memory difficulties. His symptoms have been coming on for several years and his wife initially took no notice of his memory lapses. Recently he has become disinterested in all activities, but his wife does not feel that he is depressed. His wife tells you that he is a shadow of his former self and can sit alone in a chair for hours without initiating conversation or activity. He recently had to be brought home by a friend after he was found wandering back and forward in front of his local shops. They have two sons in their forties.

The results of the blood tests, including thyroid function, erythrocyte sedimentation rate, syphilis serology and B_{12} were normal. His CT scan demonstrated some mild generalised atrophy, but there was no evidence of hydrocephalus, subdural haematoma, focal cortical atrophy or infarcts. His electroencephalogram demonstrated some diffuse slow waves but no overt epileptiform activity. The diagnosis is probable Alzheimer's disease.

His wife is finding it very frustrating as her husband does not appear to be aware of most of his problems. She would like to know what has caused his memory problems, and their son is anxious that it may affect him. Is it 'mad cow disease'?

At the neurological meeting some of these issues have been discussed recently: the risk of inheriting late onset Alzheimer's disease is not high, perhaps two to three times the risk of it occurring in a member of the general population with no family history.

Your task: to explain to the patient and his wife and son the diagnosis of probable Alzheimer's disease; its prognosis and treatment; as well as discussing the probability of inheriting late onset dementia.

Key issues to explore

> A common problem with patients who have Alzheimer's disease is that they often have little insight into how they have been affected. This cognitive anosognosia may be characterised by relatives as 'being in denial' and can cause significant problems, especially with frustration, within the family.

> The prognosis of the condition.

> The issue of symptomatic treatment with cholinesterase inhibitors.

> Risk of family members developing the disease.

Key points to establish

> The diagnosis and prognosis of Alzheimer's disease.

> Possible treatment symptomatic options.

> Genetic risks in first-degree relatives.

> Future care involving the Alzheimer's Society, the patient's GP and social services in conjunction with regular outpatient follow-up.

Appropriate responses to likely questions

Wife: *what is the diagnosis?*

Doctor: the diagnosis is almost certainly a form of dementia called Alzheimer's disease, although it is often difficult to be 100% certain of the diagnosis in life. Other treatable causes of dementia have been excluded with the tests that have been done, and any other possible diagnoses would be degenerative brain conditions similar to Alzheimer's.

Wife: *what do you mean by a degenerative brain condition?*

Doctor: I'm afraid it means that the brain gradually deteriorates as a consequence of disease, so this is more than would be anticipated simply from the ageing process, and we currently don't have any effective treatments that will stop this happening.

Wife: *how long has he got to live?*

Doctor: no one can give you a definite answer to that question, not because they are hiding anything, but because they don't know. However, he is not in any imminent danger of dying, but I'm afraid that his ability to do things for himself will slowly get worse and he is likely to need increasing care in the next few years. It should be emphasised that many patients with Alzheimer's disease are able to continue to live fulfilling and worthwhile lives for some years.

Son: *what is the chance of me developing Alzheimer's disease?*

Doctor: as your father has what we call late onset Alzheimer's disease, the risk of you developing Alzheimer's is only marginally higher than in the general population, perhaps two to three times more likely.

Son: *can I have any tests to find out whether I will get Alzheimer's?*

Doctor: no, there aren't currently any tests that will reliably predict whether people are going to get late onset Alzheimer's. It may be that such tests will become available in the future, but unless there is some sort of treatment that can be offered to stop or modify the course of disease it will require very careful thought as to whether you, or anyone else, would want to have such testing.

Wife: *is there any treatment or cure?*

Doctor: I'm afraid that there is currently no cure for Alzheimer's, despite what you may have sometimes seen in the newspapers. But there are some medications called cholinesterase inhibitors that have a mild symptomatic benefit in some patients by increasing one of the chemicals in the brain that is low in people with Alzheimer's. However, these drugs don't alter the long-term outlook. If your husband wanted to try them, he would be monitored with memory tests every 3–6 months initially. If there was ongoing deterioration, then the drug would probably not be of benefit and would probably be stopped.

Wife: *are there any more tests that can be done?*

Doctor: none that have become available outside research settings. A neuropsychological assessment

[Section 3.1] is a more formal and accurate way of assessing the degree and types of thinking problems your husband has, and it may be useful in monitoring progression of the disease and response to treatment.

Wife: *where can I get more information and help?*

Doctor: some patients and their carers find contact with the Alzheimer's Society helpful. I will write to your GP outlining our conversation and send you a copy of the letter. Your GP will be able to initiate contact with social services, nurses and other health professionals as and when they are needed.

1.3.3 Prognosis after stroke

Scenario

Role: you are the medical junior doctor working on a care of older people ward.

Scenario: Mr John Smith, a 78-year-old man, was admitted to your ward yesterday following sudden onset of right-sided weakness and speech difficulties. He is also unable to swallow safely. There has been no change in his condition over the last 24 hours: he has no movement in his right arm or leg, he cannot speak and he does not respond to simple commands. A CT brain scan has shown a large left-sided middle cerebral artery infarct. His prognosis is very poor.

Your task: to explain to Mr Smith's wife that he has had a large stroke and may not survive; and also that if he does survive, there is a high chance of severe disability.

Key issues to explore

> What does the patient's wife know already about her husband's condition?

> What are her expectations? What does Mrs Smith already know and, in particular, what does she understand by the term 'stroke'?

Key points to establish

> That you would normally obtain permission from a patient to speak to their relatives, but this is not possible due to communication difficulties.

> That Mr Smith is very unwell having suffered a large stroke; that there is a large amount of damage seen on the brain scan, and that it is not possible to reverse this damage; that everything that can be done for Mr Smith is being done and that he is quite comfortable; that he could die from this illness and that the first few days are particularly unpredictable; and that even if Mr Smith does not die as a result of the stroke it is very possible that he will have some long-term disability as a result, but that the nature and extent of this cannot be determined at this early stage.

> That Mrs Smith is introduced to key members of the stroke team and encouraged to ask as many questions as she wishes.

Appropriate responses to likely questions

Wife: *why did this happen to him?*

Doctor: there are lots of reasons why people have a stroke, especially as they get older. Your husband's scan shows a type of stroke caused by a blood clot rather than a bleed, but we don't know exactly what caused this. At the moment we need to focus our attention on looking after him, but if he shows signs of recovery then he will have more tests to see if we can find the cause.

Wife: does he need an operation?

Doctor: no, that wouldn't help. We very rarely operate on patients who have had a stroke, unless the scan shows us that the brain is under a lot of pressure: we didn't see this on your husband's scan so an operation would not help him. In fact it would almost certainly make things worse.

Wife: can he be given a new 'clot-busting' drug?

Doctor: no, I'm afraid not. You are right that there are drugs available which can dissolve blood clots – they're often used for patients who have had heart attacks – but using them for people who have had strokes is not at all straightforward because they can cause severe bleeding in the brain that makes things worse. They are sometimes used, but only in people with some sorts of stroke and who have got to hospital very quickly. In your husband's case I'm afraid they wouldn't help – they wouldn't do any good and the risk of bleeding on his brain would be very high.

Wife: is he going to live?

Doctor: I'm not hiding anything when I say I don't know. As you know he's had a big stroke, but I don't know whether or not it's going to kill him. We have to take things hour by hour and day by day at the moment, but if there's any change in his condition then – assuming it's what you would like – we will let you know immediately.

Wife: if he does survive, then what sort of disability could he have?

Doctor: again, I'm afraid that I can't give you a definite answer as to what

will happen but the stroke is on the left side of his brain, which controls the right side of his body and his speech. At the moment he is unable to move his arm and leg and he cannot speak. The extent to which these functions will recover is unpredictable, but if he stabilises and shows progress over the next few days then our team of physiotherapists, speech and language therapists and occupational therapists will make some assessments. They will then devise treatment plans with the aim of recovering as much function as possible. If he does survive, the rehabilitation programme will last many months and he still may require help to look after himself. There is a high chance that he will need to use a wheelchair, at least in the early stages and perhaps in the long term, and he may also have persistent problems with understanding and speech.

Wife: should I tell my son to fly home from his holiday?

Doctor: your husband is in a stable condition for now, but he could become worse at any time. This can happen suddenly and he could deteriorate very quickly and even die. I would suggest that you should speak to your son and ensure that he understands this; he can then make a decision based on this information as to whether or not to return.

Key point

Despite recent advances in the management of acute stroke, the prognosis remains poor with up to 20% of patients dying within 30 days of the onset of the stroke. It is important when breaking the news of a large stroke to relatives that you are realistic about the chances of survival and full recovery.

1.3.4 Conversion disorder

Scenario

Role: you are the neurology junior doctor working on the neurology ward.

Scenario: Miss Kate Beaumont was originally referred to the epilepsy clinic with a 2-year history of frequent episodes of apparent loss of consciousness. She is taking antiepileptic medication. These attacks were recently witnessed on the neurology ward while she was undergoing video-electroencephalogram (EEG) telemetry. The episodes do not have an epileptic basis on either clinical or EEG grounds. Other investigations have also been normal, and a diagnosis of non-epileptic attack disorder has been made. The neurology team have agreed that no further investigations are required. Miss Beaumont wishes to know what the cause of her attacks is and how you are going to treat them.

Your task: to explain to Miss Beaumont that the attacks are not due to epilepsy but have a psychological basis and are best managed with help from the neuropsychiatry team.

Key issues to explore

> What does the patient think is the cause of her attacks?

> What were the possible triggers more than 2 years ago that led to the attacks emerging?

> Is there any relevant past psychological history, eg depression, anxiety or self-harm?

Key points to establish

> Appropriate tests have given reassuring results and further tests are not indicated.

> The episodes will not improve with antiepileptic medication, which should be gradually withdrawn.

> The most appropriate therapy is psychological, and this is usually successful in reducing the attack frequency or stopping the attacks altogether.

Key point

The patient is not considered to be 'putting it on' or 'faking illness'. The patient has little control over the nature of the episodes.

Appropriate responses to likely questions

Patient: so you think I am putting on the attacks?

Doctor: no, not at all. The attacks that you have are real, disabling and outside of your conscious control: they could be thought of as involuntary episodes of 'switching off' or going into a 'trance'. For example, we have all had times when we do not hear our name being called when we are engrossed in a book or film, or remembering nothing of a familiar journey home. We can all therefore be unaware or have no memory of episodes that we have experienced.

Patient: why do I have the attacks?

Doctor: we don't fully understand what causes this disorder, but two-thirds of people with it have suffered some sort of traumatic experience in the past. This may be important for us to talk about further. We can't explain the link for certain, but it may be that when

people are exposed to repeated frightening incidents they learn to switch off. Initially this is a helpful thing for them to do; it protects them emotionally at the time. But it may come back later in life as these attacks, so it may be that your attacks are brought on by stress. However, sometimes people are initially unable to identify the triggers of their attacks; and when they are found they often turn out to be fleeting stressful or unpleasant thoughts that you may barely be aware of, and which have little to do with your circumstances at the time of the attack.

Patient: aren't there any more tests you can do?

Doctor: as you probably know, there are always more tests that doctors can do; but I don't think that any more tests would be helpful for you. You've had thorough tests done – including monitoring of the brain waves when you've been having an attack – and we've discussed the results with everyone in the neurology team. We think we should move on from doing tests to focus on how we can try and treat the problem.

Patient: how do you treat the attacks?

Doctor: in some patients clarification of the cause of the attacks and withdrawal of antiepileptic medication is enough for the episodes to stop or greatly improve. If your attacks do not improve then it is likely that we will need to refer you to another member of our team – the neuropsychiatrists or neuropsychologists – with whom we work very closely. They will need to see you and talk more about the cause of your attacks. Usually they suggest some form of counselling or therapy involving changing your body's response to a certain trigger or experience.

Patient: will I come to any harm from having these attacks so frequently?

Doctor: there is no evidence that the attacks that you have cause you any harm, other than minor injuries that you may already have experienced such as biting your tongue or friction burns from the carpet. It is theoretically possible to be hurt more seriously if an attack occurs at the roadside or on the stairs, but this is extremely unusual and it's very rare for patients with this sort of problem to come to serious harm because of them.

1.3.5 Explaining the diagnosis of multiple sclerosis

Scenario

Role: you are the neurology junior doctor in an outpatient clinic.

Scenario: Miss Marlene Cox is a 34-year-old woman who is coming back to the neurology clinic for the results of her recent scans. She was initially referred by her GP with numbness and tingling in the legs, and she has a past history of episodes of blurred vision 6 months ago. An MRI scan of her brain and spinal cord has shown several high-signal white matter lesions in both cerebral hemispheres and a high-signal lesion at the level of C4 typical of demyelination. Visual evoked potentials and the results of a lumbar puncture are all consistent with this diagnosis. No further investigations are required. She needs referral to the specialist multiple sclerosis (MS) service for discussion of further management.

Your task: to explain to Miss Cox that the most likely diagnosis is MS.

Key issues to explore

> What does the patient know/fear about MS?

> The prognosis and treatment options.

Key points to establish

> That the most likely diagnosis is MS.

> That there is no definitive test to make a diagnosis of MS, but that the combination of typical symptoms and results from various tests help to make the diagnosis.

> That MS can manifest in many different ways and is not always disabling. Often patients with MS that are seen in the media are those with more severe disability. There are many thousands of patients with MS who live relatively normal lives, hold down jobs and raise families.

> That there are now several treatments available: these cannot cure the condition but can help to keep patients as healthy as possible for as long as possible.

> That the patient has the contact details of someone that she can call when she leaves the clinic (the MS specialist nurse if possible).

Appropriate responses to likely questions

Patient: how can you be sure I've got MS?

Doctor: there isn't one single test that can ever prove the diagnosis of MS, but the problems that you've had – with the vision and now with the legs – coupled with the test results, the scans, the vision tests and the lumbar puncture all point to MS. I wouldn't be telling you the truth if I said anything different.

Patient: will I need to use a wheelchair?

Doctor: I'm not hiding anything when I say that I don't know whether or not you will need to use a wheelchair in the future, but hopefully you will stay

as well as you are now for a long time. As you know some patients with MS do deteriorate, but very many don't. However, it tends to be the ones with severe disease that you see in the papers or on the television. We will make sure we see you regularly so that you will be able to report any changes in your condition to us.

Patient: do I need any treatment now?

Doctor: I'm afraid that there isn't any treatment that has a magical effect in MS, but there are some treatments that can possibly help in some cases. I'm not an expert on this, but I want to suggest that I will make an appointment for you to see someone from the MS specialist service so that they can discuss things with you.

Patient: what should I do if I develop new symptoms?

Doctor: you should still see your GP as the first port of call if you are worried about any new symptoms, because not everything you experience will necessarily be caused by MS. Also, you can always contact the MS specialist nurse to discuss new symptoms or problems with medication. You may also find it helpful to keep a diary of symptoms so that when you come to clinic you are able to report any changes.

Patient: have I passed this on to my children?

Doctor: that's very unlikely. We don't know exactly what causes MS. There is a lot of research being done that is trying to establish what factors can increase the risk of developing the condition, but it is not a genetic condition that is inherited from parents. So although there is a slightly higher risk that children with an affected parent will develop the condition, the risk is still very small indeed.

Hazard
Beware of making a diagnosis of MS in patients who have had only one episode of central nervous system demyelination. This is referred to as a 'clinically isolated syndrome' and the patient may not ever have any further symptoms. Making a diagnosis of MS has many implications for the patient medically, socially and psychologically.

1.3.6 Explaining the diagnosis and limitation of treatment

Scenario
Role: you are the neurology junior doctor on the ward.

Scenario: Mrs Christine Kane is a 67-year-old woman who has been admitted recently for investigations for progressive weakness of her arms and legs, and swallowing difficulty. An MRI scan of the brain was normal and an MRI scan of the cervical spine showed very mild degenerative changes. Neurophysiology testing was suggestive of motor neurone disease (MND). She wants to know what treatment options are available to her. The neurology multidisciplinary team has agreed that the diagnosis is MND and that there is no good specific treatment for her condition, although a medication called riluzole may prolong life by a few months, but without helping symptoms.

Your task: to explain to Mrs Kane the different treatment options and their limitations in MND.

Key issues to explore

> How much does the patient want to know about the prognosis of MND?

> What does the patient understand about treatment options in MND?

Key points to establish

> That MND is a progressive neurological disorder for which there is no cure.

> Medical treatments are limited and only modestly prolong life expectancy.

> Treatments are largely symptomatic, but do improve the quality of life.

> That the patient has the contact details of someone that she can call (the MND specialist nurse if possible).

Appropriate responses to likely questions

Patient: have you discovered the cause of my weakness?

Doctor: yes, we have … the problem is with the muscles themselves. The scans of your brain and spine did not show anything unexpected, but the test of the muscles showed that that's where the problem is.

Patient: so what's the problem with the muscles, and can you treat it?

Doctor: it's a condition called motor neurone disease, or MND for short … I'd like to say something different, but I'm sorry to say that this is not good news … there are things that we can do to help symptoms, but I'm afraid that we don't have any treatments that will cure things.

Patient: how will my condition progress?

Doctor: I'm afraid that MND is a progressive condition … it causes weakness of limb muscles and can affect swallowing, as you've already noticed … and it can go on to affect other muscles as well.

Patient: what other muscles are you talking about?

Doctor: well … it can affect the muscles involved in speech, making it difficult to talk … and it can go on to affect breathing as well.

Patient: how long have I got to live?

Doctor: I'm not hiding anything when I say I'm not sure … unfortunately we don't have a cure at present … different patients progress at different rates, and it is very difficult to predict life expectancy for a single patient … on average, patients live 3–5 years from diagnosis, but some live for 10 years or more.

Patient: isn't there any medicine I can take to improve my condition?

Doctor: I'm afraid that there isn't any medicine that has a magical effect in MND. A medication called riluzole may help some patients a bit, but I'm sorry to say that it only has a slight benefit … it may improve life expectancy by a few months, but it doesn't result in day-to-day improvement of muscle weakness.

Patient: so what can be done?

Doctor: although we can't cure the problem, we can provide help. Various aids can help mobility and with things like eating and drinking. If your swallowing becomes very bad, then you can be fed through a tube into your stomach.

Patient: will I have any pain?

Doctor: pain isn't usually a big problem … sometimes patients get cramps in their muscles, and medications can help to relieve these.

Patient: what's the worst that will happen?

Doctor: we've talked about a lot of things … there's a lot to take in … are you sure you want to talk about this now, or would another time be better?

Patient: no, I'd like to know now.

Doctor: well, I suppose the worst thing is if it affects your breathing … if that happens then help with breathing machines can be needed … these can improve quality of life and in many cases will increase survival as well.

Patient: where can I get information on MND treatment?

Doctor: I will make an appointment for you to see a nurse from the MND specialist service so that he or she can discuss things with you in more detail.

1.4 Brief clinical consultations

1.4.1 Increasing seizure frequency

Letter of referral to neurology outpatient clinic

Dear Doctor,

Re: Mrs Sally-Anne Cooke, aged 30 years

This woman with previously well-controlled idiopathic epilepsy for many years has experienced worsening seizure control over the last 3 months. Her medication (sodium valproate 600 mg bd) has not changed and she seems otherwise fit and well, so I am at a loss as to an explanation. What do you think has happened and how can we improve things?

Yours sincerely,

Introduction

The most important points to establish are the level of previous seizure control, whether this has been achieved easily and by what means. A full and careful drug history is required. In the case described, the first question is whether the increased seizure frequency has occurred despite an adequate blood concentration of antiepileptics. Causes of deterioration in seizure control can be divided into those secondary to a fall in level of the available drug and those that occur despite adequate drug levels (Table 29).

Table 29 Causes of deterioration in seizure control[1]

Drug level	Causes to consider
Reduced drug level	Poor compliance Poor absorption Drug interactions Pregnancy Outdated or erroneous drug preparations
Increased seizure frequency despite stable drug levels	Poor sleep Excessive alcohol / illicit drugs Non-epileptic seizures Progression of aetiological basis of seizure disorder, ie cerebral tumour Reduced efficacy of, or development of tolerance to, antiepileptic medication, ie with benzodiazepines

1 Any cause of acute illness or metabolic disturbance can cause a temporary deterioration in seizure control.

Beginning the encounter

Doctor: hello, my name is Dr A, I understand that you have been having increased seizure frequency in the past 3 months – is that right?

Patient: yes

Doctor: before we get onto the details of that, can you tell me if you have any major medical problems, apart from epilepsy?

Patient: [gives list (with doctor politely but firmly discouraging lengthy detail).]

Doctor: how many seizures were you getting before the last 3 months? How many seizures have you been getting in the last 3 months?

Patient: before the past 3 months, I was getting one seizure every 2 months. In the last 3 months, I have been getting three seizures a month.

Doctor: are you on any tablets or medications?

Patient: [gives details (and will probably have been asked to produce a written list), which includes sodium valproate 600 mg bd.]

Focused history

Doctor: have you been taking your tablets regularly … have you forgotten to take them from time to time? Have you started on any new medication? … Some medications can alter the way the body metabolises antiepileptic drugs and affect the levels of the antiepileptic drugs in the blood, and many drugs can antagonise or potentiate the effects of antiepileptic drugs.

Doctor: are you sure that the tablets you have been taking are in date? Old tablets that have gone out of date sometimes don't work properly. Have you noticed any change in the tablets that you have been given? Very occasionally people get given the wrong tablets in the pharmacy.

Doctor: have you had any diarrhoea or vomiting, which can reduce drug absorption? Are you pregnant, which can also affect drug levels in the blood?

Are there new factors exacerbating epilepsy?

Doctor: are you getting sufficient sleep? Have you started working on a night shift or are you being kept awake by a young child, etc? How much alcohol do you drink, and has this changed recently? Are you using any non-prescribed drugs / drugs of abuse?

Doctor: have you had any acute illness, eg chest or urinary tract infection [which can lead to a deterioration in epileptic control, in which case the appropriate history would need to be explored]?

Are the new attacks epileptic?

Non-organic, 'functional' or non-epileptic attacks may occur in patients with concurrent true epilepsy. This can be a very difficult diagnosis to make.

Doctor: have the attacks changed in any way? Do they happen at particular times? How long has it taken you to come round from your recent seizures?

Key point

Some pointers to pseudoseizures are:

> change in the nature of attack

> the patient is experiencing social or financial gain

> the attacks occur in the presence of observers, often in emotional situations

> a specific pattern of injuries including carpet burns or biting of the tip rather than the sides of the tongue

> tremulous or flailing limb movements, or pelvic thrusting

> unusually rapid postictal recovery.

Could there be a new or expanding lesion?

Although not to be expected in PACES, this is a particular concern in patients in whom a structural lesion is known to be responsible for the attacks. It is essential to exclude expansion of the lesion. Warning symptoms include:

> recent headache, nausea or vomiting

> new focal neurological symptoms.

Key point

Increased seizure frequency is seen in about one-third of pregnant epileptic patients, usually in the later stages of the pregnancy and related to expansion of the blood volume and changes in plasma protein binding and metabolism. Some patients will require an increase in drug dosage.

Hazard

Addition of new antiepileptic drugs can worsen as well as improve seizure control. This is especially likely to happen if inappropriate medication is used for particular epileptic syndromes, eg carbamazepine may aggravate myoclonic jerks and absence seizures in juvenile myoclonic epilepsy.

Focused examination

Examine the mouth and tongue for injuries from biting during a seizure. Perform a rapid screening neurological examination to rule out any new focal neurological signs (eg cranial nerve abnormalities, weakness, cerebellar signs and sensory disturbance). Time will be pressing in Station 5 so a reasonable approach would be to do as follows.

Key point

A very quick screening neurological examination:

> Ask the patient if there is any problem with their vision.

> Check visual fields to confrontation.

> Check eye movements.

> Ask the patient to:

> > screw up their eyes and clench teeth

> > open their mouth, say 'Aah', put out tongue

> > hold their arms outstretched with palms up and eyes closed (watch for drift and test ability to return to horizontal position after a brief push down); give instruction to touch nose with each hand with eyes closed.

> Test finger–nose pointing.

> Ask the patient to:

> > stand up with feet together and eyes closed

> > get up and walk, including heel–toe.

Questions from the patient

Patient: why am I getting more seizures recently?

Doctor: [on the assumption that the history and examination have not revealed a clear cause] frequency of epilepsy seizures can sometimes vary without a clear cause, but it would be useful to do some tests to make sure we are not missing a treatable or reversible cause [see below].

Patient: what sort of tests?

Doctor: blood tests to measure the level of the antiepileptic drug in your blood, and other chemicals in the blood that can affect the tendency to have seizures.

Questions from the examiner

Examiner: what investigations may be useful as there is no suggestion on history or examination for the loss of epileptic control?

Doctor: it would be useful to do or consider the following:

> Glucose; electrolytes; renal, liver and thyroid function tests; serum calcium; full blood count and inflammatory markers as a 'screen'. Check pregnancy test if appropriate.

> Serum levels of antiepileptic medication. Therapeutic ranges are known for a number of antiepileptic drugs, although these should be used as a guide rather than as the sole basis for altering drug dosages.

> Imaging may be required if a new or expanding lesion is considered likely, but otherwise a brain scan is not necessary.

> If non-epileptic attacks are suspected, measurement of serum prolactin (normal threshold <360 mU/L) within 30 minutes of an attack can be helpful; this may be elevated following genuine seizures (convulsive), but not following functional seizures.

Examiner: how can seizure control be improved?

Doctor: this will depend on the cause of increased seizure frequency. The options are:

> improve compliance

> increase dose or consider additional antiepileptic medication

> more sleep, less alcohol.

Examiner: what if the patient had started on a new drug?

Doctor: this always raises the possibility of a drug interaction. If in any doubt at all, I'd always refer to the *British National Formulary* or the drug data sheet.

Further discussion

If the seizure frequency remains increased despite appropriate drug levels and lifestyle, then revisit the possibility of non-epileptic seizures. Ambulatory electroencephalogram recording during an attack may help to make this diagnosis. Remember, however, that patients can become tolerant to drugs, particularly benzodiazepines, and it may be necessary to introduce new antiepileptic medication.

In patients with focal lesions, eg hippocampal sclerosis, there is a higher chance that seizures may remain drug resistant, in which case it may be appropriate to refer them for consideration of surgical treatment.

1.4.2 Numb toes

Letter of referral to neurology outpatient clinic

Dear Doctor,

Re: Mr Nigel Thomas, aged 60 years

I would be grateful if you could see this man who has developed numbness and tingling in his toes and feet, and more recently his fingertips. He also complains that he trips up occasionally.

He works as a publican, smokes 10–20 cigarettes per day and drinks about 25 units of alcohol per week. He has no significant past medical history but takes omeprazole occasionally for symptoms of reflux.

Examination was normal, except that I could not elicit tendon reflexes in his legs.

I would value your help with diagnosis and management.

Yours sincerely,

Introduction

The combination of distal sensory symptoms and absent or depressed deep tendon reflexes makes peripheral neuropathy (polyneuropathy or mononeuritis multiplex) very likely in this case. It is essential to determine if the patient has any motor involvement, eg foot drop, as neuropathies can be predominantly motor or sensory, or most commonly both. Focal and multifocal neuropathies may also occur (see Section 2.1.1).

Key point

Particular care needs to be taken to look for a treatable or reversible causes of neuropathy.

Beginning the encounter

Doctor: hello, my name is Dr A, I understand that you have developed numbness and tingling in your hands and feet – is that right?

Patient: yes

Doctor: before we get onto the details of that, can you tell me if you have any major medical problems? Any history of diabetes, pernicious anaemia or hypothyroidism? [Doctor lists possible causes of neuropathy.]

Patient: [gives list (with doctor politely but firmly discouraging lengthy detail).]

Doctor: and are you on any tablets or medications?

Patient: [gives details (and will probably have been asked to produce a written list). Check all drugs in the *British National Formulary*: is neuropathy listed as a side effect? (Not for omeprazole).]

Focused history

Doctor: can you describe your symptoms in detail?

Peripheral nervous system dysfunction would be suggested by description of:

> tingling, numbness and burning in the patient's feet (Fig 22), together with a description of them feeling as if they were walking on cotton wool (peripheral neuropathy)

> numb fingertips (peripheral neuropathy)

> the patient catching their feet on uneven ground (foot drop/distal weakness), or having difficulty in rising from a chair and going up and down stairs (proximal weakness).

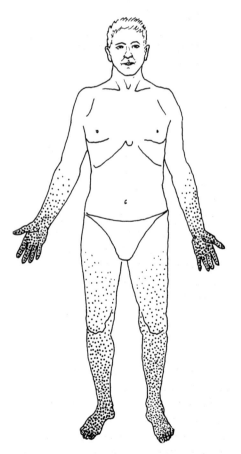

Fig 22 Sensory loss in peripheral neuropathy. All modalities should be equally affected, but the transition phase to light touch, pain and temperature sensation is not a sharp cut off – it gradually fades.

Doctor: how long have you had your symptoms? How quickly have your symptoms got worse?

The duration of symptoms and the rate of progress give clues.

> If acute, consider Guillain–Barré syndrome.

> Subacute symptoms may also indicate a neuropathy associated with vasculitis, systemic inflammatory disorders or malignancy.

> Very long-standing symptoms may be hereditary.

> Painful neuropathies may also indicate a serious underlying pathology.

For further information see Section 2.1.

Doctor: [probing for causes]

> Are you a vegetarian or vegan? [nutritional deficiency]

> How much alcohol do you drink, and have you ever drunk heavily in the past?

> Has anyone in the family had a problem like this, or any other problems with their nerves? [hereditary neuropathies are common in PACES]

> Do you smoke? Are there any other symptoms, eg weight loss? [considering paraneoplastic syndrome]

> What jobs have you done over the years? [occupational exposures]

Focused examination

You would obviously examine the patient to confirm the presence of a peripheral neuropathy. It is important to check the different sensory modalities (pinprick, temperature, vibration sense and proprioception), look for the presence or absence of deep tendon reflexes, and examine for distal or proximal limb weakness. It is important to try and determine if this is a large fibre or small-fibre neuropathy (see Section 2.1 for a fuller discussion).

Questions from the patient

Patient: what is the cause of the numbness and tingling in my hands and feet?

Doctor: it is caused by peripheral neuropathy, which is damage to the nerves of the hands and feet.

Patient: what is the cause of my peripheral neuropathy?

Doctor: [assuming no obvious cause is apparent] I'm not sure … in up to one-third of cases above the age of 50 years we don't find any convincing cause … but it is important to do tests to rule out treatable conditions [see below].

Questions from the examiner

Examiner: what investigations would you do in a patient suspected to have a peripheral neuropathy?

Doctor: [the history and examination may enable focused investigations] if there are no clear clinical leads then the following would be appropriate [see also Section 2.1]:

> *Blood tests*
In all cases: FBC, erythrocyte sedimentation rate, vitamin B_{12}/folate, creatinine and electrolytes, glucose, liver function tests, thyroid function tests and C-reactive protein. As indicated: antinuclear antibodies, extractable nuclear antigen, antineutrophil cytoplasmic antibodies, antineuronal antibodies, heavy metals, porphyrins and genetic testing.

> *Nerve conduction studies (NCS) and electromyography*
These will establish if the neuropathy is generalised or multifocal, motor and/or sensory, and axonal or demyelinating. But note that standard NCS only detect abnormalities of large fibres. A more specialised test – detection of thermal thresholds – is required to detect an isolated small-fibre neuropathy. Limited NCS of affected family members may be appropriate.

> *Cerebrospinal fluid examination*
This is not usually required for diagnosis, but may be helpful in inflammatory neuropathies with proximal involvement (elevated protein) and paraneoplastic neuropathies (elevated protein).

> *Nerve biopsy*
The superficial radial or sural nerve are most commonly biopsied. These are readily accessible pure sensory nerves, hence another nerve must be used if the problem is exclusively motor. It is best if the chosen nerve is involved clinically but not severely affected, in which case only end-stage disease process may be seen. Biopsies may show diagnostic abnormalities in vasculitis or amyloidosis, but in general the diagnostic yield is low.

> *Other investigations*
A hunt for underlying malignancy is often unrewarding, but should be pursued if there are suggestive symptoms, eg in chest or abdomen, or if routine tests reveal clues.

Hazard

A patient presenting with distal reduction in pain and temperature but with preserved proprioception and reflexes may have normal NCS. A more specialised test – detection of thermal thresholds – is needed to diagnose isolated small-fibre neuropathies.

Further discussion

Treatment – painful neuropathies (see Section 2.1) can be extremely difficult to treat. Drugs such as pregabalin, gabapentin, duloxetine, carbamazepine, lamotrigine and amitriptyline may be helpful in symptom control. The role of opioids in neuropathic pain is less clear. If all other medications fail, then a trial of opioid therapy is justified.

Meralgia paraesthetica – this is an entrapment neuropathy of the lateral cutaneous nerve of the thigh. The nerve is entrapped in the lateral end of the inguinal ligament. It causes sensory changes only, with no motor or deep tendon reflex changes. Symptoms include numbness or tingling – and occasionally a burning sensation – on the lateral aspect of the thigh down to, but not below, the knee. The lateral cutaneous nerve is vulnerable to focal compression (eg from a seatbelt); may be damaged during abdominal, pelvic or inguinal operations; or can be stretched by pelvic masses (eg pregnancy).

1.4.3 Tremor

Letter of referral to neurology outpatient clinic

Dear Doctor,

Re: Mr Alan Barnes, aged 60 years

Thank you for reviewing this accountant who has recently noticed a tremor in his right hand. He is especially worried as it is affecting his writing. His uncle developed Parkinson's disease in his seventies.

He has no significant past medical history, does not smoke and drinks 20 units of alcohol per week.

Please could you advise as to whether you feel he also has Parkinson's disease and what treatments we should offer him?

Yours sincerely,

Introduction

The main differential diagnoses of tremor are shown in Table 30. It is important to differentiate tremors which are most severe at rest, suggesting idiopathic Parkinson's disease, from tremors that are worst when the patient performs an action, suggesting benign essential tremor (BET).

Key point

Whether a tremor is maximal at rest or on action is diagnostically important.

Beginning the encounter

Doctor: hello I am Dr A. I understand you have a tremor – is that right?

Patient: yes

Doctor: before we discuss the tremor do you have any other major medical problems? Any history of stroke, high blood pressure or heart problems?

Patient: [gives list (with doctor politely but firmly discouraging lengthy detail).]

Doctor: and are you on any tablets or medications?

Patient: [gives list (and will probably have been asked to produce a written list).]

In routine clinical practice – but not in PACES – it may be possible to make the diagnosis before or as the patient enters the consulting room. If the tremor is part of Parkinson's disease or a cerebellar disorder, the patient's gait may also be affected. Observation will enable focused history taking.

Table 30	Common causes of tremor
Tremor type	**Diagnoses**
Resting	Parkinson's disease (3–6 Hz)
Action/intention	Cerebellar (3 Hz)
Postural	BET (5–8 Hz; sporadic or familial) Enhanced physiological – exacerbated by anxiety

BET, benign essential tremor.

Focused history

Doctor: please tell me about the tremor – how long have you had it? Which parts of the body are affected, is it one side or both? When do you notice it, when resting or moving?

Doctor: [probing for evidence of Parkinson's disease:]

Ask specifically about the following:

> Are your movements slower? Do activities of daily living take longer?

> Has your handwriting changed? [A presenting feature in this case, the writing typically becomes smaller and fatigues in those who have idiopathic Parkinson's disease – only if dominant side affected.]

> Is the tremor most marked at rest?

> Is there asymmetry of symptoms? [Parkinson's disease is almost always asymmetrical at onset.]

> Has your gait changed? Is your posture more stooped? Are your steps shorter? [All of these are typical of Parkinson's disease.]

> Do you feel that you 'hurry to catch up with yourself'? [festinant gait]

> Do you have difficulty turning over in bed?

Hazard
Idiopathic Parkinson's disease can only be diagnosed if upper limb bradykinesia is present.

Doctor: [probing for evidence of benign essential tremor (BET):]

BET is a fine tremor that often starts in childhood or adolescence, but presents only later when it becomes functionally debilitating. Some older patients may present with a tremor similar to BET that is due to discrete vascular lesions.

Ask specifically about the following:

> Is the tremor worse on using the affected limb? Typically it affects the arms during activities such as using a knife and fork or holding a cup, ie an action tremor.

> Is there a family history? BET can be sporadic or can occur in the context of a family history that is autosomal dominant with variable penetrance.

> Does alcohol improve the symptoms? BET often gets better with alcohol and may lead to dependence in severe cases.

Doctor: [probing for evidence of cerebellar disease:]

Tremor is rarely the only symptom or sign of cerebellar disease. The patient will more often have a broad-based staggering gait if the tremor is due to cerebellar disease (see Section 1.2.5). Past neurological and vascular history are important with an emphasis on vascular risk factors and possible demyelinating episodes, eg optic neuritis, complex intermittent sensory symptoms and paraplegia. The cerebellum is a common site for some metastases, such as bronchogenic and breast carcinoma, and therefore relevant aspects of the history should be taken to exclude possible underlying malignancy (although these are unlikely in PACES).

Doctor: [probing for evidence of physiological tremor:]

Physiological tremor is a small-amplitude, higher-frequency tremor that is enhanced by fear or anxiety. It may be pathologically enhanced by:

> thyrotoxicosis

> hypoglycaemia

> alcohol withdrawal

> drugs (beta-2 agonists, caffeine and amphetamine).

Doctor: [considering other causes of tremor:]

Consider these rare causes of tremor.

> Some 'Parkinson-plus' syndromes such as progressive supranuclear palsy ('Steele–Richardson–Olszewski syndrome') or multiple system atrophy may present with tremor, but this is not usually typical of idiopathic Parkinson's disease.

> Wilson's disease – tremor may be an early feature in 30% of cases.

> Peripheral neuropathies – fine distal tremor is occasionally seen as part of a peripheral neuropathy. Ask about numbness or tingling of hands and feet.

> Dystonic tremor – patients with dystonia may appear to have a tremor in the dystonic limb due to intermittent contraction and relaxation of the affected muscles, eg side-to-side tremor of craniocervical dystonia or 'torticollis'.

Focused examination

Face – look for hypomimia: is there paucity of facial expression with 'mask-like' facies and a reduced blink rate?

Posturing – is there any dystonic posturing of the hand or neck?

Tone – is there rigidity? Is this unilateral? Is there cogwheeling (rigidity with superimposed tremor)? Note that tone is normal in BET.

Resting tremor – is the tremor present with the arms resting on the lap? If so, is it unilateral? What is the frequency?

Postural tremor – with the hands outstretched, then elbows flexed with hands under chin (not touching), is there a postural tremor? Is it unilateral or bilateral? What is the frequency?

Is there a re-emergent tremor (no tremor at first, then starts again), which is seen in Parkinson's disease?

Intention tremor – on finger–nose testing, is there intention worsening as the finger nears the target. If there is a tremor throughout, but no terminal worsening, then this is an action tremor, not an intention tremor.

Parkinson's disease – the tremor, when present (one-third do not have tremor), is classically pill-rolling and most marked at rest, although in severe cases it will often be seen with posture and action. Rest tremor of the hands is best seen with the hands resting, palms facing inwards on the lap. The tremor may be intermittent and if it is not seen it can be elicited by mental taxation – such as 'serial threes' (see Section 1.2.10).

BET – examination may be normal except for a tremor of the outstretched arms, which may be worsened as the patient changes posture.

Cerebellar disease – produces an 'intention' tremor because it occurs with action, although when severe it can also occur at rest. The tremor is often severely functionally disabling and can render a patient virtually incapable of walking or using their arms. There will be other signs of cerebellar disease as outlined in Section 1.2.5.

Bradykinesia – is there slowness and fatigability of rapid movements? Ask the patient to open and close each hand as widely and as rapidly as possible, or to tap the thumb with each finger of the same hand in rapid succession with the widest amplitude possible. If not obviously slow, continue at least 10 times to demonstrate decrement in rate and amplitude. An extrapyramidal syndrome cannot be diagnosed without this feature. See Section 1.2.10.

Gait – is there unilateral loss of arm swing? Is there shuffling? Both are seen in Parkinson's disease.

Is the gait wide-based, as seen in cerebellar involvement? See Section 1.2.4.

Questions from the patient

Patient: what is causing my tremor?

Doctor: [assuming the diagnosis is Parkinson's disease] I think that the most likely diagnosis is Parkinson's disease … this is caused by a lack of a chemical in the brain called dopamine, which can cause tremor and some problems with movements, making them slower.

Patient: do I need any tests to prove the diagnosis?

Doctor: no, tests wouldn't help us here … Parkinson's is a clinical diagnosis made from the history and examination, and we don't need any investigations when the diagnosis is clear.

Key point

If the parkinsonian picture is atypical, eg symmetrical bradykinesia mostly affecting the lower limbs with a frontal apraxic gait, then brain imaging should be performed to exclude structural or ischaemic disease.

Patient: is there any treatment that will help?

Doctor: yes, there are several types of medication which can replace (levodopa based) or mimic (dopamine agonist) the chemical messenger dopamine that is lacking in Parkinson's disease. These are adjusted to your symptoms over time.

Questions from the examiner

Examiner: how can you differentiate the tremor in Parkinson's disease from BET?

Doctor: in Parkinson's disease, the tremor is asymmetrical (in particular, initially) and worse at rest, bradykinesia and rigidity are found in the affected limb, writing may be smaller, gait is altered so there is more shuffling and reduced arm swing. In BET, the tremor is bilateral, worse on position holding (postural) and action, there is no rigidity or bradykinesia, writing is untidy, but not smaller, the tremor frequency is faster than that seen in Parkinson's disease and walking is not affected.

Examiner: what is the treatment of BET?

Doctor: often reassurance that this is not something more serious is sufficient. If medication is desired beta-blockers, primidone, anticholinergics and clonazepam are the drugs of choice.

Further discussion

In spite of a thorough history and examination there is sometimes still doubt about the differentiation of the tremor of BET from that of idiopathic Parkinson's disease, in which case the patient is monitored over time until the diagnosis becomes clearer. A radioactive dopamine transporter (DAT) or 'DAT scan' can also be performed. This indirectly assesses the density of presynaptic dopaminergic terminals and in idiopathic Parkinson's disease there is often gross asymmetrical loss in the basal ganglia.

1.4.4 Dysphagia

Dear Doctor,

Re: Mr Dennis Blair, aged 66 years

I would be grateful if you could see this man who has an 18-month history of gradually progressive dysphagia. I initially thought that this was due to a hiatus hernia, but an upper gastrointestinal endoscopy only showed very mild oesophagitis and he was not helped by a trial of ranitidine.

He has no significant past medical history apart from migraine, takes no regular medication, has not smoked for many years and drinks very little alcohol.

I am at a loss to explain his symptoms and would be grateful for your opinion.

Yours sincerely,

Introduction

Key point

Dysphagia (difficulty in swallowing) must be distinguished from odynophagia (painful swallowing) and the globus sensation (a feeling of a lump in the throat).

It is necessary to determine if the patient's symptoms are due to an oropharyngeal or an oesophageal cause, and whether this is attributable to a mechanical, motility, neurological or muscular problem (Table 31).

Table 31 Common causes of dysphagia

Type of disorder	Oropharyngeal	Oesophageal
Mechanical	Tumour Zenker's diverticulum Neck surgery Goitre Retropharyngeal mass	Tumour Schatzki's ring Posterior mediastinal mass Peptic stricture
Motility	Achalasia Scleroderma	Achalasia Scleroderma
Neurological	Pseudobulbar palsy (eg stroke or MND) Bulbar palsy (eg poliomyelitis or MND) Myasthenia gravis	Idiopathic autonomic dysfunction Vagal neuropathy due to diabetes
Muscular	Polymyositis Myotonic dystrophy	Polymyositis

MND, motor neurone disease.

Beginning the encounter

Doctor: hello, my name is Dr A, I understand that you are having difficulty swallowing – is that right?

Patient: yes

Doctor: before we get onto the details of that, can you tell me if you have any major medical problems? Any problems with hiatus hernia, reflux oesophagitis or oesophageal stricture? [This diagnosis was clearly considered and excluded by the GP in this case.]

Patient: [gives list (with doctor politely but firmly discouraging lengthy detail).]

Doctor: and are you on any tablets or medications?

Patient: [gives details (and will probably have been asked to produce a written list).]

Focused history

Doctor: please tell me about your swallowing problem. Do you get any choking or coughing due to food or drink going down the wrong way? Aspiration is more likely to occur in patients with neurological or muscular disorders than those with mechanical problems.

Doctor: is swallowing worse with liquids than with solids? Patients with neuromuscular disorders usually complain of difficulties with liquids first, whereas those with mechanical disorders tend to complain that solid food sticks.

Doctor: do you ever get liquid coming back down your nose? Nasal regurgitation is most common in neuromuscular disorders affecting the oropharynx.

Doctor: how long have you had the problem, and is it getting worse? Progressive symptoms might indicate a worsening mechanical lesion, but if the problem is neuromuscular then the time course can also give important diagnostic clues, eg inexorable progression in motor neurone disease (MND), fluctuating course in myasthenia gravis, or a static situation following a stroke.

Doctor: is your speech affected? If so, how? This is likely to indicate a neuromuscular cause.

Doctor: do you have any muscle cramps [common in MND] or muscle weakness [obviously suggestive of a neuromuscular disorder]?

Doctor: do you have any problems with your vision … or your ability to feel things with your hands and feet … or with your bladder or bowels? If the problem is neuromuscular and yet there are no problems with vision, sensation or sphincter control, then MND is more likely.

Doctor: have you got any problems with your breathing? Respiratory difficulties might indicate MND or myasthenia gravis, but might also be attributable to aspiration.

Doctor: Have you lost any weight? This may arise because dysphagia is preventing adequate food intake, but may also indicate a malignant cause.

Are there clues to any of the other diagnoses listed in Table 31? For instance, a history of Raynaud's phenomenon may indicate scleroderma with associated oesophageal motility disorder.

A careful 'gastrointestinal' past medical history is clearly required. In this case the GP has explored these issues and the information given clearly points away from a gastrointestinal cause of dysphagia in this scenario, but if they have not then ask: 'Do you get indigestion?'; 'Do you take any treatments for indigestion?'; 'Have you ever done so?'; and 'Have you ever had a barium meal or an endoscopy test?'.

As regards neurological causes, is the patient at increased risk of stroke? Is there a family history of neurological problems?

Focused examination

This needs to begin with assessment of swallowing (there will almost certainly be a glass of water available) and the lower cranial nerves (see Section 1.2.16), with a rapid screening neurological examination if time permits (see Section 1.4.1).

Questions from the patient

Patient: why do I have difficulty swallowing?

Doctor: [assuming that the patient has a hemiparesis from a stroke and the likely diagnosis is a pseudobulbar palsy] I think it's almost certainly because the nerves to the muscles that control swallowing have been affected by your stroke.

Patient: can anything be done to improve my swallowing?

Doctor: [case of stroke] I'm afraid that we don't have any magic treatment that will make it better, but things can improve for quite a time after a stroke … what I can do is to arrange for you to get advice from a speech and language therapist about feeding and drinking, to make this as easy as possible.

Patient: why do I have difficulty swallowing?

Doctor: [assuming that the diagnosis is not clear, but seems to be neurological or muscular] I'm not absolutely sure, but it seems to be due to a problem with the nerves or muscles that control the swallowing, rather than a blockage or anything like that.

Patient: how can you find out what's wrong?

Doctor: [assuming a neurological or muscular problem] we need to get some tests done … blood tests, a scan of the part of the brain that controls the nerves that deal with swallowing and a test of the muscles themselves.

Questions from the examiner

Examiner: what investigations would you consider in this patient?

Doctor: I would consider the following:

> Blood tests – FBC (for anaemia), electrolytes (for hypokalaemia if

vomiting), and renal, liver and bone function tests (for hypoalbuminaemia as a nutritional marker); autoimmune screen (connective tissue diseases); serum immunoglobulins and electrophoresis (lymphoproliferative diseases) and thyroid function tests (thyrotoxicosis) to exclude diseases that may mimic MND; anti-acetylcholine receptor antibody (myasthenia gravis); creatine kinase, erythrocyte sedimentation rate and C-reactive protein (inflammatory muscle disease).

> Imaging – MRI is needed to exclude the presence of lesions in the brainstem if there is evidence of other cranial nerve dysfunction that suggests a structural cause.

> Electrophysiological studies – these help diagnose MND, myasthenia gravis and inflammatory muscle disease (eg polymyositis).

Examiner: is there anything else you would to do related to possible consequences of dysphagia?

Doctor: a full nutritional assessment is required for any patient whose main problem is dysphagia, and many of them will require investigation (barium swallow or endoscopy) to look for a mechanical cause.

Further discussion

The phases of normal swallowing
There are three phases of normal swallowing:

> Oral phase – this is divided into the preparatory and propulsive phases: preparatory phase – bolus of food is processed to make it swallowable; propulsive phase – bolus is propelled from the oral cavity into the oropharynx. Contractions of the tongue and striated muscles of mastication mix the bolus of food with saliva, and then propel it from the anterior oral cavity into the oropharynx.

> Pharyngeal phase – this involves a rapid sequence of events: the soft palate rises, the hyoid bone and larynx move upwards and forwards, the vocal folds move to the midline, and the epiglottis folds backwards to protect the airway. The tongue pushes backwards and downwards into the pharynx to propel the bolus down. The pharyngeal walls contract from top to bottom, helping propel the bolus downwards. The upper oesophageal sphincter relaxes during this phase and closes after passage of the food.

> Oesophageal phase – the bolus of food is propelled downwards by a peristaltic movement from the cervical oesophagus to the lower oesophageal sphincter. The lower oesophageal sphincter relaxes at initiation of the swallow; this relaxation persists until the food bolus enters the stomach.

1.5 Acute scenarios

1.5.1 Acute weakness of legs

Case history

A 27-year-old woman is referred urgently with a 3-day history of progressive weakness of her legs.

Introduction

What are the main priorities in this case?

It is critical that you think of acute spinal cord compression. In the acute stage it may be difficult to differentiate upper and lower motor neurone weakness since even in spinal cord lesions the legs may initially be flaccid. However, on the basis of the history and examination it should be possible to pick up enough clues to distinguish between an acute cord syndrome, acute neuropathy and muscle disease.

What are the causes of acute leg weakness?

See Table 32.

History of the presenting problem

What would indicate that the patient had a spinal cord syndrome?

> Is there a problem with the bladder? Any involvement suggests spinal cord or cauda equina pathology in this context.

> Is there a sensory level, or even a band of tightness (suspended sensory level) around the torso? These features would suggest a cord lesion.

If a cord lesion is likely then a sudden onset indicates a probable vascular cause (cord stroke or arteriovenous malformation). Compression or transverse myelitis would typically come on over hours to a few days.

Key point

A suspended sensory level is a band of impaired sensation below and above which sensation is normal. It may be unilateral or bilateral and is indicative of an intrinsic cord lesion.

What features would suggest Guillain–Barré syndrome?

> A history of preceding illness, particularly diarrhoea.

> Ascending symptoms.

Other rare acute neuropathies may need to be considered. Have there been any episodes of colicky abdominal pain or acute delirium/confusion (suggesting porphyria), which can also occasionally cause an acute neuropathy? Systemic features together with fever should alert you to the possibility of an infective myeloradiculitis, eg due to tuberculosis.

Key point

Back pain and weak legs

> Back pain is thought often to indicate pathology in the vertebral bodies or discs, but it may equally be a feature of transverse myelitis or an epidural abscess.

> Back and proximal muscle pain is commonly seen in early stages of Guillain–Barré syndrome.

Table 32	Causes of acute leg weakness	
Site of lesion	**Diagnoses**
Brain	Stroke, tumour (especially parasagittal) and MS
Spinal cord	Spinal cord infarction, tumour, disc protrusion, transverse myelitis, abscess, MS and poliomyelitis
Peripheral nerve	Guillain–Barré syndrome, porphyria and diphtheria
Neuromuscular junction	Myasthenia gravis, aminoglycosides and botulism
Muscle	Polymyositis, dermatomyositis, inclusion body myositis, periodic paralysis and metabolic myopathy (eg hypokalaemia)
MS, multiple sclerosis.	

What features would be suggestive of muscle or neuromuscular involvement?

> Muscle disease or neuromuscular junction disease is likely to be generalised if it is causing this particular clinical picture, so ask carefully about symptoms in the arms and cranial nerves (particularly diplopia and dysphagia), and whether fatigability has been a recent feature (myasthenia gravis).

> Is there any shortness of breath suggesting respiratory muscle involvement? This could equally indicate progressive Guillain–Barré syndrome.

> Is there any muscle pain, eg in myositis?

> Is there a rash, eg in dermatomyositis?

Other relevant history

Drugs may cause a motor neuropathy (eg dapsone) or a myopathy (eg zidovudine), impair neuromuscular transmission (eg aminoglycosides) or precipitate an acute attack of porphyria (eg phenytoin).

Neurological examination

What features would be suggestive of a spinal cord syndrome?

> Brisk reflexes, extensor plantars and a clear sensory level make localisation easy, but not all of these may be present. Look very carefully for any of them. If you find an extensor plantar, go back and re-examine for tone, power and reflexes, looking more carefully for upper motor neurone features.

> It is crucial to examine carefully for a sensory level or a suspended sensory deficit, as either of these strongly suggests the spinal cord is the site of any lesion.

Key point

> The presence of cranial nerve signs does not necessarily mean the lesion is in the brainstem. There may be multiple lesions, as in multiple sclerosis (MS) (acute cord syndromes are a common way for MS to present), and cranial nerve palsies are common in Guillain–Barré syndrome.

> Look at the patient's back for evidence of trauma, and also for superficial vascular markings/ malformations that may indicate an underlying vascular malformation as a cause of cord stroke. Auscultate over the spine for bruits: these are very rare, but if you do not check you will never hear one!

Hazard

Although a sensory level points to the spinal cord as the site of pathology, it is notoriously inaccurate at localising the level. You should therefore use all possible clinical signs to help you, eg a patient with a sensory level at the umbilicus (T10) – and who also has brisk arm reflexes – is likely to have a lesion in the cervical cord above C5, rather than at T10. The significance of this is that it is the cervical cord that requires imaging, not the thoracic cord. It is generally much better to start imaging at the top (cervical) and work down, rather than the other way around.

What features would be suggestive of Guillain–Barré syndrome?

In the presence of a suggestive history, the finding of a symmetrical weakness of the legs (this may be more proximal or more distal, as this is a demyelinating neuropathy), minimal sensory loss and areflexia is virtually diagnostic (see Section 2.1.2).

What features would be suggestive of muscle or neuromuscular disease?

> The presence of more extensive weakness, in particular of proximal arm muscles and neck flexors.

> Muscle tenderness suggesting myositis.

> A heliotrope rash over the eyelids or extensor surfaces of joints suggesting dermatomyositis.

> Fatigability of muscle power, ptosis or bulbar features, suggesting myasthenia gravis.

Investigation

An MRI scan should be undertaken to rule out a compressive lesion that is amenable to neurosurgical decompression. A scan reported as normal should exclude a compressive lesion but does not rule out the spinal cord as the site of the lesion: cord stroke and (sometimes) inflammatory lesions may be difficult to visualise.

Further comments

Treatment depends on the underlying disorder.

> Urgent intervention is needed in acute spinal cord compression and may include surgical decompression, high-dose steroids and radiotherapy depending on the type of the lesion.

> Disc protrusions causing cord compression need surgical removal.

> In epidural metastasis treatment is with high-dose steroids and radiotherapy, with the prognosis depending on the patient's condition at diagnosis and the radiosensitivity of the particular tumour.

> In epidural abscess, surgical decompression, drainage and intravenous antibiotics are needed in cases of spinal cord compromise.

> Neurosurgical intervention may be useful for some spinal tumours.

For management of other conditions see the relevant sections on individual diseases.

1.5.2 Acute ischaemic stroke

Case history

You are called to the care of older people ward to see a 78-year-old woman who was admitted the previous day with palpitations. The ward staff found her slumped in bed, conscious but not communicating. You suspect she has had a stroke.

Introduction

How common is stroke?
Stroke is the fourth single leading cause of mortality in the UK and is the leading cause of long-term acquired adult disability in most countries. It is the most common life-threatening neurological condition and is responsible for around 5% of the expenditure of the entire NHS budget. Ischaemic infarction is responsible for about 85% of all strokes, with the remainder being caused by intracranial haemorrhage (15%) and other rare causes.

What is the prognosis?
The prognosis following a stroke is poor, with up to 20% of patients dying within the first 30 days after a first-in-a-lifetime stroke. The risk of dying following a stroke is highest immediately after the event and then falls over the next few weeks and months, although the risk of dying in the years following a stroke remains elevated compared with that in stroke-free individuals.

Key point

The key to improving the outcome from stroke is to recognise it as a medical emergency and act quickly to make an early accurate diagnosis.

How can ischaemic and haemorrhagic strokes be told apart?
It can be very difficult to tell a stroke caused by cerebral ischaemia from one due to primary intracerebral haemorrhage. Neuroimaging, in particular CT scanning, is the only way of making the distinction securely. It is crucial to make the distinction so that treatment and secondary prevention can be accurately targeted.

History of the presenting problem

Some features in the history help to make the diagnosis of stroke. The symptoms should be of sudden onset and maximal within minutes to hours. If the symptoms are more gradual in onset, then this should raise the suspicion of an alternative diagnosis such as a space-occupying lesion or cerebral infection. Symptoms should be predominantly negative, eg loss of power, loss of sensation and loss of speech rather than positive, eg involuntary movements or pins and needles.

Other relevant history

Who is at risk of having a stroke?
There are certain 'non-modifiable' vascular risk factors associated with an increased risk of any vascular occlusive event (eg ischaemic stroke, myocardial infarction and peripheral vascular disease). These are increasing age, male sex, history of a previous vascular event and a family history of vascular event(s). It is important to establish the presence of any modifiable vascular risk factors in order to reduce the future risk of stroke. These include hypertension, diabetes mellitus, smoking, hypercholesterolaemia, cardiac arrhythmias, physical inactivity and obesity.

Examination: general features

Is the patient in a stable condition?
Following an acute stroke, patients are not usually critically unwell and are generally haemodynamically stable and fully conscious. However, if the stroke is large and causing mass effect or if there is significant brainstem involvement, then the patient may present in coma or deteriorate rapidly. Remember:

> Check their airway, breathing and circulation. If the patient is not maintaining their airway, protect with an oropharyngeal tube and high flow oxygen. Call for early anaesthetic support.

> Check the Glasgow Coma Scale – see Section 1.5.5.

> Check vital signs – temperature, pulse rate, blood pressure (BP) and respiratory rate. Raised BP is common following a stroke (whatever the cause).

> Check for neck stiffness – this raises the possibility of intracranial infection (and haemorrhage).

> Look specifically for signs of atrial fibrillation, cardiac valve disease, cardiac failure and carotid bruits.

Neurological examination

A neurological examination will enable accurate identification of the site of the lesion, but in routine clinical practice this degree of accuracy has no value over and above a bedside system of classification, such as the Oxfordshire Community Stroke Study (OCSS) classification (see Section 1.2.9). Therefore, perform a rapid neurological examination based on the OCSS classification and concentrating on motor, sensory, visual and cognitive domains.

Cranial nerves:

> Check for facial asymmetry.

> Check for Horner's syndrome (may suggest carotid artery dissection, or vertebral artery dissection presenting with a lateral medullary syndrome).

> Check visual fields – is there hemianopia? This can be difficult to ascertain in a patient who is not communicating: hold their eyelids gently open and present a visual threat from the left and then from the right side – does the patient shut their eyes in response to one stimulus but not the other?

> Check for papilloedema (this suggests an alternative diagnosis such a space-occupying lesion, although malignant hypertension complicated by stroke is another possibility).

> Look for deviation of the eyes and check eye movements if possible (ophthalmoplegia suggests brainstem involvement).

> Check palatal elevation and gag reflex (this is commonly affected following a stroke and can lead to aspiration pneumonia. If there is any suspicion that swallowing is affected the patient must be made nil by mouth and a nasogastric tube inserted until an assessment can be made by a speech and language therapist).

Limbs:

> Look at the posture of the patient. Are they slumped to one side, suggesting a weakness and/or inattention on that side?

> Tone – in the acute setting this may be normal or even low, only becoming increased on the affected side after hours or days.

> Power – this will be reduced in the affected limbs. There may be complete hemiplegia or a hemiparesis, in which case the weakness may be in a pyramidal distribution (arm flexors weaker than extensors and leg extensors weaker than flexors). Quadriparesis suggests brainstem or spinal cord pathology.

> Reflexes – in the acute setting these may be normal, but they soon become increased on the affected side.

> Coordination – this may be impossible to assess if the patient is very weak. Any suggestion of ataxia should raise the possibility of a cerebellar or brainstem lesion.

> Sensation – it may be impossible to ascertain whether or not sensation is preserved in a patient who is obtunded/not communicating. Sensory disturbance in affected limbs may range from inattention, to a subjective impression of reduced light touch and pin-prick sensation on the affected side, to a complete loss of all sensory modalities.

Speech (see Section 1.2.17):

> It is important to assess the patient's ability to communicate as this will help diagnostically and also have major bearing on their recovery.

> Check for dysarthria (a disorder of articulation with normal speech content).

> Check for dysphasia (a disorder of language) indicating a lesion in the dominant (usually left) hemisphere: there may be receptive or expressive problems, or both.

> Dysphasia should be distinguished from acute confusion or cognitive impairment.

Investigation

Key point
An urgent CT brain scan should be the first test ordered.

The diagnosis of stroke is made on clinical grounds, but investigations help to localise the problem, distinguish the pathology and establish the cause. Necessary tests include:

> CT scan – all patients presenting with stroke or stroke-like symptoms should be scanned immediately, primarily to exclude intracranial haemorrhage, also to look for the hyperdense middle cerebral artery (MCA) sign.

> Blood tests – FBC, electrolytes, renal/liver/bone function tests, glucose, inflammatory markers and cholesterol should be taken in the first instance.

> Chest X-ray – check for signs of aspiration pneumonia, cardiac failure, left atrial enlargement or widened mediastinum.

> Electrocardiogram (ECG) – is the patient in atrial fibrillation or any other cardiac arrhythmia? Check for signs of a previous myocardial infarction.

> MRI scan with diffusion-weighted imaging is useful to obtain in all patients with an established diagnosis of stroke. This is for confirming the diagnosis and to determine the extent of the ischaemic infarct. The MRI scan should be performed within 2 weeks of an acute stroke presentation.

Further investigation will depend on the individual case and may include:

> Echocardiogram – if the clinical examination suggests a cardiac valve abnormality or cardiac failure. Normally a transthoracic echocardiogram is sufficient but in younger patients presenting with strokes transoesophageal echocardiogram should be considered.

> 24–48-hour ECG – If the patient has a history of palpitations or for any reason it is suspected that they have a cardiac arrhythmia.

> Carotid Doppler ultrasound scan – in all patients with an anterior circulation stroke who make a reasonable recovery.

> MRI fat-suppressed axial T1-weighted scan from the skull base down to C4 if carotid dissection is a possibility (Fig 23).

Management

Key point

The management of acute stroke is best provided in specialised stroke units.

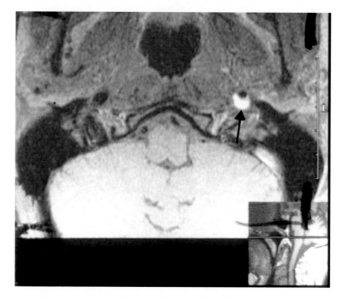

Fig 23 Axial T1-weighted MRI through the neck. Arrow indicates crescentic shape of blood in the wall of the left internal carotid artery.

Key point

Intravenous thrombolysis is the standard treatment for all eligible acute ischaemic stroke patients (presenting within 4.5 hours of the event, and without contraindications). Acute ischaemic stroke patients presenting with the hyperdense MCA sign (indicating presence of thrombus within the artery) should be immediately considered for mechanical thrombectomy following computerised tomography angiography (CTA) of the head and neck.

Management is as follows:

> Place of care – patients should be transferred to a specialised stroke unit as soon as possible.

> Specific treatment – once intracranial haemorrhage has been ruled out, patients should be treated with intravenous thrombolysis if eligible and provided there are no contraindications (see below). Within 24 hours post-thrombolysis, patients should be started on an antiplatelet agent (aspirin 300 mg once daily for the first 2 weeks, and then aspirin 75 mg once daily).

> Swallowing, hydration and feeding – early assessment of swallowing is crucial in improving outcome, and a nasogastric tube should be inserted if swallowing is not safe. Hydration should be maintained either with intravenous fluids or via a nasogastric tube. Feeding should be started early unless there is any contraindication to doing so, eg vomiting or the possibility of surgery.

> Hyperglycaemia – this may need to be managed with a sliding scale of insulin.

> **Hazard**
> Hypertension – this is common in the acute setting, but because of the disturbance of cerebral autoregulation much harm can be done by inappropriate treatment. Most authorities would recommend giving antihypertensive agents to a patient who has just had a stroke only if hypertension were extreme (>240/140 mmHg) or there were other pressing indications, eg aortic dissection.

> Nursing care – turning regularly to prevent pressure sores is required for patients with severe hemiparesis.

> Venous thromboembolism prophylaxis – thromboembolic stockings and prophylactic doses of low-molecular-weight heparin reduce the incidence of deep vein thrombosis and subsequent pulmonary embolism.

> Rehabilitation – early assessment by physiotherapists and occupational therapists is vital to provide a personalised, integrated programme of therapy to aid recovery.

Further comments

How do stroke units benefit patients?
A systematic review of randomised trials that compared the outcome for acute stroke patients cared for in a specialist stroke unit with those who were cared for in general medical wards showed that care on a stroke unit reduces mortality, physical dependency and the need for institutionalisation: the result is an overall odds reduction of 23% in patients treated on a stroke unit for the outcomes of death or living in an institution within 6–12 months of randomisation. This benefit probably arises because stroke units contain knowledgeable and enthusiastic multidisciplinary teams that implement well-coordinated care. Stroke units are potentially the most effective treatment available for acute stroke, principally because they can be applied to most stroke patients. The *National Service Framework for Older People* (a UK government document) states that all patients who have a stroke should have access to integrated stroke care services.

What are the benefits and risks of thrombolysis?
A Cochrane review published in July 2014 included 27 trials involving 10,187 patients and various thrombolytic agents. The review concluded that thrombolytic therapy given within up to 6 hours of onset of symptoms reduced the proportion of dead or dependent people. Patients treated within 3 hours of onset of symptoms benefit the most despite an increase in symptomatic intracerebral haemorrhage within the 10 days post-thrombolysis.

A meta-analysis of nine randomised trials included 6,756 patients and compared intravenous thrombolysis (alteplase) with placebo. This study showed significant improvement in functional outcome when treated within 4.5 hours of stroke onset. Earlier treatment was associated with bigger benefit (odds ratio (OR) 1.75, 95% confidence interval (CI) 1.35–2.27).

> **Hazard**
> *Why are we not using thrombolysis more often?*
> Thrombolysis is a complex treatment to administer, requiring a trained team, access to rapid neuroimaging and high-dependency monitoring facilities. In addition, the proportion of acute stroke patients who are eligible to receive thrombolysis is very small because intracranial haemorrhage must be excluded and the drug started within 4.5 hours of onset of symptoms. Therefore, despite the clear benefits seen in randomised trials, the impact of thrombolysis on the burden of stroke is likely to be limited in practice.

What is the role of mechanical thrombectomy in acute ischaemic stroke?
Recent randomised clinical trials have proven the benefit of endovascular mechanical thrombectomy in the management of acute stroke patients. This establishes a new standard of treatment in management of acute ischaemic stroke patients. Mechanical thrombectomy is provided in addition to thrombolysis in ischaemic stroke patients presenting with major vessel occlusion confirmed on neuroimaging such as CTA. The treatment should be provided within 6 hours of acute stroke onset with proximal intracranial anterior circulation occlusion (distal internal carotid artery to proximal middle cerebral artery occlusion).

Complications of acute stroke

These include the following:

> Cerebral oedema – this is the commonest cause of death and is usually associated with deterioration in the condition of the patient 4–5 days after the onset of stroke.

> Haemorrhagic transformation.

> Seizures – may complicate up to 10% of strokes (whatever the cause).

> Syndrome of inappropriate antidiuretic hormone secretion (SIADH) – this typically occurs at around 7–9 days after the onset and should be monitored for by checking serum sodium frequently in the early stages after stroke.

> Pressure sores.

> Venous thromboembolism.

> Infective – aspiration pneumonia, urinary tract infection.

> Depression – this is particularly common following left anterior circulation lesions and may complicate up to 50% of all strokes.

Key point

The Royal College of Physicians *National Clinical Guidelines for Stroke*, 4th edn (2012) is a useful document for all aspects of stroke care. NHS trusts have a responsibility to ensure that local guidelines for the management of acute stroke are produced and followed.

1.5.3 Subarachnoid haemorrhage

Case history

You are asked to see a 19-year-old man in the resuscitation area of the emergency department. His mother tells you that he had been out for the night and came home early complaining of severe headache and nausea. He went straight to bed and when she checked on him later he had vomited and was drowsy, so she called an ambulance. There was no history of headaches and no prodromal illness.

Introduction

Your first priority is to rule out subarachnoid haemorrhage (SAH).

What causes subarachnoid haemorrhage?

Most non-traumatic SAHs (around 80%) are caused by ruptured saccular (berry) aneurysms, which are usually found at arterial bifurcation sites along the circle of Willis. Other causes of SAH are much less common and include arteriovenous malformations, arterial dissection, cerebral amyloid angiopathy, cerebral venous sinus thrombosis and hypertension.

The commonest sites for aneurysms are:

> bifurcation of the internal carotid and posterior communicating artery (30–35%)

> anterior communicating artery (30–35%)

> middle cerebral artery bifurcation (20%)

> basilar artery bifurcation (5%)

> posterior circulation arteries (5%).

It is a common misconception that aneurysms are congenital, in fact they develop during the course of life.

What is the differential diagnosis?

Studies have shown that up to 30% of patients with SAH are misdiagnosed at presentation. It is important to rule out other causes of severe headache, nausea and neck stiffness such as meningitis, encephalitis and migraine. This should be possible with good history taking and examination skills.

What is the prognosis?

The prognosis following SAH is poor, with mortality around 40% within the first 24 hours of aneurysmal rupture and another 25% die from complications within 6 months. Figures from neurosurgical units tend to be somewhat better than this, probably because they never see the most severely affected patients. A good clinical outcome is expected in 90% of patients admitted in a good clinical condition, ie with a Glasgow Coma Scale (GCS) score of 14 or 15. Although the clinical course of SAH is unpredictable and clinical signs do not reliably determine which patients will have a worse outcome, it is generally accepted that an impaired level of consciousness at presentation is a poor prognostic indicator.

History of the presenting problem

The key feature in diagnosing SAH is a history of severe, sudden onset headache 'like a blow to the head'. The headache usually begins when the patient is active, and sexual activity may precipitate an SAH (as well as other more benign headaches). There is little in the history that will distinguish aneurysmal versus non-aneurysmal bleeding, except perhaps a history of trauma. Other presenting symptoms include drowsiness, neck pain or stiffness, nausea and vomiting, back pain, seizures (10–20% of cases) and focal neurological symptoms such as limb weakness.

Other relevant history

Are there any identifiable risk factors for developing SAH, such as smoking or heavy drinking? A family history of SAH could be relevant: the risk in first-degree relatives of individuals who have suffered SAH is increased three- to fivefold, and particular note should be taken of a family history of adult polycystic kidney disease.

Examination: general features

Is the patient stable?
Patients with SAH are often critically unwell and may be haemodynamically unstable with a depressed level of consciousness. To confirm their stability assess the following:

> Start by checking the patient's airway, breathing and circulation. If they are not maintaining their airway, then the first priority must be for this to be protected with an oropharyngeal tube and high flow oxygen. Call for early anaesthetic support.

> Check their GCS score – see Section 1.5.5.

> Check vital signs – temperature, pulse rate, BP and respiratory rate. The combination of hypertension and bradycardia should alert you to the possibility of raised intracranial pressure.

> Check for neck stiffness.

> Look specifically for:

 > head injury

 > hypertension

 > signs of alcohol excess or drug abuse

 > connective tissue diseases (unlikely)

 > abdominal masses (polycystic kidneys, although this is very unlikely).

Neurological examination

Cranial nerves:

> Check the fundi, looking for papilloedema and retinal haemorrhages (thought to result from an acute increase in intracranial pressure that causes obstruction to the venous outflow from the eye).

> Check for visual field defects, which may be monocular (caused by anterior communicating artery aneurysms compressing the optic nerve after rupture) or hemianopic (caused by rupture of a posterior communicating artery aneurysm).

> Check the pupil responses – small unreactive pupils may signify hydrocephalus as a consequence of raised intracranial pressure.

> Check eye movements. Third nerve palsy is a well-recognised sign after a rupture of a posterior communicating artery aneurysm. Ophthalmoplegia may suggest brainstem involvement. Bilateral sixth nerve palsies may occur due to increased intracranial pressure.

Limbs:

> Examine the patient looking for hemiparesis (occurs in 15% of patients with ruptured aneurysms).

> Check for cerebellar signs, which may suggest vertebral artery dissection as an aetiological factor.

Investigation

Investigation of the patient with suspected SAH is divided into tests needed to assess the patient's general medical condition such as FBC, electrolytes, renal/liver/bone function tests, glucose, inflammatory markers, clotting studies, chest X-ray (also to check for aspiration) and electrocardiogram (ECG), as well as those aimed at detecting the underlying cause with a view to treatment.

> CT scan – this is the immediate investigation of choice and should be done without contrast, taking very thin cuts through the base of the brain to optimise the chance of seeing a small collection of blood (Fig 24). The sensitivity of modern scanners to detect SAH is very high: 98–100% if the scan is performed within 12 hours of onset of symptoms and 93% in the first 24 hours.

> A patient in whom SAH is strongly suspected but a CT scan is negative should have a lumbar puncture. Laboratories vary in which cerebrospinal fluid (CSF) test they perform in cases of suspected SAH: some look for xanthochromia, whereas others look for elevated bilirubin in the context of normal serum bilirubin. Both of these tests may be negative if the CSF is examined in the first 12 hours after onset. It is not always possible to distinguish true haemorrhage from a 'traumatic tap', in particular, the three tube method that looks for decreasing numbers of erythrocytes in successively collected specimens is not always reliable.

Further imaging studies may be appropriate in patients with confirmed SAH if intervention is contemplated. This can be done invasively (digital subtraction angiography) or non-invasively (usually with computerised tomography angiography (CTA)) and helps to assess vascular anatomy, the site of bleeding (and possibly the location of the aneurysm that bled) and the presence of other aneurysms (about 20% of those with SAH have multiple aneurysms). Non-invasive imaging may be preferred in very unstable patients.

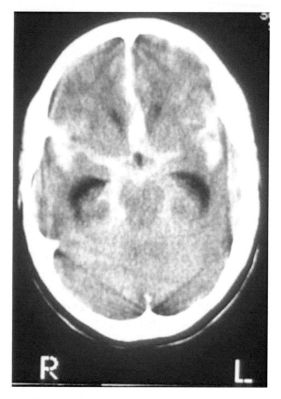

Fig 24 Non-contrast CT scan showing blood in the subarachnoid space and early ventricular dilatation.

Management

The management of SAH involves general and specific measures aimed at stabilising the patient and intervening to control a haemorrhage or prevent complications.

General measures

> Transfer to a high dependency or intensive care bed as soon as possible.

> Strict bed rest.

> Management of hypertension.

Key point

Hypertension in the acute phase of SAH can be left untreated, unless there are signs of end-organ damage. Existing antihypertensive drugs can be continued.

Specific measures

Nimodipine (60 mg PO every 4 hours or intravenous infusion at a rate of 0.5–2 mg/hour) should be given, provided the patient is not hypotensive. This helps to prevent or treat the ischaemic deficit that may occur due to vascular spasm.

Endovascular treatment of aneurysms is being used increasingly and is much less invasive than surgery. The aneurysm can be packed with coils, which ideally results in the lumen becoming occluded by thrombus. Success of the procedure is dependent on having an experienced neuroradiologist and favourable characteristics of the aneurysm, such as it having a narrow neck.

Surgery to clip the aneurysm, which may prevent rebleeding and has been shown to improve the outcome, may be required if the patient is not suitable for endovascular intervention. Although

the timing of surgery has not been shown to be a critical factor in determining the outcome, most neurosurgeons favour early intervention. Indications for surgery in patients with confirmed aneurismal bleeding (and a technically accessible aneurysm) are:

> GCS score ≥12

> GCS score <12 with space-occupying intracranial haemorrhage or hydrocephalus.

Hazard

If patients with large intracranial collections of blood become increasingly drowsy, they are candidates for immediate surgical evacuation of the haematoma.

Long-term measures

After surgery or endovascular intervention it is important to address vascular risk factors. Patients must be advised to refrain from driving and contact the Driver and Vehicle Licensing Agency (DVLA) – their license is usually returned after 3 months if they have made a full recovery. They should be strongly advised to refrain from smoking and heavy alcohol consumption.

Further comments

Complications of SAH include the following:

> delayed cerebral ischaemia secondary to vasospasm

> rebleeding – this occurs in around 50% of patients and is associated with a much worse prognosis

> hydrocephalus – this should be suspected in patients with a declining conscious level; early ventricular drainage may be required.

1.5.4 Status epilepticus

Case history

A 33-year-old man with known epilepsy is brought into the emergency department by ambulance. He has had at least six convulsive seizures in quick succession over the last 45 minutes.

Aetiology	No previous history of epilepsy (%)	Previous history of epilepsy (%)
Cerebrovascular disease	20	19
Cerebral tumour	16	10
Intracranial infection	15	6
Other acute event	14	3
Cerebral trauma	12	17
Acute metabolic disturbance	12	5
No cause identified	11	41

Table 33   Causes of status epilepticus

Introduction

What is the definition of status epilepticus?

Status epilepticus is defined as a condition in which epileptic activity persists for 30 minutes or more. This may take the form of either a prolonged seizure or recurrent attacks without recovery in between. From a pragmatic point of view, emergency treatment and investigations should be initiated for any convulsion lasting longer than 10 minutes.

What are the potential causes?

About 50% of patients with status epilepticus do not have pre-existing epilepsy. In this group, the commonest causes of status epilepticus are cerebral tumour and stroke (Table 33). Of patients with epilepsy, 5% will have at least one episode of status epilepticus at some point, commonly due to drug withdrawal, intercurrent illness or progression of the underlying disease.

What is the outcome of status epilepticus?

The 30-day mortality rate in status epilepticus is 10–20% and is determined by the aetiology and duration of the status. It is also increasingly recognised that, in addition to the morbidity resulting from the underlying cerebral pathological process and physiological derangement during status, persistent seizure activity may further damage the brain.

History of the presenting problem

It is clearly not possible to obtain any history from a patient in status epilepticus, but after rapid initial examination and instigation of treatment (see below) you should:

> Talk with any witnesses that are available – family/friends that have accompanied the patient; or ambulance/paramedical staff. Is the patient known to have epilepsy? Do they have any other medical conditions, eg diabetes? What were the circumstances surrounding the beginning of epileptic fitting – in particular, has the patient been unwell recently (and in what way); have they had any injury to their head; or have they been using alcohol or drugs?

> Read all records completed by ambulance staff or others.

Examination

> Check airway, breathing and circulation. Monitor oxygenation with pulse oximeter, but note that this may not read accurately while a patient is convulsing.

> Look for evidence of head injury.

> Note if there are any focal features to the status epilepticus: are both sides of the body convulsing; and are the eyes (if they can be seen) deviated to one side?

> Look for clues that the patient may have epilepsy or diabetes, eg Medic-Alert bracelet, a bottle of antiepileptic drug (AED) or an appointment card for neurology outpatient clinic.

Investigation

Immediate

Check finger-prick blood glucose concentration and immediately give intravenous glucose/dextrose if it is <2.5 mmol/L. It is unlikely that a blood glucose concentration >1.5 mmol/L will cause status epilepticus, but correct to give a therapeutic trial if there is even a remote possibility because neglected hypoglycaemia can be fatal or cause permanent neurological damage.

Check FBC, clotting screen, glucose (laboratory), electrolytes (hyponatraemia), renal/liver/bone function tests (renal failure, hepatic failure and hypocalcaemia) and hypomagnesaemia. Take a venous blood sample for storage. Check arterial blood gases (consider poisoning if there is unexplained metabolic acidosis).

When fitting controlled

Perform a CT (or MRI) brain scan if cause of status epilepticus not clearly established.

Check the following:

> Electrocardiogram (ECG) – note that abnormalities mimicking cardiac ischaemia can be seen with some intracranial pathologies, eg subarachnoid haemorrhage.

> Chest X-ray – look for signs of aspiration.

> Other tests as dictated by clinical circumstances, eg thick film for malaria, blood cultures and lumbar puncture.

Management

Treatment should be started immediately (Tables 34 and 35; Fig 25).

Early status epilepticus (0–30 minutes)
Supportive

Ensure airway maintenance and high flow oxygen with, if necessary, a nasopharyngeal airway if masseter trismus prevents placement of an oral airway.

Hazard

Do not try to force an oropharyngeal airway into a patient who is fitting: only two things will result – damage to the patient's teeth, tongue or mouth; and damage to your fingers.

Insert intravenous lines for fluid replacement and drug administration (preferably with 0.9% sodium chloride rather than 5% glucose solutions).

Hazard

Drugs should not be mixed: if two AEDs are needed (eg phenytoin and diazepam) then two intravenous lines should be sited. The lines should be in large veins because many AEDs cause phlebitis and thrombosis at the site of infusion.

Table 34 General measures for the patient presenting with status epilepticus based on National Institute for Health and Care Excellence (NICE) guidelines (published in 2004)

Stage	Measures
First stage (0–10 minutes)	Secure airway and resuscitate
	Administer oxygen
	Assess cardiorespiratory function
	Establish intravenous access
Second stage (0–30 minutes)	Institute regular monitoring
	Consider the possibility of non-epileptic status
	Emergency AED therapy
	Emergency investigations
	Administer glucose (50 mL of 50% solution) and/or intravenous thiamine (250 mg) as high-potency intravenous Pabrinex if any suggestion of alcohol abuse or impaired nutrition
	Treat acidosis if severe
Third stage (0–60 minutes)	Establish aetiology
	Alert anaesthetist and the ICU
	Identify and treat medical complications
	Pressor therapy when appropriate
Fourth stage (30–90 minutes)	Transfer to ICU
	Establish intensive care and EEG monitoring
	Initiate intracranial pressure monitoring where appropriate
	Initiate long-term, maintenance AED therapy

AED, antiepileptic drug; EEG, electroencephalogram; ICU, intensive care unit.

Duration of seizure	Treatment
Before admission	Diazepam 10–20 mg given rectally, repeated once 15 minutes later if status continues to threaten; or midazolam 10 mg given buccally *If seizures continue, treat as below:*
Early status	Lorazepam (IV) 0.07 mg/kg (usually a 4 mg bolus, repeated once after 10–20 minutes; the rate is not critical) *If seizures continue 30 minutes after first injection, treat as below:*
Established status	Phenytoin infusion at a dose of 15–18 mg/kg at a rate of 50 mg/minute *or* fosphenytoin infusion at a dose of 15–20 mg phenytoin equivalent/kg at a rate of 50–100 mg phenytoin equivalent/minute *and/or* Phenobarbitone bolus of 10–15 mg/kg at a rate of 100 mg/minute (usually 700 mg over 7 minutes in an adult)
Refractory status	General anaesthesia, with propofol, midazolam or thiopental Anaesthetic continued for 12–24 hours after the last clinical or electrographic seizure, then dose tapered

Table 35 Emergency AED therapy for convulsive status epilepticus based on NICE guidelines (published in 2004)

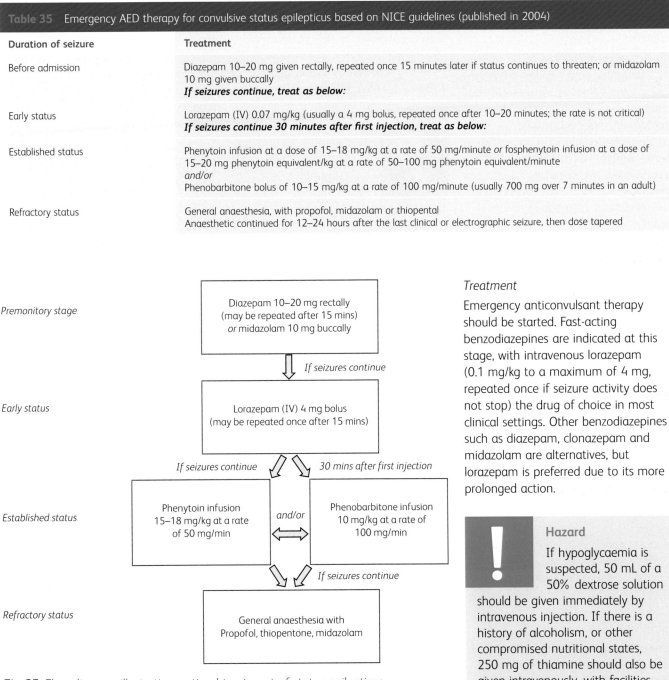

Fig 25 Flow diagram illustrating optimal treatment of status epilepticus.

Treatment

Emergency anticonvulsant therapy should be started. Fast-acting benzodiazepines are indicated at this stage, with intravenous lorazepam (0.1 mg/kg to a maximum of 4 mg, repeated once if seizure activity does not stop) the drug of choice in most clinical settings. Other benzodiazepines such as diazepam, clonazepam and midazolam are alternatives, but lorazepam is preferred due to its more prolonged action.

> **! Hazard**
>
> If hypoglycaemia is suspected, 50 mL of a 50% dextrose solution should be given immediately by intravenous injection. If there is a history of alcoholism, or other compromised nutritional states, 250 mg of thiamine should also be given intravenously, with facilities for treating anaphylaxis. Routine glucose administration in non-hypoglycaemic patients should be avoided, as there is some evidence that this can aggravate neuronal damage.

Prevent injury to the patient by nursing with the cot sides up.

Monitoring

Ensure there are regular neurological observations and recording of vital signs, eg ECG monitor. Metabolic abnormalities may cause status epilepticus or develop during its course, hence frequent repeated biochemical/haematological and arterial blood gas analysis is required in patients who are not improving.

Established status epilepticus (30–60/90 minutes)

Supportive

The physiological changes of uncompensated status epilepticus may require specific therapy. Active treatment is most commonly required for hypoxia, hypotension, raised intracranial pressure, pulmonary oedema and hypertension, cardiac arrhythmias, cardiac failure, lactic acidosis, hyperpyrexia, hypoglycaemia, electrolyte disturbance, acute hepatic or renal failure, rhabdomyolysis or disseminated intravascular coagulation.

Key point

It is frequently suggested that in the presence of acidosis the administration of bicarbonate may prevent shock, and mitigate the effects of hypotension and reduced cerebral blood flow. However, in most cases this is unnecessary: adequate support of respiration and abolition of motor seizure activity is more effective.

Monitoring

If seizures continue in spite of the measures taken above, the patient must be transferred to an intensive care environment.

Treatment

There are three alternative treatment options: fosphenytoin, phenytoin and phenobarbitone (Table 35). All are given by intravenous loading followed by repeated oral or intravenous supplementation, eg phenytoin infusion at a dose of 15–18 mg/kg at a rate of 50 mg/minute, titrated to serum levels.

There are numerous alternative treatment options. Although once popular, continuous benzodiazepine and chlormethiazole infusions are hazardous (on a general medical ward) and are not now recommended. There have been uncontrolled studies of intravenous sodium valproate at doses of at least 15 mg/kg followed by an infusion of 1 mg/kg per hour, but experience remains limited.

Key point

Establish the aetiology

The range of causes of status epilepticus depends primarily on the patient's age and the presence or absence of established epilepsy (Table 33). The investigations required depend on clinical circumstances, with CT/MRI scans and cerebrospinal fluid examination often required. The latter should be carried out only with facilities for resuscitation available as intracranial pressure is often elevated in status epilepticus. If the status epilepticus has been precipitated by drug withdrawal, the immediate re-commencement of the withdrawn drug will usually rapidly terminate the status epilepticus.

Refractory status epilepticus (after 60/90 minutes)

If seizures continue for 60–90 minutes after the initiation of therapy, the stage of refractory status epilepticus is reached and full anaesthesia is required.

Supportive

Full intensive care support should continue.

Monitoring

In prolonged status epilepticus or in comatose ventilated patients, motor activity can be barely visible. In this situation, continuous electroencephalogram (EEG) monitoring using a full EEG or a cerebral function monitor is necessary, and at the very least intermittent daily EEGs should be recorded, aiming for a particular EEG pattern termed burst suppression (Fig 26).

Continuous intracranial pressure monitoring is sometimes needed, especially in children experiencing persisting, severe or progressive elevated intracranial pressure.

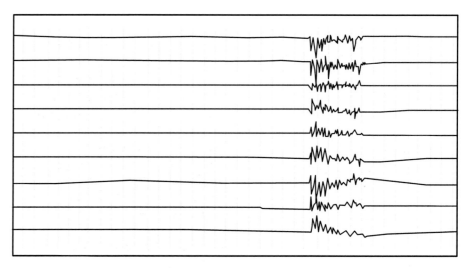

Fig 26 Electroencephalogram recording of burst suppression. Burst suppression provides an arbitrary physiological target for the titration of barbiturate or anaesthetic therapy. Drug dosing is commonly set at a level that will produce burst suppression with inter-burst intervals of 2–30 seconds.

Treatment

Anaesthesia can be induced by barbiturate or non-barbiturate drugs, although few have been subjected to formal evaluation and all have drawbacks. Most commonly used are the intravenous barbiturate thiopental, the intravenous non-barbiturate propofol or continuous midazolam infusion.

Long-term, maintenance, anticonvulsant therapy must be given in tandem with emergency treatment. The choice of drug depends on previous therapy, the type of epilepsy and the clinical setting. If phenytoin or phenobarbitone has been used in emergency treatment, maintenance doses can be continued orally (through a nasogastric tube), guided by serum-level monitoring. Other maintenance AEDs can also be started with oral loading doses. Care needs to be taken with nasogastric feeds, which can interfere with the absorption of some AEDs (especially phenytoin).

Anaesthesia should be slowly withdrawn once the patient has been free of seizures for 12–24 hours and provided that there are adequate plasma levels of concomitant antiepileptic medication.

> **Hazard**
>
> *Magnesium*
> Although effective in preventing eclampsia, there is no evidence that increasing magnesium serum concentrations to supranormal levels has any benefit in cases of status epilepticus. Indeed, such a policy can result in motor paralysis, difficulty in detecting clinical seizure activity and hypotension. However, serum magnesium can be low in alcoholics and patients on medication for HIV, and in these patients intravenous loading with magnesium sulphate may help with seizure control and prevention of arrhythmias.

Further comments

Is it possible to avert status epilepticus at a very early stage?

In patients with established epilepsy, status epilepticus seldom develops without warning. Usually there is a prodromal phase (the premonitory stage) during which seizures become increasingly frequent or severe. The earlier treatment is given the better, and urgent drug treatment will usually prevent the evolution into true status epilepticus. Diazepam has generally been the drug of choice. Alternatives include midazolam, which has the advantage over other benzodiazepines in that it can be administered by intranasal, buccal and intramuscular routes, with buccal midazolam (10 mg in 2 mL) seeming to be the most promising. The acute administration of either diazepam or midazolam will cause drowsiness or sleep, and occasionally cardiorespiratory collapse. Therefore, patients should be carefully supervised. If regular antiepileptic treatment has been reduced or stopped by the patient or doctor, then this should be reinstated.

Are there forms of status epilepticus other than convulsive?

The term 'typical absence status epilepticus' should be reserved for prolonged absence attacks with a continuous or discontinuous 3 Hz spike and wave occurring in patients with primary generalised epilepsy. There is no evidence that absence status induces neuronal damage and thus aggressive treatment is not warranted. Treatment can either be intravenous or oral, with intravenous benzodiazepines so effective that the response is diagnostic.

Complex partial status epilepticus
Complex partial status epilepticus has to be differentiated not only from other forms of non-convulsive status epilepticus, but also from post-ictal states and other neurological and psychiatric conditions. It presents in a variety of ways, but typically with a confusional state with variable clinical symptoms. An EEG can be helpful, but often the scalp EEG changes are non-specific and the diagnosis is chiefly made on clinical grounds. Treatment with oral or rectal benzodiazepines is recommended; oral clobazam has proven to be an effective treatment. Treatment of the underlying cause (eg encephalitis or metabolic derangement) is paramount and can often lead to resolution of the status epilepticus.

> **Hazard**
> **Non-epileptic status (pseudo-status)**
>
> Due to the inherent morbidity and mortality of the management of status epilepticus, this is an extremely important diagnosis to make before escalation of AED treatment and admission to the intensive care unit. Often, however, the diagnosis is made only when EEG monitoring has been established.

1.5.5 Encephalopathy/coma

Case history
A 70-year-old man is found collapsed in his home by a neighbour and is brought in by ambulance. He is unconscious with a Glasgow Coma Scale (GCS) score of 8. You are called down to the emergency department to review him.

Introduction

What are the causes of encephalopathy/coma?

There is a wide differential diagnosis to encephalopathy, ie impairment of cerebral function associated with loss or disturbance of consciousness. A systematic approach to assessing the patient is required. A list of common causes of encephalopathy and coma is shown in Table 36.

History of the presenting problem

It is clearly not possible to obtain any history from a patient who is unconscious, but after rapid initial examination and instigation of immediate treatment (see below) you should:

> Talk with any witnesses that are available – family/friends that have accompanied the patient; or ambulance/paramedical staff. In this case, has the neighbour come to hospital with him, and if so, what were the circumstances in which they found him? Do they know if the patient has epilepsy? Does he have any other medical conditions, eg diabetes? Has he been unwell recently (and in what way); has he had any injury to his head; and has he been using alcohol or drugs?

> Read all records completed by ambulance staff or others.

Examination: general features

> Check airway, breathing and circulation. Monitor oxygenation with a pulse oximeter.

> Check vital signs: temperature, pulse, blood pressure (BP) and respiratory rate.

> Look for evidence of head injury or neck stiffness: consider intracerebral bleeding or meningitis (much less likely).

Table 36	Causes of coma and encephalopathy[1]
Causes	**Diagnoses**
Vascular	Ischaemic or haemorrhagic stroke; subarachnoid, subdural or extradural haemorrhage
Metabolic	Hypoglycaemia, uraemia, hepatic encephalopathy, carbon dioxide and carbon monoxide, hypoxia, acidosis (eg diabetic), hyponatraemia, hypernatraemia/calcaemia or hypothyroidism
Drugs	Alcohol, opioids, benzodiazepines and other CNS depressants
Epilepsy	Post-ictal/status epilepticus
Infection	CNS sepsis, eg meningoencephalitis or an abscess
Hypothermia	
Trauma	Head injury

1 Any cause of severe hypotension can lead to encephalopathy/coma, in which case the primary aim must be to diagnose and correct the cause of hypotension – at which point the patient's conscious level can be reassessed. If it remains depressed, then the diagnoses listed in this table need to be considered.
CNS, central nervous system.

> Look for clues that the patient may have diabetes, epilepsy or other medical condition, eg a Medic-Alert bracelet, prescription/medications or an appointment card for an outpatient clinic.

Neurological examination

Check GCS score (Table 37).

If the patient can communicate then an assessment of cognitive status should be made (see Section 1.2.17).

Investigation

Urgent in all patients

> Check finger-prick blood glucose concentration and immediately give intravenous glucose/dextrose if <2.5 mmol/L (see Section 1.5.4).

> Conduct a CT brain scan if the coma is worsening (GCS score falling); this is also required (less urgently) if stable coma with focal neurological signs or diagnosis remains uncertain.

Routine in all patients

> Check FBC, clotting screen, glucose (laboratory), electrolytes and renal/liver/bone function tests.

> Electrocardiogram (ECG) – note that abnormalities mimicking cardiac ischaemia can be seen with some intracranial pathologies, eg subarachnoid haemorrhage (SAH).

> Chest X-ray – look for signs of aspiration.

Consider depending on clinical context
Lumbar puncture (LP) – if the diagnosis is not established and a CT scan shows no evidence of raised intracranial pressure. Also consider arterial blood gases; sepsis screen, including (when appropriate) thick film for malaria; MRI brain scan; and electroencephalogram.

Table 37	The Glasgow Coma Scale[1]	
Domain	**Finding**	**Score**
Best eye-opening response	Spontaneously	4
	To speech	3
	To pain	2
	None	1
Best verbal response	Orientated	5
	Confused conversation	4
	Words	3
	Sounds	2
	None	1
Best motor response (in any limb)	Obeys commands	6
	Localisation to painful stimuli[2]	5
	Withdraws to pain[2]	4
	Flexor (decorticate) response to pain[2]	3
	Extensor (decerebrate) response to pain[2]	2
	No response	1

1 Add scores in the three domains: minimum 3 and maximum 15, with coma defined as 8 or less.
2 Do not use methods of applying painful stimuli that cause bruising or bleeding: rubbing the sternum with your knuckles and applying pressure to the nail bed with a pencil or biro are recommended.
Are there any focal neurological features? Look in particular for facial asymmetry, ocular deviation and lateralising responses when assessing GCS score. The presence of focal signs suggests a focal rather than metabolic cause. Place particular emphasis on those signs listed in Table 38.

Hazard

Contraindications to lumbar puncture

Do not perform LP if there is:

1 clinical suspicion of raised intracranial pressure – such as drowsiness/coma, papilloedema or focal neurological signs – unless a CT scan shows no features of raised intracranial pressure; or

2 a CT scan shows mass lesion or other evidence of raised intracranial pressure.

Risk is of transforaminal herniation or 'coning'.

Management

Key point

Management of coma

> Give 50 mL of 50% dextrose intravenously if finger-prick blood glucose <2.5 mmol/L.

> Give 0.4–1.2 mg naloxone intravenously if there is clinical suspicion of opioid overdose (small pupils and low respiratory rate).

General supportive care

The most important priority is always to maintain the airway and ensure adequate ventilation. Unless there is suspicion of an injury to their cervical spine, nurse the patient in the recovery position with high flow oxygen delivered by face mask. In general, if the patient's GCS score is <8 then an anaesthetist should be called immediately to monitor and protect the airway.

> Monitor the patient's pulse (continuous ECG), BP, respiratory rate, oxygenation (pulse oximeter) and temperature.

> Give them intravenous fluids to maintain hydration and correct any electrolyte disturbance; also a urinary catheter to monitor urine output and protect their skin from soiling.

> Turn the patient over regularly to prevent pressure area damage.

> Give them low-molecular-weight heparin to prevent thromboembolism (unless there is clear contraindication).

Specific care

As determined by cause of encephalopathy/coma.

> Anticonvulsants should be commenced for prolonged (>5 minutes) or recurrent seizures (see Section 1.5.4).

> Broad-spectrum antibiotics should be given if there is even a slight chance of bacterial meningitis.

Hazard

Do not forget that *Listeria* meningitis is the second commonest cause of bacterial meningitis in older people and this responds to high-dose amoxicillin and not so well to third-generation cephalosporins.

Table 38 Important neurological signs in patients with coma

Sign	Finding	Interpretation
Fundoscopy	Haemorrhages	Trauma or SAH
	Hypertensive/diabetic retinopathy	Increased risk of cerebrovascular disease
	Papilloedema	Raised intracranial pressure
Pupillary reflexes	Dilated pupil/third nerve palsy	False localising sign
	Meiotic pupil	Opioids or pontine lesion (Horner's syndrome)
Doll's head and caloric eye movements	Abnormal	Midbrain/pontine dysfunction
Corneal reflex	Absent	Pontine dysfunction
Gag reflex	Absent	Medulla dysfunction
Jaw jerk	Brisk	Suggests suprapontine lesion
Tone	Increased	Extrapyramidal/pyramidal disease (not acute)
Limb movements	Asymmetrical	Focal lesion in pyramidal tract
Reflexes	Asymmetry or hyperreflexia	Pyramidal tract lesions
Plantars	Extensor	Pyramidal tract lesions

SAH, subarachnoid haemorrhage.

> Consider herpes encephalitis when there is a preceding history of personality change, seizures or immunosuppression and give the patient empirical high-dose aciclovir. Other viral, bacterial and atypical organisms should be considered in the immunosuppressed patient, in which case close consultation with the local microbiologist is essential.

> If encephalopathy is prolonged (>24 hours), then start nasogastric feeding.

Further comments

The prognosis of coma due to CNS suppressant drugs, metabolic/infective encephalopathies and seizures is often very good and patients may make a full recovery.

Patients in prolonged coma/encephalopathy with a persistent GCS score of <8 have a particularly poor prognosis – 50% will die and only a small proportion will regain independent living.

Brainstem death is the legal definition of death in the UK (Table 39).

Table 39 Diagnosis of brainstem death[1]

Conditions	Criteria
Preconditions	Diagnosis must confirm irreversible aetiology
	Patient must be in unresponsive coma (spinal reflexes do not exclude diagnosis)
Exclusions	Drugs, eg narcotics, hypnotics or muscle relaxants
	Metabolic or endocrine causes of coma
	Hypothermia (<35°C)
Clinical criteria	No pupillary response to light
	Absent corneal reflexes
	Absent vestibulo-ocular reflexes (no nystagmus with instillation of 20 mL of cold fluid into unblocked ears)
	No motor response within cranial nerve distribution to painful stimulation of face, trunk or limbs
	Absent gag reflex
	Absent cough reflex
	Absence of spontaneous respiration (after ventilating with oxygen to prevent hypoxia, disconnect from ventilator and allow $PaCO_2$ to rise to >7kPa)

1 The diagnosis of brainstem death must be confirmed by two competent medical practitioners who test the patient either separately or jointly on two occasions, usually 1–6 hours apart (other conditions also apply).

2 Diseases and treatments

2.1 Peripheral neuropathies and diseases of the lower motor neurone

2.1.1 Peripheral neuropathies

Pathophysiology

Peripheral nerves contain bundles of nerve fibres, both large-diameter myelinated fibres and small-diameter non-myelinated fibres. The large myelinated fibres carry both efferent motor signals and afferent sensory signals (proprioception and vibration sense). The small non-myelinated fibres carry afferent pain and temperature as well as autonomic signals. The peripheral nerve can react to injury or insult in one of four ways: axonal degeneration, demyelination, Wallerian degeneration and neuronal cell body disease (neuronopathy).

Axonal degeneration

This is the commonest pathological process encountered in peripheral neuropathies, particularly those associated with systemic, toxic, nutritional and metabolic disorders. The commonest aetiology is diabetes mellitus (Table 40) which is the commonest cause of neuropathy in the UK (three-quarters of these cases being a distal symmetrical sensory or sensorimotor polyneuropathy). Large-diameter fibres are predominantly involved, and the longest fibres are affected first by this dying back process.

Demyelination

Destruction of the myelin sheath, leaving the axon intact, leads to segmental demyelination, which is commonly secondary to an immune-mediated disorder (see Table 41). Demyelination may occur distally or proximally and is patchy.

Wallerian degeneration

This is the name given to the degenerative process of the distal stump seen after nerve transection (or an equivalent insult). Regeneration from the proximal stump is slow and variable.

Neuronopathy

Neuronopathy describes a disease process that specifically attacks the neuronal cell bodies. In the case of motor nerves this occurs within the anterior horn of the spinal cord, and in the case of sensory nerves it occurs within the dorsal root ganglion.

Examples of motor neuronopathies include motor neurone disease, spinal muscular atrophies and poliomyelitis. The sensory ganglion cell may be the primary site of injury in paraneoplastic neuropathies (see Section 2.11.1) or in Sjögren's syndrome.

Clinical presentation

The commonest type of neuropathy is the distal symmetrical sensorimotor axonal type. Patients will first complain of tingling, burning or band-like sensations in the toes or soles of the feet. As the symptoms progress the sensory disturbance will extend onto the dorsum of the foot and the ankle reflexes will be lost; there may also be weakness of dorsiflexion of the toes and ankle and possibly muscle wasting. Patients may complain of a feeling of walking on cotton wool or on stumps. Progression may lead to foot drop and a high steppage gait; and knee reflexes will be lost. Sensory symptoms in the

Table 40	Classification of diabetic neuropathies	
Type	**Diagnoses**
Symmetrical polyneuropathies	Distal sensory or sensorimotor polyneuropathy
	Large-fibre neuropathy ('diabetic pseudotabes')
Asymmetrical polyneuropathies	Cranial neuropathy (single or multiple)
	Limb mononeuropathy (single or multiple)
	Trunk mononeuropathy (single or multiple)
	Proximal diabetic neuropathy/diabetic amyotrophy

Table 41	Causes of neuropathies
Category	**Diagnoses**
Sensorimotor polyneuropathy	Alcohol
	Diabetes mellitus
	Hypothyroidism
	GBS
	CIDP
	HMSN
	Vasculitis
	Paraneoplastic
	Paraproteinaemic
Sensory polyneuropathy	Diabetes mellitus
	Hypothyroidism
	Drugs, eg isoniazid and vincristine
	Vitamin B_{12} deficiency
	Paraneoplastic
	Amyloidosis
	HIV
	Leprosy
Motor neuropathy	GBS/CIDP
	MMN
	Porphyria
	Lead
	Diphtheria
Focal/multifocal neuropathies	Connective tissue disorders
	Vasculitis
	Granulomatous disorders, eg Wegener's granulomatosis and sarcoidosis
	Carcinomatous infiltration
	Nerve compression, eg common peroneal nerve palsy
	HIV
	Leprosy
	HNLPP
	Diabetes mellitus
	Fabry disease
Painful	GBS
	Vasculitis
	Amyloidosis
	HIV
	Leprosy
	Malignant infiltration
	Diabetes mellitus
	Uraemia
Demyelinating	GBS/CIDP
	MMN
	Paraproteinaemic
	HIV
	Drugs (amiodarone)
	HMSN 1
Axonal (small fibre)	Amyloid
	Leprosy
	HIV
	Diabetes mellitus (rare)
	HSAN
	Fabry disease
	Tangier disease
Axonal (large fibre)	Vasculitis
	Paraneoplastic
	Toxins
	Diabetes mellitus
	Porphyria
	Uraemia
	Vitamin B_{12} deficiency
	HMSN 2
	Friedreich's ataxia
Autonomic	GBS/CIDP[1]
	HIV
	Paraneoplastic[1]
	Porphyria[1]
	Diabetes mellitus
	Toxins[1]
	HSAN
	Amyloidosis

1 Predominantly acute.
CIDP, chronic inflammatory demyelinating polyneuropathy; GBS, Guillain–Barré syndrome; HIV, human immunodeficiency virus; HMSN, hereditary motor and sensory neuropathy; HNLPP, hereditary neuropathy with liability to pressure palsies; HSAN, hereditary sensory and autonomic neuropathy; MMN, multifocal motor neuropathy with conduction block.

fingertips do not develop until those in the leg have ascended to at least the knee. The patient's gait may become unsteady due to proprioceptive loss. Progression continues smoothly, moving centrally up the arms and legs in a symmetrical fashion, eventually affecting the anterior torso. In extreme cases involvement of the intercostal and diaphragmatic muscles leads to ventilatory disturbance.

Variations from this clinical picture are discussed below.

Axonal versus demyelinating neuropathies

Although the pathological process cannot be reliably distinguished clinically, the following may act as pointers:

> Concurrent proximal and distal involvement suggests a demyelinating process. Remember that axonal degeneration is a distal dying back process, and demyelination can occur anywhere on the nerve.

> Loss of all reflexes early in the process, rather than sequential loss as described above, might suggest demyelination.

Asymmetry

Asymmetry of clinical findings suggests a multifocal process affecting individual nerve trunks or roots.

Large-fibre versus small-fibre neuropathies

In small-fibre neuropathies, the following are more likely:

> No significant weakness (motor fibres are large myelinated axons).

> Preserved reflexes (the fibres subserving the afferent limb of the muscle stretch reflex arc are large myelinated axons, as are the efferent motor fibres).

> Preserved balance (proprioceptive information is conducted in large myelinated axons).

> Reduced pin-prick and temperature sensation.

> Sometimes autonomic disturbance.

Arms versus legs

It is unusual for the first symptoms of a peripheral neuropathy to be in the arms, and this should bring the diagnoses suggested below to mind.

Neuropathies that can present in the arms before legs:

> Guillain–Barré syndrome (GBS) / chronic inflammatory demyelinating polyneuropathy (CIDP)

> porphyria

> spinal muscular atrophy

> hereditary motor and sensory neuropathy (HMSN)

> vitamin B_{12} deficiency (sensory symptoms).

Investigation

Peripheral neuropathies are often investigated with a blanket screening process. It is hoped that the preceding description of different types of neuropathy makes it clear that in some circumstances investigations can be targeted. Where this is not the case, blood screening is performed to consider the common or treatable causes of peripheral neuropathy.

Key points

Carpal tunnel syndrome

> Bilateral carpal tunnel syndrome may initially be mistaken for a peripheral neuropathy.

> Patients complain of nocturnal paraesthesia, numbness or burning sensations, often describing how they shake their hands or hang them over the side of the bed for relief.

> Symptoms may be confined to the thumb, index, middle and lateral half of the ring finger, but are often more diffuse, extending to the elbow and sometimes to the shoulder.

> Look for reduced sensation on the lateral part of the palm and splitting of the ring finger; and in more severe cases wasting of the thenar eminence and weakness of the abductor pollicis brevis.

> In mild cases the diagnosis is made on the history and confirmed electrophysiologically.

Other upper limb entrapment neuropathies

See Fig 27 and Sections 1.2.2 and 1.2.6.

Lower trunk of brachial plexus

Mainly affected by cervical rib syndrome, altered anatomy, cervical outlet syndrome, brachial neuritis or Pancoast tumour of the lung apex.

Axillary nerve

Damaged by fracture of humeral neck, dislocation of shoulder and deep intramuscular injections (Fig 27).

Radial nerve

May be damaged at the following sites:

> Axilla – damaged by weight bearing on a crutch or resting the arm over back of chair while asleep or intoxicated.

> Spiral groove of humerus – vulnerable to direct blow laterally (during anaesthesia or while drunk), medially or after mid-shaft humeral fracture (which may be either immediate or delayed as callus forms).

> Supinator muscle – the radial nerve (posterior interosseous nerve) passes through the supinator and may be damaged by occupational overuse or acute haemorrhage into muscle during trauma.

Ulnar nerve

May be damaged at the following sites:

> Elbow – often damaged by repeated minor trauma and prolonged bed rest (patient resting on elbows), or delayed following fractures in childhood leading to minor anatomical abnormality (tardy ulnar palsy).

> Palm – deep branch damaged by trauma to the heel of the hand or idiopathically due to a ganglion. Confusing clinically as often there is no sensory loss and it is often mistaken for motor neurone disease (Fig 28).

Median nerve

May be damaged at the following sites:

> Elbow – rarely damaged by direct trauma but may be involved in elbow fracture as deeply placed.

> Forearm – the anterior interosseous branch of the median nerve is a rarely damaged nerve that lies very deep; flexors of index finger and thumb are affected by it (ie pinch grip). Haemorrhage into the muscle during physical exertion is the most common cause of damage.

> Wrist – see carpal tunnel syndrome above (Fig 28).

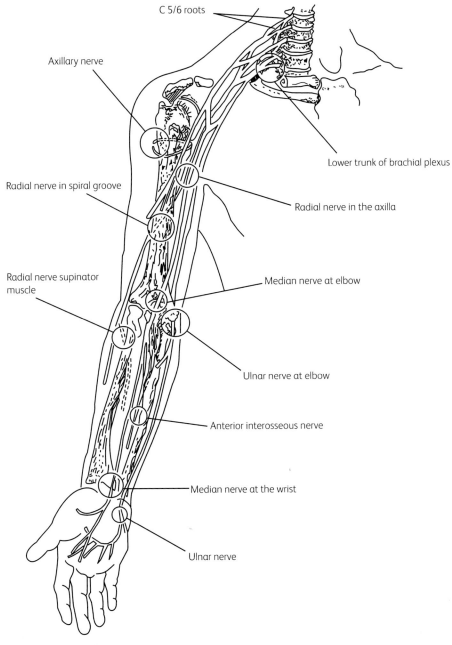

C 5/6 roots

Axillary nerve

Radial nerve in spiral groove

Radial nerve supinator muscle

Lower trunk of brachial plexus

Radial nerve in the axilla

Median nerve at elbow

Ulnar nerve at elbow

Anterior interosseous nerve

Median nerve at the wrist

Ulnar nerve

Fig 27 Neurological anatomy of the arm showing main locations of damage.

Therefore a patient presenting with distal reduction in pain and temperature as well as preserved proprioception and reflexes may have normal NCS. A more specialised test – detection of thermal thresholds – is required to detect an isolated small-fibre neuropathy.

If relevant, limited NCS of affected family members should be performed.

Cerebrospinal fluid examination
This is not usually required for diagnosis, but it may be helpful in inflammatory neuropathies with proximal involvement (elevated protein).

Paraneoplastic neuropathies may also be associated with elevated protein.

An elevated white cell count in a patient with suspected GBS should raise the possibility of HIV-associated inflammatory neuropathy.

Hunt for underlying malignancy
This is often unrewarding, but should be guided by other symptoms, eg chest, abdomen and blood film.

Nerve biopsy
Nerve biopsy is an invasive procedure and should only be carried out in a specialist centre. You need to consider whether management is being helped, as diagnostic yields are often low. It is usual to biopsy either the superficial radial or sural nerve: readily accessible pure sensory nerves. If the process is exclusively motor, another nerve must be used. As with other tissue sampling it is preferential that the chosen nerve is involved clinically, but not severely affected – in which case only end-stage disease process may be seen with little or no diagnostic value. Biopsies may show diagnostic abnormalities in vasculitis or amyloidosis. In the case of hereditary neuropathies, the availability of genetic testing is making the role of nerve biopsies less important.

Blood tests
FBC, erythrocyte sedimentation rate, vitamin B_{12}/folate, urea and electrolytes, glucose, liver function tests, thyroid function tests and C-reactive protein. Special blood tests include: antinuclear antibodies, extractable nuclear antigens, antineutrophil cytoplasmic antibodies, antineuronal antibodies, heavy metals, porphyrins and genetic testing.

Nerve conduction studies and electromyography
These tests should be able to inform you about whether the neuropathy is:

> generalised or multifocal

> motor and/or sensory

> axonal or demyelinating.

Standard nerve conduction studies (NCS) (see Section 3.3) only detect abnormalities of large fibres.

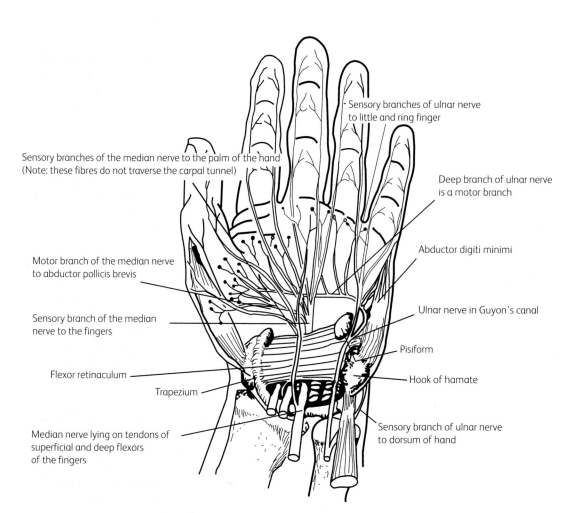

Fig 28 The anatomy of the median and ulnar nerves in the hand.

Labels in figure:
- Sensory branches of ulnar nerve to little and ring finger
- Sensory branches of the median nerve to the palm of the hand (Note: these fibres do not traverse the carpal tunnel)
- Deep branch of ulnar nerve is a motor branch
- Abductor digiti minimi
- Motor branch of the median nerve to abductor pollicis brevis
- Ulnar nerve in Guyon's canal
- Sensory branch of the median nerve to the fingers
- Pisiform
- Flexor retinaculum
- Hook of hamate
- Trapezium
- Median nerve lying on tendons of superficial and deep flexors of the fingers
- Sensory branch of ulnar nerve to dorsum of hand

Management

Depends on the underlying cause.

Remove any insult or correct any metabolic/endocrine abnormality as appropriate. While this may prevent further nerve damage, axonal recovery in particular is slow.

Inflammatory

Unlike GBS, CIDP may respond to steroids. Like GBS, both plasma exchange and intravenous immunoglobulin (IVIG) have equal efficacy. Some clinicians will try a 6–8-week course of high-dose oral prednisolone and reserve IVIG for steroid non-responsive cases. Others use IVIG as a first-line treatment. Treatment courses may need to be repeated if the condition relapses and some patients become treatment dependent, requiring regular IVIG to maintain well-being.

Vasculitic neuropathy

Initial treatment with high-dose oral prednisolone or if severe, a short course of intravenous methyl prednisolone followed by maintenance oral steroids. The use of IVIG is anecdotal but would appear sensible and is becoming more widely used. Systemic, necrotising vasculitides may require cyclophosphamide.

Paraneoplastic neuropathy

See Section 2.11.1.

2.1.2 Guillain–Barré syndrome

Disease

This is defined as an acute (post-infectious) inflammatory demyelinating polyneuropathy, affecting 2:100,000 per annum. It is usually monophasic, but relapses have been described.

Pathology

This is an inflammatory condition, leading to multifocal demyelination of spinal roots and peripheral nerves. Demyelination may occur anywhere along the lower motor nerve pathway, but the ventral (motor) roots, proximal spinal nerves and lower cranial nerves are most often affected, which accounts for the pattern of clinical features. Much evidence suggests that Guillain–Barré syndrome (GBS) is an organ-specific autoimmune disorder mediated by autoreactive T-cells and humoral antibodies to peripheral nerve antigens. Preceding infections, particularly *Campylobacter jejuni*, may trigger this response through molecular mimicry.

Clinical presentation

Approximately 60–70% of sufferers report an illness in the preceding weeks (often 1–4 weeks prior to the onset). This is usually an upper respiratory tract illness or diarrhoea, and many pathogens have been implicated (Table 42).

The onset is subacute, usually over a few days, but can be rapid with complete paralysis in hours. However, the progression of symptoms may continue for up to 4 weeks (but no longer, by definition).

The main complaints are of ascending sensory symptoms (symptoms are more prominent than sensory signs) and ascending, or occasionally proximal, weakness. In most cases the legs are affected first and to a greater degree than the arms, but occasionally the arms can be worst affected. Muscle pain is common, frequently manifesting as deep intrascapular or lower back pain, or even initiating bilateral sciatica.

Physical signs

The main signs are of symmetrically reduced tone, areflexia, a varying degree of glove-and-stocking sensory disturbance (often mild), and lower motor neurone weakness. Facial involvement and ophthalmoplegia may be present.

Autonomic features occur in approximately half the patients (fluctuations in blood pressure, heart rate, ileus and urinary retention).

Key point

The clinician must be aware that fixed pupils can occur with autonomic involvement and this must not be confused with brainstem pathology.

Other clinical variants of GBS:

> Miller Fisher syndrome (ataxia, areflexia and ophthalmoplegia)

> cranial nerve variant (polyneuritis cranialis)

> pure sensory variant

> pharyngeal–cervical–brachial variant

> acute autonomic variant

> axonal variant (motor and sensory)

> acute motor axonal variant.

Investigations

If the condition is suspected clinically, your priorities are to monitor for potential complications, particularly respiratory and cardiac. Further investigations may confirm the diagnosis but are unlikely to be available immediately. Initial management therefore has to be based on clinical suspicion.

Measurement of respiratory function

Monitor forced vital capacity (not peak flow) at regular intervals, the frequency depending on the severity of the weakness or the rate of change.

Cardiac monitor

Doctors are aware of the respiratory complications of GBS but neglect the autonomic complications. Dysrhythmias can be fatal without intervention.

Cerebrospinal fluid

Cerebrospinal fluid (CSF) may be normal in the first few days. Later protein rises as a consequence of inflammation in the proximal roots (within the subarachnoid space). If pleocytosis is present, consider other diagnosis (see differential diagnosis below).

Nerve conduction studies

In GBS peripheral nerve demyelination starts proximally at the nerve roots. Distal conduction velocities and distal motor latencies are therefore normal early in the illness, even in the face of profound weakness. The earliest electrophysiological abnormality is prolongation, impersistence or absence of the F-wave. The electromyogram (EMG) will show denervation in later stages.

Antiganglioside antibodies

Gangliosides are sialylated glycosphingolipids found on nerves. Anti-GQ1b antibodies appear to be present in all cases of GBS with associated ophthalmoplegia, particularly the Miller Fisher variant (triad of ataxia, areflexia and ophthalmoplegia).

Identification of the infective agent

> Results can often be negative, but may help with prognosis if they are positive.

> Stool culture for *Campylobacter jejuni*.

> Serology for atypical pneumonias.

> CSF viral analysis.

Table 42 Common pathogens implicated in Guillain–Barré syndrome (GBS)	
Cause	Diagnoses
Viral	Cytomegalovirus
	Epstein–Barr virus
	HIV
	Hepatitis A
Bacterial	Mycoplasma
	Campylobacter jejuni
Immunisation	Tetanus toxoid
	Rabies
	Swine influenza

Differential diagnosis

The differential diagnosis of acute/ subacute weakness is broad but important. Given a good history together with examination features that are clear then GBS is the commonest cause, but also consider the following:

> Other acute neuropathies including porphyria.

> Metabolic disturbances (severe hypophosphataemia, hypokalaemia and hypermagnesaemia) should be excluded.

> Myasthenia gravis may cause subacute onset weakness. Look for fatigability.

> Occasionally central nervous system disease, such as acute brainstem stroke, spinal cord compression or transverse myelitis, may cause confusion, but a careful history and examination should prevent this mistake from being made.

> Poliomyelitis is now a less common differential. The presentation is usually strikingly asymmetrical, which helps differentiate it from the symmetrical picture of GBS.

> Typical features of GBS associated with CSF pleocytosis (over 50 cells/μL) raise the possibility of meningoradiculitis caused by HIV, Lyme disease, tuberculosis or cytomegalovirus infection.

Treatment

The following points need to be considered:

> Patients who are deteriorating should be transferred to a unit that is able to deal with neuromuscular respiratory failure and autonomic dysfunction.

> Consider elective ventilation early if the patient is tiring.

> Cardiac arrhythmias should be treated as appropriate.

> Antihypertensive drugs must be used with extreme caution in the presence of autonomic dysfunction.

> Note that tracheal suction may trigger hypotension or bradycardia in the presence of autonomic dysfunction.

> Treat pain with non-steroidal anti-inflammatory drugs (NSAIDs) or opiates.

> Feed patients via nasogastric tube or percutaneous endoscopic gastrostomy if necessary.

> Administer prophylactic subcutaneous heparin and thromboembolic stockings for immobile patients.

> Provide:
> > regular chest physiotherapy
> > regular turning
> > early physiotherapy
> > psychological support for the patient and their family.

Specific treatment

A 5-day course of intravenous immunoglobulin (IVIG) (0.4 g/kg/day) is as efficacious as plasma exchange, but with fewer side effects. Plasma exchange followed by IVIG does not confer a significant advantage. Patients with mild GBS do not require treatment.

Key point

IVIG is easily administered. This should not dissuade the clinician from early transfer of the patient to a centre with a good intensive care unit if the patient deteriorates clinically. If a patient requires treatment, they require transfer!

Prognosis

GBS begins with a period of deterioration, then a plateau phase, followed by a period of recovery. In series, up to 30% of patients require ventilation. Mortality remains about 5% despite treatment. On the whole this is a self-limiting disease. In very broad terms, one-third of patients make a full recovery (although they may remain areflexic), one-third are left with mild disability and one-third have moderate to severe disability.

Key point

Preceding illness with *Campylobacter jejuni* can result in a severe axonal variant with a poor prognosis.

2.1.3 Motor neurone disease

Aetiology

The causes of motor neurone disease (MND) are unknown, but many hypotheses have been suggested. Mutations in the cytosolic Cu/Zn superoxide dismutase gene on chromosome 21 accounts for 20% of cases of familial amyotrophic lateral sclerosis (ALS) and 2% of all cases of ALS. Glutamate is a major excitatory neurotransmitter, and overstimulation of glutamate receptors is associated with neurotoxicity in MND. Oxidative stress with free radical damage is also implicated in the pathogenesis of MND. Dysregulation of the vascular endothelial growth factor (VEGF), protein aggregation in the motor neurone, mitochondrial dysfunction and neuroinflammation modulated by non-neuronal cells may also play a part.

Epidemiology

The incidence of MND is 1–3 per 100,000 people, with the mean age of onset being 55 years. The male to female ratio is 3:2 and 10% of cases are familial, usually of an autosomal dominant inheritance. Most cases of MND are of the ALS type that has both upper motor neurone (UMN) and lower motor neurone (LMN) involvement. The other clinical variants, progressive muscular atrophy (PMA) with its purely LMN involvement and primary lateral sclerosis (PLS) with its purely UMN involvement, may just represent ends of the spectrum of ALS.

Clinical presentation

Muscle weakness is the most common presenting complaint, with onset in the arms more common than in the legs. Occasionally, one limb may become involved on its own. Some patients notice muscle twitching or fasciculations, muscle cramps and easy fatigability.

> **Hazard**
>
> Fasciculations are virtually never the sole presenting feature of MND.

In 20% of patients, bulbar symptoms are the initial problem, eg dysarthria, dysphagia, difficulty chewing or coughing, and eventually sialorrhoea. Weight loss may occur. Rarely, respiratory muscle weakness causing breathlessness is the first symptom.

Physical signs

Cranial nerve examination may reveal lower cranial nerve involvement, eg facial weakness (seventh), depressed gag reflex (ninth/tenth), poor palatal movement (tenth) and a wasted, fasciculating tongue (twelfth and bulbar palsy). A brisk jaw jerk (fifth), increased gag reflex or a spastic tongue indicates pseudobulbar palsy.

In the limbs, UMN involvement produces spasticity, weakness, hyperreflexia and Babinski sign, whereas LMN involvement produces atrophy (Fig 29) fasciculations, flaccidity, weakness and hyporeflexia.

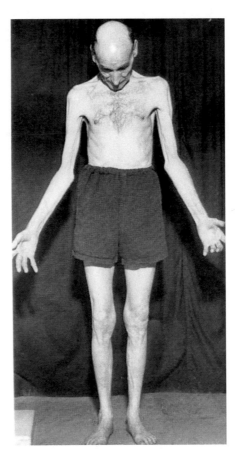

Fig 29 Wasted muscles in motor neurone disease.

> **Key point**
>
> > In MND there is no extraocular or sphincter disturbance, and sensory examination is normal.
>
> > You should never examine for fasciculations when the tongue is protruded, as you will often see 'abnormalities' that are not really present.

Investigation

See Sections 1.4.4 and 1.2.8.

Further points on investigation are as follows:

> Anti-GM1 ganglioside antibodies and an electromyelogram are important in ruling out multifocal motor neuropathy (MMN).

> An MRI scan excludes cervical spine and foramen magnum lesions, eg syringomyelia, syringobulbia and cervical spondylosis.

Differential diagnosis

Misdiagnosis of MND is a common clinical problem with serious implications. Certain differentials should always be considered:

> Spondylotic cervical myelopathy – although this is a potentially treatable condition, there is increasing doubt as to whether it can actually mimic MND as it almost always causes only spastic paraparesis.

> It is important to diagnose MMN because it is potentially treatable with intravenous immunoglobulin (IVIG) or cyclophosphamide. It is associated with LMN signs only and anti-GM1 ganglioside antibodies (although these are not specific).

> X-linked bulbospinal neuronopathy (Kennedy's disease) – this is associated with perioral fasciculation, LMN signs only, gynaecomastia, testicular atrophy, diabetes mellitus and a CAG expansion in the androgen receptor locus.

> Benign fasciculations, hexosaminidase A deficiency (Tay–Sachs disease), lymphoproliferative disorders and thyrotoxicosis may all mimic MND and should be excluded in atypical cases.

Treatment

Symptomatic treatment and supportive care are the mainstays of management in MND. The patient's right to self-determination should be respected at all times.

Riluzole, a sodium channel blocker that inhibits abnormal glutamatergic neurotransmission in the central nervous system (CNS), has only modest effects on disease progression. A patient's FBC and liver function needs to be monitored when it is used.

Prognosis

Death usually ensues in 3–5 years from aspiration pneumonia and respiratory failure.

Key point

Poor prognosis factors include:

> older patients

> shorter duration between onset and diagnosis

> ALS (rather than PLS or PMA)

> low amplitude muscle action potentials.

2.2 Diseases of muscle

A wide range of sporadic and hereditary insults can affect muscle. These include:

> systemic disorders of metabolism

> local and systemic inflammatory conditions

> hereditary disorders of a muscle itself

> abnormalities of membrane ion channels.

Presentation may be with weakness, cramps, pain or a combination of these. The age of onset, presence or otherwise of a positive family history, nature of presentation and distribution of muscle involvement are all instructive pointers to the aetiology. A classification of muscle disorders is given in Table 43.

2.2.1 Metabolic muscle disease

Disorders of carbohydrate metabolism (glycogen storage diseases)

Pathophysiology

Fig 30 describes the biochemical pathway by which glycogen metabolism and glycolysis occurs within muscle cells. Deficiencies of the enzymes shown have all been associated with metabolic muscle disease. Clinically, enzyme

Table 43	Classification of muscle disease	
Cause	**Diagnoses**	
Metabolic	Disorders of carbohydrate metabolism	
	Disorders of lipid metabolism	
	Mitochondrial myopathies	
Inflammatory	Polymyositis	
	Dermatomyositis	
	Inclusion body myositis	
Inherited myopathies	Disorders of dystrophin	
	Limb girdle muscular dystrophies	
	Facioscapulohumeral dystrophy	
	Emery–Dreifuss muscular dystrophy	
	Myotonic dystrophy	
	Others	
Channelopathies	Periodic paralysis	
	Myotonia	

deficiencies can be divided into those associated with exercise intolerance and those causing progressive muscle weakness. The most important disease of each group is described below.

McArdle's disease

Also called myophosphorylase deficiency or type V glycogenosis. The same clinical picture is seen with phosphorylase b kinase deficiency (Fig 30). This was first described by Dr Brian McArdle in 1952.

Genetics

Myophosphorylase gene is encoded on 11q.13. It is usually autosomal recessive but autosomal dominant inheritance has been described.

Clinical presentation

Carbohydrate stores within muscle are necessary in the early stages of exercise prior to added energy supply being provided by lipid metabolism. Disorders

of carbohydrate metabolism therefore present with exercise intolerance after minimal exercise. A 'second wind' phenomenon may be described if the patient exercises gently through the initial barrier enabling diversion of their blood flow to muscle and the onset of fatty acid metabolism.

Symptoms

Often presents in the second and third decade, although in retrospect there may have been poor exercise tolerance as a child. Symptoms include:

> muscle pain after minutes of exercise

> painful muscle contractures

> episodes of dark urine (myoglobinuria secondary to rhabdomyolysis).

Physical signs

Usually no abnormal signs when resting. Patients may develop a mild myopathy late in the disease.

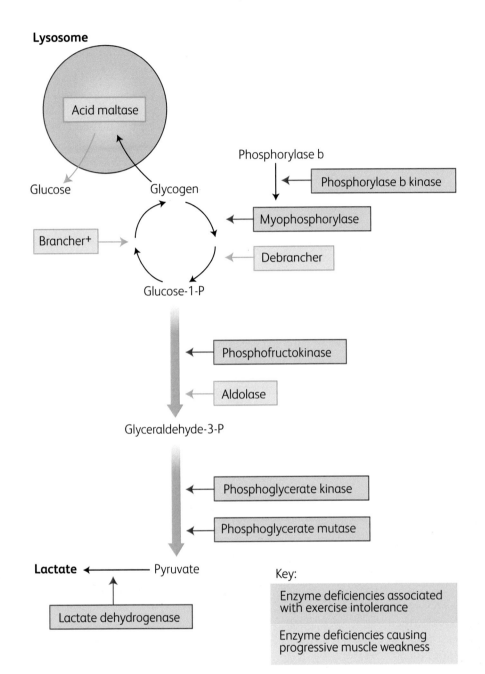

Lysosome

Acid maltase

Glucose   Glycogen

Brancher+

Glucose-1-P

Phosphorylase b

Phosphorylase b kinase

Myophosphorylase

Debrancher

Phosphofructokinase

Aldolase

Glyceraldehyde-3-P

Phosphoglycerate kinase

Phosphoglycerate mutase

Lactate ← Pyruvate

Lactate dehydrogenase

Key:

Enzyme deficiencies associated with exercise intolerance

Enzyme deficiencies causing progressive muscle weakness

Fig 30 Simplified diagram of glycogen metabolism and glycolysis.

Investigation

Consider the following:

> Provocative exercise tests to demonstrate increased creatine kinase (CK) or a failure to increase lactate (ischaemic lactate test) may precipitate muscle necrosis and are potentially harmful.

> Electromyelogram (EMG) – this may be normal. Painful contractures are electrically silent.

> Muscle biopsy – routine histology may be normal or may show some necrosis. This may show increased glycogen. Specific muscle biochemistry confirms enzyme deficiency.

> Genetic sequencing of the *PYGM* gene which encodes myophosphorylase can be done to detect the presence of common mutations of this gene. It is less invasive than a muscle biopsy.

Acid maltase deficiency

Also called Pompe disease or type II glycogenosis. First described by Dr J.C. Pompe in 1932.

Clinical presentation

There are four types: infantile, late infantile, juvenile and adult, the severity decreasing the later the age of onset. Cardiac involvement is almost invariable in the severe infantile type but is less frequent in the adult form.

Symptoms

Progressive weakness. There may be respiratory involvement, often as the prominent feature.

Physical signs

Muscle weakness *with or without* signs of cardiac or respiratory involvement.

Investigation

The following will confirm the diagnosis:

> Measurement of acid alpha-glucosidase enzyme activity in dried blood specimens is an optimal and reliable diagnostic test for acid maltase deficiency.

> CK may be normal or moderately raised.

> EMG is usually myopathic with neurogenic changes and complex repetitive discharges late in the disease.

> Muscle biopsy demonstrates evidence of increased glycogen storage.

Treatment

Mainly supportive only. Recombinant human enzyme alpha-glucosidase has recently been designated an orphan drug, but its efficacy is limited.

Disorders of lipid metabolism: carnitine palmitoyltransferase deficiency

Pathophysiology

Lipid metabolism, in particular the oxidation of fatty acids, takes over from carbohydrate metabolism on sustained exercise. The enzyme carnitine palmitoyltransferase (CPT) catalyses the coupling of carnitine to long-chain fatty acids, a reaction that must occur for the transfer of fatty acids across the mitochondrial membrane.

Clinical presentation

Presents in young adults.

Symptoms

Suspect this diagnosis if the following are features:

> bouts of weakness after prolonged exercise

> myoglobinuria (more severe than in the glycogenoses)

> respiratory involvement may be associated with severe attacks.

The patient may subconsciously adapt to his/her circumstances, preferring sprinting to long-distance running and snacking on sweet food to improve stamina.

Physical signs

Examination may be normal.

Investigations

Note:

> CK is normal unless soon after an attack.

> Muscle biopsy shows increased lipid storage.

> Biochemical analysis of muscle will show the enzyme defect.

Treatment

Avoid precipitating factors.

Disorders of lipid metabolism: mitochondrial disorders

The respiratory chain of mitochondria is responsible for oxidative metabolism within cells. Diseases of mitochondrial function tip the cell towards anaerobic mechanisms and lactic acidosis. Mitochondrial myopathies are one group in a range of diseases of mitochondrial dysfunction, the mitochondrial cytopathies.

Mitochondria and their disorders are inherited through the maternal line. However, some aspects of their function are under nuclear control, therefore some mitochondrial disorders may have a defect of nuclear, rather than mitochondrial, DNA.

2.2.2 Inflammatory muscle disease

Polymyositis and dermatomyositis have been covered elsewhere and will not be repeated here.

Inclusion body myositis

Inclusion body myositis (IBM). This can be sporadic or hereditary.

Sporadic inclusion body myositis

Clinical presentation

Look for:

> IBM affects men more than women. It is more common in those over the age of 50.

> Painless weakness and wasting, with selective involvement of long finger flexors and anterior thigh muscles (quadriceps). May be asymmetrical.

> Relentless progression.

Investigation

Look for:

> Creatine kinase mildly elevated (normal ranges are 24–195 U/L for males and 24–170 U/L for females).

> Imaging – MRI can show the pattern of wasting and therefore distinguish sporadic from hereditary IBM (see below).

> Electromyelogram as in polymyositis, with spontaneous activity and myopathic features.

> Muscle biopsy shows myopathic changes with endomysial CD8$^+$ T-cell infiltrate. Rimmed vacuoles and characteristic tubulofilamentous are inclusions. Interestingly, there is an abnormal accumulation of proteins within the diseased muscle fibres including β-amyloid, amyloid precursor protein and prion protein.

Treatment

IBM does not respond to steroids, despite the inflammatory changes. This may suggest that the inflammation is a secondary phenomenon.

Hereditary inclusion body myositis

This is far less common than the sporadic type, and can be differentiated as follows:

> usually autosomal recessive and linked to chromosome 9

> dramatic sparing of quadriceps

> no inflammation on biopsy.

2.2.3 Inherited dystrophies (myopathies)

These are a diverse group of hereditary muscle disorders.

Disorders of dystrophin

Pathophysiology

The key to understanding why a defect in dystrophin, or certain other proteins (see autosomal recessive limb girdle muscular dystrophy, or LGMD, below), can have such a devastating effect on muscle is the dystrophin–glycoprotein complex (DGC) shown in Fig 31. This is a protein complex found within the sarcolemma that couples the contractile apparatus of the cell to the extracellular matrix through laminin 2. Each member of the DGC is an integral component, with deficiency of any one leading to disease.

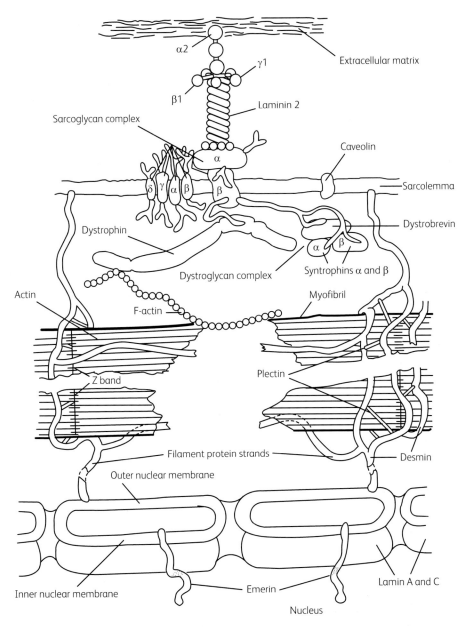

Fig 31 The dystrophin-associated glycoprotein complex is found in the muscle fibre membrane and is connected to the supporting and contractile apparatus of the muscle fibre.

Duchenne muscular dystrophy
Clinical presentation
Look for:

> X-linked.

> Presents in early childhood, often in second year, with clumsiness.

> Proximal weakness and falls develop over the next few years.

> Pseudohypertrophy of the calf muscles is noticed.

> Wheelchair bound by the early teens, with the loss of mobility contributing to contractures and scoliosis.

> Cardiac involvement usually occurs and is characterised by cardiomyopathy.

> Death is from respiratory or cardiac involvement.

Key point

Gower's manoeuvre: the use of the upper limbs to push up on the knees to assist with rising from the floor.

Investigations
Use:

> Creatine kinase (CK) – often >10,000 mU/mL (normal ranges are 24–195 U/L for males and 24–170 U/L for females).

> Electromyelogram (EMG) – myopathic.

> Muscle biopsy – severe dystrophic changes with characteristic hyaline fibres; absence of dystrophin on immunocytochemistry.

> DNA analysis – Xp21, molecular diagnosis available.

Treatment
.The use of corticosteroids is controversial, but some feel they are beneficial. Other than this, treatment is primarily supportive, although gene therapy may offer better outcomes in the future.

Becker muscular dystrophy
Features include:

> X-linked.

> A milder form of Duchenne muscular dystrophy caused by a deficiency or defect in, rather than absence of, dystrophin.

> Presents late in the first decade of life.

> Patients may not be wheelchair bound until their third decade.

> Cardiomyopathy may be severe.

> Female carriers of an abnormal dystrophin gene may have a raised CK (normal range for females 24–170 U/L) and cardiomyopathy.

Limb girdle muscular dystrophy

Various limb girdle muscular dystrophies (LGMDs) have historically been lumped together to distinguish them from the X-linked muscular dystrophies (above) and facioscapulohumeral dystrophy (below). Recent developments have enabled molecular classification of these disorders. Only the briefest of synopsis will be given here.

Autosomal dominant limb girdle muscular dystrophy

Also known as LGMD1; features are as follows:

> Less severe than autosomal recessive LGMD, often with adult onset.

> Most cases have been identified in a few large families.

> Numerous different genetic loci had been identified.

Autosomal recessive limb girdle muscular dystrophy (AR LGMD or LGMD2)

Also known as AR LGMD or LGMD2; features are as follows:

> Often presents in childhood and can be clinically similar to the dystrophinopathies.

> Many subtypes have been identified, including those with deficiencies of the proteins calpain and dysferlin, and the sarcoglycans (see Fig 31).

Facioscapulohumeral dystrophy
Clinical presentation

An autosomal dominant condition with incomplete penetrance and sporadic cases. Clinically, it varies from mild facial weakness to severe generalised weakness involving particularly the face, scapular fixators, triceps, biceps, hip flexors and anterior thigh/calf muscles. The deltoid is often well preserved. Typically it commences around the early teens with only slow progression, but this is extremely variable.

Genetics

Tandem repeat deletion is identified at 4q35. The longer the deletion, the more severe the illness with earlier onset and more rapid progression. Anticipation is seen in families (ie it becomes worse in successive generations), suggesting an increasing deletion size with each generation. Penetrance varies, being 95% in males and 65% in females. The deletion appears to be located close by (possibly within regulatory DNA), but not within an actual gene.

Emery–Dreifuss muscular dystrophy

This rare disease is characterised by the following:

> Xq28, deficiency of emerin.

> Similar phenotype also recognised with normal emerin and autosomal dominant inheritance.

> Early contractures and cardiac complications.

> Female carriers may develop cardiac problems.

Myotonic dystrophy
Clinical features

Myotonia is best demonstrated by getting the patient to open and close the fist rapidly, or by percussing the thenar eminence with a tendon hammer, which causes the thumb to flex across the palm. It is difficult to demonstrate in the tongue as the mouth is warm, and myotonia is best demonstrated in the cold.

A mild, progressive myopathy starting distally. Facial involvement with ptosis.

Look for the following associated features:

> cardiac conduction abnormalities

> frontal balding

> cataracts

> gonadal atrophy

> glucose intolerance

> mental retardation.

Investigations

Genetics – Autosomal dominant gene at 19q13.1 in which there is an abnormal large expansion of CTG trinucleotide repeats. The disorder shows anticipation (ie worse in successive generations) and may have been undiagnosed in older generations in whom signs may have been restricted to cataracts and mild ptosis.

Other investigations – DNA analysis should be first line and it is no longer necessary to subject patients to EMG. However, an EMG will demonstrate characteristic myotonic discharges (likened to a dive-bomber or motorcycle revving up).

Treatment

Mainly supportive.

2.2.4 Channelopathies

A group of disorders characterised by episodic paralysis or myotonia due to mutations of either the calcium or sodium channel gene.

2.2.5 Myasthenia gravis
Aetiology/pathophysiology

Myasthenia gravis (MG) is a disorder of neuromuscular transmission caused by antibodies to postsynaptic proteins, mainly nicotinic acetylcholine receptor (AChR) and muscle-specific tyrosine kinase (MuSK). About 15% of patients (50% in ocular myasthenia) are seronegative; 75% of patients have thymic abnormalities (usually hyperplasia), but thymomas are only seen in 10% of cases. The thymus, with its antigen-presenting cells (T-cells and B-cells) is therefore thought to play a key role in the pathophysiology of MG.

Epidemiology

The prevalence of MG is estimated at approximately 200 cases per 1,000,000 members of the population. It has a bimodal age distribution: the second and third decades in women and the seventh and eight decades in men.

The female to male ratio is 2:1. MG is often associated with other autoimmune diseases, eg Graves' disease.

Clinical presentation

Patients most commonly present with ptosis and diplopia (70%), not with fatigue. Oropharyngeal weakness (difficulty chewing, swallowing and talking) is the initial symptom in 15% of patients and limb weakness in 10%. The severity of symptoms fluctuates during the day, being less severe in the morning and more severe as the day goes on. Exacerbation of symptoms may occur in intercurrent infections, pregnancy, menses and with certain drugs, eg aminoglycosides, beta-blockers, calcium antagonists, procainamide, quinidine and neuromuscular blocking agents. D-penicillamine may induce MG.

Hazard

Since many drugs have been observed to worsen weakness, all patients with MG should be monitored when a new drug is started.

MG remains purely ocular in 15% of patients, and the rest develop generalised weakness, usually within 2 years. After 10–15 years the weakness becomes fixed with little fluctuation.

Physical signs

In MG the weakness shows fatigability. Repetitive testing is therefore needed to fully appreciate this feature. The pattern of weakness does not conform to the distribution of any particular nerves. In the eyes there is ptosis and extraocular muscle weakness, particularly of the medial rectus with sparing of the pupillary reflexes. There may be facial weakness that characteristically gives a 'myasthenic snarl' on attempted smiling, dysarthria, hoarseness, nasal speech, dysphagia and difficulty chewing.

Key point

Weakness of neck flexors is often a good indicator of weakness. However, any limb or trunk muscles may be weak. Deep tendon reflexes are normal. Patients are occasionally diagnosed as hysterical because of the odd distribution of weakness and the fatigability.

Investigation

The following may be useful:

> The edrophonium chloride (Tensilon) test is positive in about 90% of those with MG. It is performed as follows: first identify what it is that you are going to measure, the best results being obtained with diplopia, ptosis and dysarthria. The patient is pretreated with 400 µg atropine IV, then given edrophonium in doses of 2 mg, 3 mg and 5 mg with at least 1–2 minutes between each injection. Observe for a transient response.

> Serum anti-AChR antibodies are present in 80% of patients with generalised MG and 50% with ocular MG. Anti-AChR antibody concentrations do not reliably predict disease severity in individual patients.

> Plasma from patients with generalised MG who do not have detectable anti-AChR antibodies contains various other immune factors, and about 50% have an immunoglobulin G antibody against MuSK. The majority of patients with anti-MuSK antibodies have prevalent involvement of facial and bulbar muscles.

> Anti-striated muscle antibodies are associated with thymoma.

> An autoantibody screen and thyroid function tests should be done because of the association of MG with other autoimmune diseases.

> Single-fibre electromyography is the most sensitive diagnostic test in MG.

It shows an increased jitter in those with MG, but this also occurs in other neuromuscular transmission disorders.

> Electromyography shows a decremental response to repetitive nerve stimulation in muscles.

> A chest X-ray (Fig 32) and CT thorax should be done to look for a thymoma.

Key point

Single-fibre electromyography is performed by simultaneously recording the evoked responses from two muscle fibres of the same motor unit. In a normal muscle, action potentials recorded from two such muscle fibres are not synchronous. This variation in interpotential interval is defined as 'jitter'. Because of the variable neuromuscular transmission, this jitter is increased in disorders of the neuromuscular junction.

Differential diagnosis

Genetic forms of myasthenia are not immune mediated, but are caused by mutations of the AChR. These need to be excluded. The Lambert–Eaton myasthenic syndrome (LEMS) usually occurs in association with malignancy, mostly small-cell lung cancers. Autoantibodies against voltage-gated calcium channels are thought to result in insufficient release of acetylcholine upon depolarisation of the presynaptic membrane. Unlike in MG, muscle strength increases after exercise (post-exercise facilitation), deep tendon reflexes are depressed (but increase with exercise), extraocular muscles tend to be spared, autonomic dysfunction may be prominent and there is incremental response to repetitive nerve stimulation (see also Sections 1.4.4 and 1.2.14).

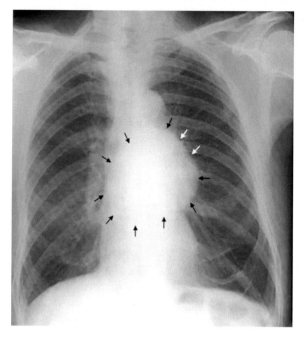

Fig 32 Thymoma, indicated by arrows. (Courtesy of Ray KK, Ryder RE and Wellings RM. *An Aid to Radiology for the MRCP*. Oxford: Blackwell Science, 2000.)

Treatment

Drugs

Anticholinesterases produce temporary improvement. Immunosuppressives are effective but take weeks or months to work. Steroids should be started at low doses to prevent exacerbation of weakness after initiation.
Plasma exchange or intravenous immunoglobulin (IVIG) is used for temporary but rapid benefit in those with sudden worsening of MG.

> **Key point**
> Patients with anti-MuSK antibodies tend to respond less well to anticholinesterases, but the majority do relatively well with immunosuppressive agents.

Thymectomy

Thymectomy should be considered for most patients. But remember:

> The maximum response is seen 2–5 years after surgery.

> The best response is seen in young patients, although benefit can occur in late disease and older patients should certainly be considered.

> Thymectomy is not generally recommended for patients with purely ocular disease, but occasionally dramatic benefit is also seen in this patient group.

> Occasionally thymic tissue is left behind, so repeat surgery should be considered for chronic or relapsing disease if this is felt to be the case.

Complications

The most serious consequence of MG is neuromuscular respiratory failure.

> **Key point**
> Respiratory failure may be due to the disease itself and/or inadequate doses of anticholinesterases (myasthenic crisis) or overdose of anticholinesterases (cholinergic crisis). It ought to be simple to tell the two apart, but in practice it can be difficult. Therefore the safest option is to discontinue all anticholinesterases temporarily and ventilate the patient if necessary.

2.3 Extrapyramidal disorders

2.3.1 Parkinson's disease

Pathophysiology

Idiopathic Parkinson's disease is a neurodegenerative disease and is characterised by death of the dopaminergic cells in the substantia nigra which project to the striatum. It has been found that α-synuclein is the major constituent of Lewy bodies, which are proteinaceous inclusions within the degenerating dopaminergic cells. Other groups of neurons also eventually die and this is possibly responsible for the lack of response of some of the symptoms of idiopathic Parkinson's disease to dopamine replacement.

Aetiology

The precise cause of sporadic idiopathic Parkinson's disease is unknown. A small proportion of cases are familial and associated with genetic mutations, eg α-synuclein and parkin. Unknown environmental influences are almost certainly important. Mitochondrial and proteasomal function as well as cell trafficking and signalling are impaired, but the exact mechanisms and triggers that cause neurodegeneration remain elusive.

Epidemiology

> Prevalence increases with age: ~1% in over-sixties (~0.1% in the general population).

> No geographical differences exist, and it is equally as common in males as in females.

> Previous epidemiological studies indicated a lower incidence in smokers, but it is unclear whether smoking is actually protective.

Clinical presentation

See also Section 1.2.4 and Section 1.2.10.

Common presenting features

The core triad of symptoms:

> rigidity

> bradykinesia

> tremor (only present in two-thirds of cases).

Common features are:

> gait disturbance – festinant, stooped and flexed with poor turning

> asymmetrical slowness (bradykinesia)/ decreased dexterity

> asymmetrical stiffness ('lead pipe' or 'cogwheel' rigidity) in limbs

> deterioration in handwriting – fatiguing and smaller or 'micrographic'

> asymmetrical resting tremor.

Non-motor features

These include:

> depression

> anosmia

> erectile and urinary dysfunction

> constipation.

Later problems

These features would not normally be part of the presenting or early clinical picture:

> loss of balance/falls

> dementia/visual hallucinations

> swallowing difficulties, drooling and severe speech impairment.

If present early then these should act as red flags that this may not be idiopathic Parkinson's disease, but may be a Parkinson plus syndrome.

Treatment complications

These may become the dominant clinical features later in the disease:

> 'Motor fluctuations' – this encompasses a range of clinical problems and usually starts with 'wearing off' of medication at the end of doses of levodopa.

> Later in the disease, there are sudden changes between 'on' state (medication working with symptom relief) and 'off' state (medication ineffective).

> 'Peak dose' and 'end of dose / beginning of dose' dyskinesias – usually choreoathetoid movements of all limbs and the neck and face. Dystonia during 'off' periods, especially of the feet, may also become problematic. These usually develop after a few years of levodopa treatment.

> Gait 'freezing', even when otherwise 'on'.

> Hallucinations (usually visual) and psychosis, which may be drug related or due to an underlying Parkinson's disease-associated dementia. Can also be seen with some medications.

 Key point

Idiopathic Parkinson's disease is a clinical diagnosis, and in the context of a typical history and examination no investigations are required.

Investigations

If the diagnosis or response to dopaminergic therapy is unclear, a formal levodopa or apomorphine challenge can help; and if it is markedly positive it strongly suggests idiopathic Parkinson's disease, although a small proportion of patients with other syndromes may respond partially. Where the diagnosis is still unclear, the passage of time can make the diagnosis clearer.

Functional imaging of the basal ganglia using single-photon emission CT (SPECT) or radioactive dopamine transporter DAT (ioflupane iodine-123 injection) can be very helpful by showing greatly reduced and asymmetrical striato-nigral dopaminergic activity. However, these do not differentiate well between idiopathic Parkinson's disease and Parkinson's plus syndromes. In some cases the correct

diagnosis may not be made until post-mortem.

In younger patients, serum and urinary copper studies should be performed to exclude Wilson's disease, and the Westphal variant of Huntington's disease (with genetic counselling and testing) should also be considered (see Section 1.3).

Differential diagnosis

The common causes of parkinsonism are listed in Table 44.

 Hazard

In older people, cerebrovascular disease is only very rarely a cause of true parkinsonism when an infarct damages the nigrostriatal pathway. Diffuse small-vessel cerebrovascular disease causes 'vascular parkinsonism' which can be misdiagnosed as idiopathic Parkinson's disease (see Section 1.2.4) and can coexist with idiopathic Parkinson's disease.

Drug-induced parkinsonism is an important cause not to miss as it is usually treatable. The other neurodegenerative conditions causing parkinsonism, multiple system atrophy (MSA) and progressive supranuclear palsy (PSP) are rarer than idiopathic Parkinson's disease, but certain clinical features should alert the clinician to the possibility of an alternative diagnosis to idiopathic Parkinson's disease.

Clinical features that are atypical in the diagnosis of idiopathic Parkinson's disease include:

> early instability or falls

> poor response to levodopa

> rapid progression

> pyramidal or cerebellar signs

> dementia early in the disease

Table 44 Common causes of parkinsonism

Diagnosis	Characteristics
Idiopathic Parkinson's disease	Asymmetrical resting tremor, rigidity and bradykinesia
Drug-induced parkinsonism	History of dopamine antagonists, no tremor and symmetrical
Steele–Richardson–Olszewski disease (PSP)	Frontal disease prominent with falls, symmetrical parkinsonism, characteristic supranuclear gaze palsy and staring face
MSA	Symmetrical parkinsonism with cerebellar, pyramidal and autonomic features
BET	Tremor mainly affects actions and posture in the upper limbs
Vascular parkinsonism	Frontal apraxic gait with pyramidal signs and dementia

BET, benign essential tremor; MSA, multiple system atrophy; PSP, progressive supranuclear palsy.

> down-gaze supranuclear palsy (up-gaze palsy is non-specific and occurs in older people)

> severe dysphonia, dysarthria and dysphagia

> respiratory stridor

> myoclonus.

Treatment

See Section 2.12 for background to neuropharmacology.

Levodopa

Levodopa remains the gold-standard treatment for Parkinson's disease, and is the most effective and best tolerated of the anti-parkinsonian drugs.

To understand the rationale for the various different treatment strategies in Parkinson's disease, it is necessary to consider levodopa metabolism (Fig 33). Of peripheral levodopa, 70% is converted to dopamine via the dopa-decarboxylase (DDC) pathway. This causes stimulation of peripheral dopamine receptors, which results in nausea and vomiting and reduces the bioavailability of the drug to the brain. Levodopa preparations, therefore,

contain a DDC inhibitor (eg Sinemet contains levodopa and carbidopa; Madopar contains levodopa and benserazide). This increases central nervous system bioavailability from 1% to 10%. Inhibition of DDC shifts peripheral metabolism of levodopa to other pathways, such as metabolism by catechol-*O*-methyltransferase (COMT).

There are several preparations of levodopa which have certain clinical uses. A dispersible form of Madopar can be useful for patients first thing in the morning when they may be extremely rigid and slow. It may act quicker than tablet preparations, and a liquid may be easier to swallow than a tablet. Each dose of standard levodopa 100 mg takes approximately 30–60 minutes to

take effect and lasts for up to 4 hours. A controlled-release preparation lengthens this period of action slightly and may be useful to take last thing at night to help the patient sleep and to enable them to mobilise in the night to go to the bathroom.

Despite giving a DDC inhibitor in the levodopa preparation, peripheral dopaminergic side effects, such as nausea and postural hypotension (usually only a problem when starting treatment), can be controlled by coadministration with the peripheral dopaminergic antagonist domperidone (the only safe antiemetic to give to parkinsonian patients).

Central effects such as hallucinations, confusion and dyskinesias can become a problem in the later stages of the disease and may be dose limiting. It used to be advocated to delay levodopa therapy to try and delay the onset of long-term complications. However, now levodopa is used more in early disease, but the dose is kept low, by using combination therapies with dopamine agonists (where appropriate). This is to reduce the long-term complications such as dyskinesia.

Dopamine agonists

These act directly on the postsynaptic dopamine receptors and mimic the effect of endogenous dopamine. They are used in early disease as monotherapy, but are not as potent as levodopa. They can be effective 'levodopa-sparing' agents and have longer half-lives than levodopa. Dopamine agonists can be useful in the

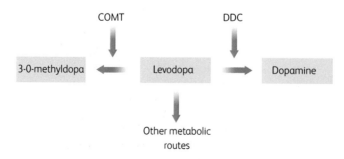

Fig 33 Pathway of levodopa metabolism in the periphery. COMT, catechol-*O*-methyltransferase; DDC, dopa-decarboxylase.

later stages of disease, when motor fluctuations and dyskinesias become a problem.

Ropinirole, pramipexole and rotigotine (patch) are the dopamine agonists generally used. Bromocriptine, cabergoline and pergolide were widely used in the past, but they are ergot-based and can produce fibrotic reactions in the lung and heart over time. Their use has therefore been phased out.

The side-effect profile of agonists is similar to levodopa, although they tend to be less well tolerated – especially by older patients who may develop psychosis, confusion and hallucinations. There have been some reports of sudden onset falling asleep at the wheel, which is relevant when prescribing for patients who are still driving. The other major problem with dopamine agonists (and to a lesser extent levodopa itself) is an increase in obsessive and compulsive behaviours such as gambling, hypersexuality, excessive eating and shopping. Patients should be warned of this prior to initiation, and monitored for this. If it occurs the drug should be reduced and stopped.

Apomorphine is a very potent dopamine agonist and is usually given subcutaneously because a very high rate of first-pass metabolism excludes the oral route. It may be given by intermittent injections or, in cases of severe disease, by a continuous infusion or an 'apomorphine pump'. It is extremely effective in improving severe motor fluctuations and dyskinesias in late-stage disease. Domperidone is usually given at the start of treatment to avoid nausea and postural hypotension, but most patients can stop it after a few weeks. Autoimmune haemolytic anaemia is a rare but serious complication, and thus 3-monthly FBC and Coombs' tests should be performed on all patients on apomorphine.

Amantadine

This is an *N*-methyl-D-aspartate receptor antagonist, but its exact mechanism of action in idiopathic Parkinson's disease is unclear. Amantadine was previously used in early disease but fell out of favour. However, its main use is in dyskinetic patients as it reduces dyskinesia.

Side effects include confusion, hallucinations and leg oedema.

Monoamine oxidase B inhibitors

There are two monoamine oxidase B (MAO-B) inhibitors used in Parkinson's disease. They reduce dopamine breakdown and can prolong the action of levodopa when used in combination. MAO-Bs are used as a monotherapy in early disease (mild effect) and as an adjunct to levodopa in later disease especially for wearing 'off'. They are generally well tolerated, but there is the possibility of the rare serotonergic syndrome (confusion, fever, myoclonus). This can occur if taken together with serotonergic drugs such as selective serotonin reuptake inhibitors (SSRIs) and other drugs such as lithium, opiates or St John's wort. (See notes on rasagiline below.)

Selegiline (Deprenyl/Eldepryl)

This is an irreversible MAO-B inhibitor. Two interesting issues have arisen surrounding this drug.

First, experimental data in animals suggests that it is 'neuroprotective', ie slowing disease progression, but this has not been substantiated in humans. The DATATOP study suggested it resulted in a delay in the need to commence levodopa, but interpretation of this trial has been questioned and long-term follow-up showed no lasting benefit.

Secondly, does selegiline increase mortality? The 1995 report by the UK Parkinson's Disease Research Group concluded that increased mortality was seen in patients taking a combination of selegiline and levodopa compared with levodopa alone. However, further studies suggest that any true increase in mortality is likely to be less than the 60% reported in this paper, and no excess was seen in the long-term DATATOP follow up.

Two of selegiline's active metabolites are amphetamine and methamphetamine, and it is thought these may increase side effects seen with selegiline.

Rasagiline

This is a newer irreversible MAO-B selective inhibitor. The original studies suggest it could have neuroprotective effects, however, this is yet to be properly proved. It comes as a single dose of 1 mg per day. It is felt to be better tolerated than selegiline, and has become the main MAO-B inhibitor in the UK.

In the rasagiline trials no safety problems were found in those on SSRIs. However, MAO-B use with fluvoxamine and fluoxetine is not recommended (they block cytochrome P450 oxidase increasing risk of side effects).

Catechol-*O*-methyltransferase inhibitors

Catechol-*O*-methyltransferase inhibitors are used to optimise the effects of each dose of levodopa and are therefore useful clinically when the patient complains of end-of-dose 'wearing off'.

There are two available to use. Entacapone is available as a tablet on its own, or in combination with levodopa and a DDC in one tablet called Stalevo (this can be prescribed with differing dosages of levodopa and DDC). This is felt to improve compliance as entacapone has to be given with each dose of levodopa. Tolcapone is available, but is restricted due to its hepatotoxicity; it is felt to be more potent than entacapone. It can only be used if other options are not tolerated or effective, and there are strict monitoring guidelines in place.

Side effects include:

> potentiation of levodopa side effects

> gastrointestinal disturbance.

A reduction in levodopa dose may be necessary.

Anticholinergics (trihexyphenidyl or benzhexol (Artane))

Anticholinergics probably have a modest effect on tremor. They are rarely used. They are avoided in older people because of neuropsychiatric side effects.

Side effects include:

> confusion (particularly in older patients)

> dry mouth

> constipation

> may worsen dyskinesias.

Surgery

Stereotactic surgery is used in selected patients, either by lesioning a specific target or more commonly by implanting a high-frequency stimulator (deep brain stimulation). Lesioning is irreversible, can only be performed unilaterally and may be more hazardous. By contrast, stimulation is reversible and can be performed bilaterally, but is much more expensive.

The targets are:

> thalamus for tremor

> subthalamus and zona incerta for all symptoms, including dyskinesia.

General measures

The treatment of Parkinson's disease requires a multidisciplinary approach with the specialist nurse, speech therapist, occupational therapist and physiotherapist; all of whom are often able to contribute just as much as the doctor to improve a patient's quality of life.

Prognosis

Most patients with idiopathic Parkinson's disease have a near-normal life expectancy. Disease progression is extremely variable and it is important to reassure patients that it can run quite a benign course. Some patients may become disabled after many years, especially if hallucinations/psychosis and dementia limit treatment; whereas

others will lead a fairly normal life, ultimately succumbing to other medical problems.

2.4 Dementia

2.4.1 Alzheimer's disease

Aetiology/pathology

Familial autosomal dominant Alzheimer's disease (AD) with early onset (usually between early forties and mid-fifties) is caused in the majority of cases by mutations in one of three genes:

> presenilin 1 on chromosome 14

> presenilin 2 on chromosome 1

> amyloid precursor protein (APP) on chromosome 21.

Genetic testing for these mutations may be indicated in the investigation of memory disorder (Section 1.1.4).

The epsilon4 allele of apolipoprotein E (encoded by a gene on chromosome 19) is the most important genetically determined risk factor for the development of AD, but as this is neither necessary nor sufficient for a diagnosis of AD it currently has no role in diagnostic evaluation (although commercially available).

The neuropathological changes of AD are cerebral atrophy (especially of the medial temporal lobes), amyloid plaques with a central core composed of β-amyloid, neurofibrillary tangles composed of tau (Fig 34), and β-amyloid in blood vessels (or 'amyloid angiopathy'). An important step in the pathogenesis of AD is the cleavage of β-amyloid peptides from the larger precursor protein, APP, which results in the accumulation of β-amyloid. In genetically determined cases, this seems to occur many years before frank neurodegeneration and onset of symptoms. The mechanism(s) of toxicity of β-amyloid and the association of β-amyloid with neurofibrillary tangles remain unclear.

Epidemiology

AD is the most common form of dementia. Familial AD accounts for <5% of cases. Increasing age is the most important risk factor, but patients with Down's syndrome (trisomy 21) are

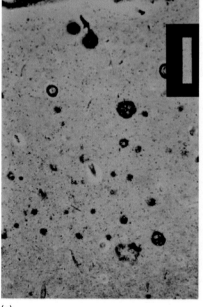

(a)   (b)

Fig 34 β-Amyloid **(a)** and neurofibrillary tangles **(b)** in Alzheimer's disease (AD).

also susceptible to developing AD neuropathology and progressive dementia which is related to a gene dosage effect as the APP gene lies on chromosome 21.

Clinical presentation

Older clinicopathological diagnostic criteria for AD have been superseded in recent years by clinicobiological diagnostic criteria based on biomarkers (see Investigation).

The earliest feature of AD is usually forgetfulness for recent events and repeating questions and conversations (ie amnesia). In contrast to this typical form of AD, other variants are also described, as atypical AD, including:

> posterior variant – either occipitotemporal with predominant visuoperceptive impairments, or biparietal with predominant visuospatial impairments

> logopenic variant (of primary progressive aphasia) – with predominant linguistic deficits, especially in single word retrieval and repetition of sentences

> frontal variant – with predominant behavioural change, apathy or disinhibition.

Occasionally AD presentation overlaps with corticobasal degeneration, hence corticobasal syndrome.

As AD progresses, patients may develop:

> cognitive decline – disorientation (initially to time), impairment of verbal fluency, loss of computational ability

> functional problems – difficulty with activities of daily living such as money, medications, transport

> behavioural change – inattentiveness and agitation, personality change

> neuropsychiatric features – depression, psychosis with delusions or hallucinations

> neurological signs – extrapyramidal signs (eg rigidity), myoclonus, pyramidal signs (eg hyperreflexia), epileptic seizures, mutism and incontinence. In familial (presenilin 1 mutation) patients spastic paraparesis or cerebellar signs may occur.

Progression of AD is slow and gradual over several years, although more rapid forms have been described.

Investigation

> Cognitive screening instruments (eg Mini-Mental State Examination, Montreal Cognitive Assessment, Addenbrooke's Cognitive Examination) may be used to examine cognitive function but these are not diagnostic tests. Informant-related screening tests are also available (eg IQCODE, AD8).

> Structural brain imaging – CT or, preferably, MRI brain scan may show cerebral atrophy, especially of the medial temporal lobes (Fig 35).

> Biomarkers – AD biomarkers are increasingly used, namely

cerebrospinal fluid Aβ1-42 (low) and total-tau and phospho-tau (both raised); and positron emission tomography (PET) imaging with amyloid ligands (eg PiB, florbetapir). However, these investigations are not widely available outside research settings, and hence the aforementioned investigations retain a place.

Change over time in cognitive screening test performance or in brain imaging may be helpful in establishing diagnosis if there is initial diagnostic uncertainty.

Differential diagnosis

Key point

Reversible or treatable causes of dementia must be ruled out at onset of presentation, eg hypothyroidism, vitamin B_{12} deficiency, neurosyphilis and space-occupying lesions (such as hydrocephalus and subdural haematoma). See also Table 3.

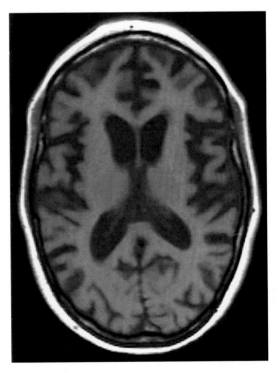

Fig 35 Global cerebral atrophy in Alzheimer's disease (AD).

Vascular dementia

Classically, multi-infarct dementia has been characterised by stepwise deterioration due to sequential large-vessel infarcts or haemorrhages. More commonly recognised is subcortical ischaemic vascular dementia due to diffuse subcortical white matter ischaemia, often in association with vascular risk factors, which may progress gradually and insidiously. Other features include:

> impaired executive function, eg planning actions

> greater visuospatial and visuoperceptive than memory deficits

> frontal gait disorder (*marche à petit pas*)

> emotional lability, pseudobulbar palsy

> urinary dysfunction

> relative preservation of personality.

An MRI scan of the brain may demonstrate diffuse white matter disease and lacunar infarcts with or without large-vessel strokes in the same patient. However, minor degrees of peripheral punctuate high-signal white matter change on an MRI scan should not automatically be equated with 'vascular dementia' since such change is common with increased age without cognitive correlate.

Key point

Cerebrovascular disease and Alzheimer-type pathology often coexist in older patients with dementia, constituting the condition of mixed dementia.

Frontotemporal dementia

The main features of frontotemporal lobar degenerations are predominantly either behavioural or linguistic dysfunction.

In behavioural variant frontotemporal dementia the key features are:

> early behavioural disinhibition – socially inappropriate behaviour, loss of manners, impulsiveness.

> early apathy or inertia

> early loss of sympathy or empathy

> early perseverative, stereotyped or compulsive/ritualistic behaviour

> hyperorality and dietary change

> neuropsychological profile of executive deficits with relative sparing of memory and visuospatial functions (Section 3.1).

Two linguistic variants of frontotemporal dementia are recognised:

> Progressive non-fluent aphasia or the agrammatic variant – characterised by impoverished speech output but with relative preservation of other cognitive domains and activities of daily living.

> Semantic dementia or the semantic variant – characterised by impaired comprehension manifest as difficulties with confrontation naming (anomia) and single word comprehension; there may be alexia for irregularly spelled words (surface dyslexia).

An MRI scan of the brain may confirm focal frontotemporal atrophy, sometimes strikingly asymmetrical.

Dementia with Lewy bodies

The main features are:

> fluctuating cognitive deterioration – 'unstable platform of attention'

> visual hallucinations – formed (eg animals, people), not distressing; insight into their unreality is often retained, hence they are sometimes called pseudohallucinations

> extrapyramidal signs – may be subtle or even absent; rigidity and bradykinesia are more common than tremor

> anosmia

> Rapid eye movement (REM) sleep behaviour disorder – 'dream enactment', loss of usual nocturnal atonia; excessive daytime somnolence

> syncope

> hypersensitivity to neuroleptic medications (dopamine antagonists).

The cognitive and neurobehavioural features which develop in many patients with Parkinson's disease are similar. An arbitrary 1-year rule is used to differentiate the conditions, depending on whether motor or cognitive features manifest first.

Other irreversible causes

These include:

> alcoholic dementia

> other parkinsonian disorders – progressive supranuclear palsy, corticobasal degeneration

> Huntington's disease (see also Sections 1.1.5 and 1.3.1)

> Creutzfeldt–Jakob disease (see Section 2.10).

Reversible or treatable causes of dementia

Although heavily emphasised in older texts, truly reversible causes of dementia are extremely rare but nevertheless must be ruled out. Hypothyroidism and vitamin B_{12} deficiency are usually cited but the evidence base for these as causes of reversible dementia is thin. Reversible causes of dementia are:

> neurosyphilis

> space-occupying lesions (eg tumour, subdural haematoma)

> idiopathic normal pressure hydrocephalus

> a circumscribed amnesic disorder, Wernicke–Korsakoff syndrome, due to dietary thiamine deficiency. This is most often seen in alcoholics and may be reversed with prompt thiamine repletion.

See also Table 3 (Section 1.1.4).

Treatment

AD is not a curable disease, but quality of life can be maintained with the appropriate supportive care for both patient and principal caregiver. A familiar environment reduces confusion and disorientation in patients with AD. Education and support of patient and caregiver is important. The Alzheimer's Society has excellent resources.

Depression commonly coexists with AD and it is important that it is recognised and treated vigorously. Other behavioural disturbances (eg agitation, aggression, hallucinations) may also require treatment, ideally with behavioural treatments rather than neuroleptics since these are associated with increased cerebrovascular mortality.

> **Hazard**
>
> ! Tricyclic drugs have anticholinergic side effects that may worsen cognitive deficits. Selective serotonin reuptake inhibitors (SSRIs) are a better choice.

Symptomatic treatment is available with cholinesterase inhibitors licensed for mild to moderate disease (donepezil, galantamine, rivastigmine), and the partial N-methyl-D-aspartate (NMDA) receptor antagonist memantine, licensed for moderate to severe disease. Effects are at best modest and not disease modifying, although time to nursing home placement may be delayed, perhaps because of an effect on behavioural features.

Therapies directed against β-amyloid have shown great promise in animal models, but clinical trials have been disappointing, although hopes remain high for antibodies against this protein, especially if given very early in the disease course. Stories of 'cures' for Alzheimer's which appear intermittently in the popular media raise inappropriate hopes in some patients and their relative/carers.

Cholinesterase inhibitors are also licensed for Parkinson's disease dementia, and may have beneficial effects in dementia with Lewy bodies and in vascular dementia.

Prognosis

Mean survival in AD is about 8 years after disease onset but many younger patients can now survive with a good quality of life for many years if they receive the appropriate management. Bronchopneumonia is the usual cause of death following a period of immobility.

2.5 Multiple sclerosis

Aetiology/pathophysiology/pathology

The aetiology of multiple sclerosis (MS) is not completely understood. In genetically predisposed individuals, one or more environmental triggers (which may include viral exposures) lead to autoimmune dysfunction causing inflammation, demyelination and axonal loss in the white matter of the central nervous system. Relative vitamin D deficiency may also increase the risk, due to its role in immune system regulation.

Epidemiology

The prevalence of MS increases with increasing distance from the equator; this may be related to ultraviolet (UV) exposure and the role of vitamin D. People who migrate from a high-risk to a low-risk area at or after the age of 15 retain the risk of their birthplace; below the age of 15 they do not. The mean age of onset is 30, being slightly earlier in women than in men and in relapsing–remitting MS (RRMS) than progressive MS. The female to male ratio is 3:2. Polygenic inheritance in MS is supported by twin studies (MZ and DZ concordance of 25% and 5%, respectively) and more recent genome-wide association studies (GWAS) data (most of the relevant genes being involved in autoimmunity).

Clinical presentation

Common symptoms are weakness, sensory disturbances (numbness or tingling), blurred vision or loss of vision (optic neuritis), unsteadiness, incoordination, dysarthria, sphincter or sexual dysfunction and fatigue. Gradually progressive MS evolves over months–years. Acute relapses present with subacutely evolving symptoms over several days, plateauing within 2 weeks and improving gradually over days–weeks, sometimes months.

Lhermitte's sign (an electric shock-like sensation down the spine or limbs on neck flexion) and Uhthoff's phenomenon (a worsening of symptoms when there is an increase in body temperature, such as when getting into a hot bath) may occur, and are fairly specific to demyelination.

Later in the disease course cognitive impairment is common, though usually mild.

Classification of MS

A first attack of demyelination, eg optic neuritis or partial myelitis, is termed a 'clinically isolated syndrome' (CIS): a single clinically evident episode of demyelination in the brain, optic nerve or spinal cord without any preceding episodes. MS cannot be diagnosed because there has not yet been multiple attacks to give dissemination in time or space. An abnormal MRI brain scan at this point (ie showing lesions consistent with demyelination) does not change the diagnosis to MS, but does increase the probability of a further attack (relapse) which would then confirm MS. If the scan is abnormal the risk of this is 50% over the subsequent 2 years, increasing to 80% at 20 years (ie 20% of patients with abnormal scans will *not* go on to develop MS). If the presenting scan is normal, the risk of a relapse over the next 20 years is only 20%.

Those patients experiencing a second (or more) attack are classed as having RRMS (Fig 36).

Over a period of years, relapses occur with variable frequency, severity and degrees of recovery. In the majority of patients, disability eventually starts to accumulate in a gradual fashion and relapses become much less common. This is termed 'secondary progressive MS' (SPMS). Age, rather than disease duration, appears to be a significant risk factor for developing SPMS.

A minority of patients develop slowly progressive MS from onset, and never experience acute relapses. This is termed primary progressive MS (PPMS) and is relatively more common in older, male patients (Fig 36).

Physical signs

Cranial nerves

Pale optic discs (indicating optic atrophy), scotoma, relative afferent pupillary defect in optic neuritis, internuclear ophthalmoplegia (best seen on horizontal saccades) and objective facial numbness or weakness.

Motor and sensory

Upper motor neurone signs (eg spasticity, pyramidal weakness, hyperreflexia and extensor plantar responses), impaired pain, temperature, vibration and joint position sense.

Cerebellar

Nystagmus, upper limb intention tremor, scanning dysarthria, dysdiadochokinesis and gait ataxia.

Investigation

MRI

An MRI scan is the investigation of choice, with good sensitivity (and if interpreted correctly, good specificity). Demyelinating lesions are typically located in the periventricular white matter (Fig 37), corpus callosum, brainstem and cerebellar hemispheres. In chronic MS, there are confluent plaques, cortical atrophy and ventricular enlargement. Enhancement with contrast is a sign of an acute lesion and indicates disruption of the blood–brain barrier.

Spinal lesions are also seen well on MRI, and are usually small, occupying <1 vertebral level and often just one side of the cord.

If the clinical picture and MRI are both typical for MS, no further investigations may be necessary. In other situations, blood testing, lumbar puncture and evoked potentials can be helpful.

Key point

Unfortunately, a lesion load on MRI correlates poorly with disability scores. This is probably due to the fact that some lesions may be silent and some may be in strategic areas. This is likely to be more clinically relevant than the overall amount of inflammation at any given time.

Cerebrospinal fluid

The white cell count and total protein are usually normal, although a mild lymphocytosis (up to 30 cells) or slightly elevated protein are sometimes seen. Oligoclonal bands (bands in the IgG region) are found in cerebrospinal fluid (CSF) but not serum (indicating intrathecal synthesis) in 90% of cases of clinically definite MS. However, oligoclonal bands may also be detected in many inflammatory conditions affecting the central nervous system (CNS) or after CNS infection. If the oligoclonal bands in the CSF are matched by those in the serum, this is indicative of systemic inflammation and can occur in a wide range of conditions such as systemic lupus erythematosus, paraneoplastic disease and infections such as HIV.

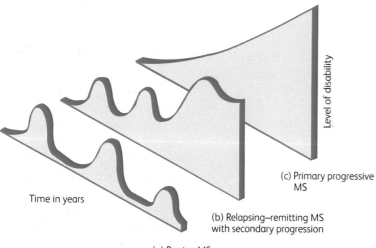

Level of disability

Time in years

(c) Primary progressive MS

(b) Relapsing–remitting MS with secondary progression

(a) Benign MS

Fig 36 Diagrammatic representation of the different clinical courses seen in MS. **(a)** Benign multiple sclerosis (MS) – there is no accumulation of disability between relapses for >10 years. **(b)** Relapsing–remitting MS becoming secondary progressive. At first, complete recovery is made between relapses. Then, a failure to recover fully from relapses leads to gradual accumulation of residual disability. Finally, the disability accumulates without clear relapses. **(c)** Primary progressive MS. Gradual accumulation of disability without relapses.

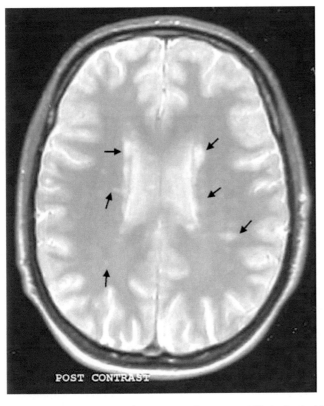

Fig 37 Periventricular white matter lesions in MS, indicated by arrows. (From Ray KK, Ryder RE and Wellings RM. *An Aid to Radiology for the MRCP*. Oxford: Blackwell Science, 2000.)

Visual, somatosensory and brainstem auditory evoked potentials

Visual-evoked potentials are a non-invasive test which may lend further support to the diagnosis of MS, particularly in patients who have had visual symptoms or those who do not wish to undergo lumbar puncture for CSF examination. These physiological studies may be abnormal in 50–80% of patients, but somatosensory- and brainstem-evoked potentials are usually only employed in difficult cases.

Differential diagnosis

The diagnosis of MS in the context of a young adult with two or more episodes of CNS dysfunction is usually straightforward. However, apparent monophasic illnesses may be caused by many pathologies including stroke, infections of the nervous system, other inflammatory disease of the nervous system and tumours.

Neuromyelitis optica (NMO) is an autoimmune, relapsing demyelinating disorder associated with serum antibodies to Aquaporin-4. It is rare but can mimic MS. Relapses tend to be severe and treatment is different to that in MS so identification is important.

Progressive MS may be more difficult to diagnose clinically, but the most important diseases to exclude are potentially treatable causes of the symptoms, such as compressive spinal cord lesions, vitamin B_{12} and copper deficiency, arteriovenous malformations and Arnold–Chiari malformation with syringomyelia. The differential diagnosis in this category is broad and includes inflammatory and granulomatous CNS disease, CNS infections (eg human T-cell lymphotropic virus, HTLV1) and hereditary disorders (such as hereditary spastic paraparesis, adrenoleukodystrophy and metachromatic leukodystrophy).

Treatment

Treatments in MS are divided into symptomatic and disease-modifying treatment (DMT), plus management of acute relapses.

Symptomatic treatments
Spasticity

This can impair mobility and may cause painful spasms. The treatment options are as follows:

> None – do not treat spasticity found on examination just for the sake of it.

> Non-medication – stretching and other exercises, avoidance of triggers (constipation, pressure sores).

> Medication:

> > baclofen (γ-aminobutyric acid agonist), oral or intrathecal

> > gabapentin

> > tizanidine (α-2 agonist)

> > benzodiazepines

> > botulinum toxin (carefully selected cases).

Although baclofen and tizanidine can be effective initially, the patient may require increasing doses if there is progression of disease. This often means the treatment becomes limited by side effects, particularly drowsiness and excessive reduction in tone (worsening mobility). Involvement of neuro-rehabilitation specialists may be very helpful.

Bladder disturbance

This is a common problem occurring in 50–80% of patients. Assessment is as follows:

> Establish whether the bladder empties using pre- and post-micturition

ultrasound (the patient will not reliably be able to tell whether the bladder empties or not).

> If the residual volume is <100 mL, then use oxybutynin 2.5 mg two to three times daily (anticholinergic side effects are less likely to be a problem at this dose). Consider also antidepressants with anticholinergic action. Desmopressin nasal spray used at night may be helpful for nocturnal symptoms. Intra-vesical botulinum can be highly effective, though some patients will need to perform intermittent self-catheterisation afterwards.

> If the residual volume is >100 mL, it is not advisable to use these drugs until outflow obstruction has been overcome. Intermittent self-catheterisation is the best and simplest way to achieve this, but special training is needed.

Sexual dysfunction

This is common but often not discussed with patients. You need to ask specifically about this, as patients are unlikely to volunteer the information. Sildenafil (Viagra) may be helpful for men and, perhaps, women. Patients should also be directed to self-help resources, or referred to an appropriate sexual health clinic.

Fatigue

This is a very common symptom, occurring in 70–80% of patients and is often out of proportion to the degree of physical disability, which may be relatively mild. Fatigue interferes with the patient's ability to perform the activities of daily living. Amantadine is often used but only works in a minority. It is important to look for correctable causes of fatigue, so check the patient's haemoglobin level and thyroid function tests, and enquire about sleep quality, mood and other medications that may exacerbate fatigue. Regular exercise is helpful.

Depression

This occurs in 50–60% of patients at some stage during their illness, so is important to identify and treat it.

Tremor

This may be severe enough to impair the activities of daily living. Various drugs have been tried (antiepileptics, clonazepam and isoniazid) with only limited success. Thalamotomy may help in refractory disease.

Paroxysmal symptoms

These include trigeminal neuralgia, pain, paraesthesiae, ataxia, dystonia and weakness, and they are thought to be due to ephaptic transmission of nerve impulses at sites of previous disease activity. All are characteristically sudden and brief, each attack only lasting seconds but can be frequent. Drugs used to treat neuropathic pain can be of some benefit (eg amitriptyline, gabapentin and pregabalin), but carbamazepine is often the best treatment.

Treatment of acute attacks (relapses)

A relapse is defined as an episode of neurological symptoms that happens at least 30 days after any previous episode began, lasts at least 24 hours, is not attributable to another cause, and occurs in the absence of an infection or fever.

Beware 'pseudo-relapse' in chronic, progressive MS; transient worsening of old symptoms eg due to fatigue, infection (eg urinary tract infection (UTI)), stress and constipation.

Relapses are often self-limiting, but the following options are available to help speed recovery:

> High-dose intravenous methylprednisolone (1 g daily for 3 days). Methyl prednisolone is increasingly given orally (500 mg OD for 5 days). Consider gastric protection with a proton pump

inhibitor (PPI). Steroids may shorten an acute attack, but do not change the final degree of recovery and have no effect on underlying gradual progression (if present).

> Rest may be just as effective.

> Physiotherapy at the time of the relapse is often of benefit.

Disease-modifying treatment (DMTs)

Disease-modifying drugs alter the course of MS, at least in terms of reducing the severity and frequency of relapses. At present there are no treatments to slow or prevent gradually progressive forms of MS (PPMS or SPMS).

A range of DMTs are available, with varying levels of potency, mode of delivery, short-term side effects and long-term risks.

> Beta interferons (IFN) and glatiramer acetate (GA) – these are given by self-injection, are usually well tolerated and serious side effects are very rare. They are only partially effective, suppressing about 30% of relapses.

> Teriflunomide – an oral DMT with similar efficacy to IFN and GA. Requires frequent blood monitoring (liver function tests (LFTs)), may cause hair thinning and teratogenicity, with a very long half-life limiting use in young women.

> Dimethylfumarate – an oral DMT that reduces relapses by about 50%. It is usually well tolerated, but flushing and diarrhoea affect some patients. Serious side effects seem to be rare.

> Fingolimod – an oral DMT with higher efficacy than IFN or GA (approximately 60% reduction in relapses) and approved for use in patients relapsing despite IFN or GA. It is usually well tolerated, although bradyarrhythmias and macular oedema may occur. There are rare

reports of progressive multifocal leucoencephalopathy (PML) with long-term use.

> Natalizumab – a monoclonal antibody given by monthly intravenous (IV) infusion. Suppresses relapses by ~70%, is usually very well tolerated but there is a risk of PML with long-term use (in JC virus-positive patients the risk is ~1:200 after 2 years or more of treatment). Most patients now survive PML, though with serious residual disability.

> Alemtuzumab – a monoclonal antibody (anti-CD52) that is given by IV infusion, resulting in prolonged suppression of T- and B-lymphocytes for 12 months. Given at year 1 and 2, most patients require no further treatment. It reduces relapses by ~80%. Generally it is well tolerated, although some patients develop other autoimmune problems such as Graves' disease or idiopathic thrombocytopenia purpura (ITP), regular monitoring for which are required.

> **Hazard**
> Disease-modifying treatments (DMTs) – the side effects of immunosuppression are a significant drawback.

Prognosis

The following factors may be associated with a better prognosis:

> diplopia, optic neuritis or sensory symptoms at onset

> female, rather than male, sex

> earlier age of onset

> long first remission.

2.6 Headache

2.6.1 Migraine

Migraine is the most common primary headache disorder. There are two major subtypes: migraine with and without aura.

Pathophysiology

The cardinal features of migraine are headache in the distribution of the trigeminal nerve and upper cervical roots, in association with transient neurological symptoms.

The pain is mediated through the trigeminal nerve fibres that innervate the large intracranial extracerebral vessels, transmitted via 5-hydroxytryptamine $(5HT)_{1B}$ serotonin receptors. These fibres project into the trigeminal nucleus ($5HT_{1D}$ serotonin receptors) where they may receive projections from high cervical nerve fibres. This interaction accounts for the characteristic distribution of pain: the pain is likely to be related to episodic dysfunction of brainstem or diencephalic systems that modulate the trigeminovascular system.

Epidemiology

> Lifetime prevalence is 5–10% for men and 15–25% for women.

> The first attack is experienced in the first decade by 25% of patients, and is less common after 50 years of age.

Clinical presentation

Common features include:

> Migraine headache is episodic, with complete resolution between attacks and each attack lasting from a few hours up to 3 days.

> Pain is often temporal and may be unilateral or bilateral. It is typically described as throbbing but may be constant.

> Patients with migraine will often describe how they take to their beds with the curtains closed. Although this is in marked contrast to the patient with cluster headache (see Section 2.6.3), aggravation by light, noise and movement experienced by those with migraine is common to many other types of headaches. Stress (and relaxation from stress), exercise, missing meals, menstruation, alcohol and various foodstuffs are often considered by patients to precipitate their attacks.

> Headache may be accompanied by nausea (90%) and vomiting (75%).

> The aura occurs prior to, but occasionally with or after, the headache, and is most often visual (90%). By definition the aura should last between 5 minutes and 60 minutes. Transient hemianopic disturbance, fortification spectra and spreading scintillating scotomata (but not blurring or non-specific spots) are symptoms of a migrainous aura. In addition, patients may describe unilateral paraesthesia, or even mild weakness, of their face and hand, and also occasionally aphasia.

Migraine variants include:

> Hemiplegic migraine – in true hemiplegic migraine the weakness is more marked than that occasionally encountered in the common aura, and it may long outlast the headache, possibly lasting up to several days (usually <72 hours). For this diagnosis to be made, there needs to be a clear family history or a good history of preceding migraine with aura. It may be sporadic or familial, with some families carrying a dominant gene on chromosome 19. Traditionally, hemiplegic migraine responds well to flunarizine, a calcium channel blocker, suggesting that the disorder is a channelopathy.

> Basilar migraine – this is accompanied by an aura in which there is frequently visual disturbance that is characteristically bilateral and associated with vertigo, ataxia, dysarthria, bilateral sensorimotor features and occasional drowsiness.

> Ophthalmoplegic migraine – the headache is associated with extraocular muscle palsies, particularly the third and rarely the sixth, which develop as the headache subsides.

> Retinal migraine – this is associated with monocular blindness, disc oedema and peripapillary haemorrhages. Vision may not recover for weeks or even months.

> Acephalgic migraine – this causes diagnostic problems, in that the presence of a typical migrainous aura without headache can be mistaken for transient cerebral ischaemia. A previous history of migraine with aura makes the diagnosis easier, but migraine equivalents can occur de novo in older patients. Characteristically, the symptoms evolve over a few minutes or longer, compared with transient ischaemic attacks (TIAs; see Section 2.8).

Investigations

Investigations do not contribute to the diagnosis of migraine, but if a secondary cause of headache needs to be excluded then an investigation may be appropriate (as discussed in Section 1.1.1).

Differential diagnosis

The main differentials are:

> episodic tension-type headache

> cluster headache

> chronic migraine (often in association with analgesia overuse) and other forms of chronic daily headache (see later in this section) can be very difficult to distinguish.

Key point

The aura, if it involves prominent sensorimotor features or speech disturbance, may be confused with stroke or TIA. Migraine auras typically spread over many minutes or longer, whereas TIA symptoms do not spread. Furthermore, migraine auras are more likely to be positive phenomena (flashing lights, coloured spots and tingling) than TIAs. Occipital lobe simple partial seizures cause hemianopic visual disturbances, although these are typically multicoloured migratory blobs rather than monochromatic scintillations or angulated lines.

Treatment

Objectives and principles

> To minimise impact on the patient's lifestyle, as the tendency to headaches cannot be cured.

> To explain and reassure.

> To identify and avoid predisposing factors (stress, depression and anxiety) and triggers (alcohol, missed meals and change in sleeping habits) within reason. However, some of these may be unavoidable and so the patient should be encouraged to have regular habits.

Acute treatment

Step 1

Simple analgesia (aspirin 900 mg or paracetamol 1,000 mg) or non-steroidal anti-inflammatory drugs (NSAIDs), with or without an antiemetic such as metoclopramide 10 mg or domperidone 20 mg. Consider suppositories (especially diclofenac plus domperidone) if nausea and vomiting is a persistent problem.

Hazard

It is extremely important to ask patients how much simple analgesia they take, particularly any compounds containing codeine or paracetamol. Medication-overuse headache may occur if simple analgesia is taken on >8–10 days in every month. However, NSAIDs appear to be less implicated and are an option, eg naproxen 500 mg bd for 2 weeks to help patients wean off other analgesia. A similar problem is seen with triptan overuse. Medication-overuse headache is important to diagnose as migraine preventatives are ineffective unless the simple analgesia is withdrawn to acceptable limits.

Step 2

Consider using:

> Specific antimigraine drugs (triptans, 5HT$_{1B/1D}$ agonists). Different drugs may suit different patients, so it may be worth trying each one.

> At 2 hours the response rates (headache improving from severe/moderate to mild/absent) are approximately 50–65%, and the proportion of patients who are headache free is approximately 20–35%.

> Recurrence of symptoms occurs within 24 hours in 20–40% of patients for all triptans.

> Oral preparations are available, together with subcutaneous, nasal spray (sumatriptan) and a rapidly dispersible wafer that is placed on the tongue (rizatriptan). Subcutaneous or wafer preparations can be used if vomiting affects oral administration.

> Naratriptan is of slower onset, but there may be lower recurrence rate with this drug.

Step 3

Before proceeding to step 3 review the diagnosis and then compliance.

As a one-off emergency treatment, intramuscular chlorpromazine 25–50 mg may improve headache that is not otherwise responding.

Prophylactic treatment

Patients are the best judge of when to commence a prophylactic agent, although generally agents tend to be considered for patients with two to three severe attacks per month. Continue with a prophylactic agent for 2–3 months, as long as it is tolerated, before deciding whether it has worked or not. Because migraine is cyclical, prophylactic agents that are effective should be continued for no more than 6 months.

These agents may be tried:

> Atenolol 25–100 mg bd or propranolol LA 80–160 mg bd.

> Sodium valproate 600–2,000 mg daily.

> Candesartan 16 mg daily.

> Pizotifen 0.5–1.5 mg nocte.

> Amitriptyline 10–100 mg nocte.

> Topiramate 50–100 mg daily.

> Gabapentin 1,800–3,600 mg daily.

> Methysergide 1–2 mg tds. Often not considered because of associations with retroperitoneal fibrosis (1 in 2,000 risk), but if it is used in short courses, eg 6 months of treatment followed by a 1-month drug-free period, then this side effect can be avoided.

> For menstrual migraine (ie those attacks in which the onset of migraine can be predicted in relation to onset of menstruation) a 100 µg oestrogen patch starting 3 days before until 4 days after menstruation may be helpful in preventing attacks.

In pregnancy

Paracetamol is the safest option for acute headache and prochlorperazine is the safest option for nausea.

Most migraines improve, but should a prophylactic agent be required then propranolol has the safest record.

Migraine and hormone replacement therapy

Hormone replacement therapy (HRT) is not contraindicated in the migraineur. Menopause may exacerbate migraine, so HRT may help the symptoms. Worsening migraine on commencement of HRT occasionally happens, but may be helped by changing the dose or formulation of the HRT.

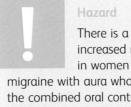

Hazard

There is a small increased risk of stroke in women with migraine with aura who are taking the combined oral contraceptive pill, particularly in the presence of other vascular risk factors.

Prognosis

If migraine starts in childhood:

> About 50% of males and 30% of females are migraine free at 30 years of age.

> Over 50% of sufferers still get migraines at 50 years of age.

> In half of these cases the migraine is less severe.

If migraine starts in adulthood 70% lose migraine or experience significant improvement over 15 years.

2.6.2 Trigeminal neuralgia
Disease

Trigeminal neuralgia (TN) occurs predominantly in patients over the age of 40 years. It is attributed to compression of the sensory root of the trigeminal nerve, either by an aberrant blood vessel (Fig 38) or occasionally by tumours in the cerebellopontine angle. In addition, TN may be seen in multiple sclerosis (MS), with demyelination in the trigeminal sensory root.

Clinical presentation

> Patients characteristically describe a severe paroxysmal pain in the distribution of the trigeminal nerve (usually mandibular or maxillary: the ophthalmic branch is affected only rarely).

> The pain is described as lancinating or electric-shock-like, and lasts only for seconds.

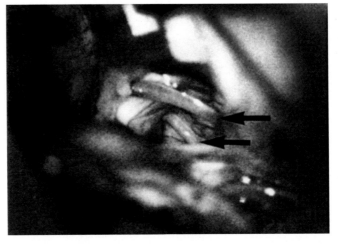

Fig 38 Perioperative view of the trigeminal nerve root entry zone in contact with two divisions of the superior cerebellar artery (indicated by black arrows) in a patient with trigeminal neuralgia. The arteries can be seen to indent the nerve. (From Hamlyn PJ. *Neurovascular Compression of the Lower Cranial Nerves.* Amsterdam: Elsevier Science, 1999 with kind permission of PJ Hamlyn and Elsevier Science.)

- Occasionally, the paroxysms are so frequent that they blur into one, giving the impression of lasting longer. There may also be a residual ache in between bouts.

- Attacks may occur in clusters, but are clearly differentiated from cluster headache by the quality of the pain.

- Triggers are common, with almost any stimulus setting off an attack. Consequently, many patients are unable to wash, shave, chew or even talk during an attack.

- Pain is unilateral in over 95% of cases, and bilateral TN should raise the possibility of MS.

Physical signs

There are usually no physical signs. However:

- The presence of a reduced corneal response, reduced sensation in the affected distribution or ipsilateral hearing loss should raise the possibility of a structural lesion.

- A larger compressive lesion may lead to weakness of the muscles of mastication, ipsilateral ataxia or other cranial nerve palsies.

Hazard

If TN occurs in a patient under the age of 40 years this should raise the possibility of MS or a structural lesion.

Investigation

In the event of a structural lesion being suspected, MRI should be performed as this will detect demyelination as well as extra-axial mass lesions. Magnetic resonance angiography (MRA) can be useful in locating a vascular compression (eg superior cerebellar artery compressing the trigeminal root); however, the sensitivity remains low.

Differential diagnosis

When the patient describes the classical history of TN, the diagnosis is easy to make. If there is a chronic element to the pain then the differential broadens (see Section 1.1.2).

Treatment
Medical
Consider:

- Carbamazepine is the drug of choice, with a response rate of 75%. Start with 100 mg daily and increase at weekly or 2-weekly intervals, up to a dose of 1,600 mg in divided doses. Lower doses usually suffice.

- If carbamazepine does not work, consider gabapentin, pregabalin, lamotrigine, baclofen, phenytoin or clonazepam, but the chances of success are much lower with these drugs.

Key point

The chances of medical treatment succeeding if carbamazepine fails are relatively small, so consider surgical options early.

Surgical

For patients with medically intractable TN, neurosurgical intervention should be considered. The options are as follows:

- Peripheral nerve block with alcohol or phenol injections may be used, but the effect is temporary (lasting 18–24 months). The injections may cause facial numbness.

- Percutaneous denervation, either by glycerol injection or radiofrequency thermocoagulation of the trigeminal ganglion. This may cause facial and corneal numbness. Anaesthesia dolorosa, a severe dysaesthesia which is generally unresponsive to therapy, occurs as a complication in 5–10% of cases.

- Microvascular decompression via a posterior fossa approach. The surgeon separates the trigeminal sensory root from the compressing aberrant blood vessel using a non-absorbable sponge. This approach is more likely to cause

death, stroke, facial weakness or hearing loss, but is less likely to be associated with recurrence, dysaesthesias or anaesthesia dolorosa. Microvascular decompression provides the highest rate of long-term patient satisfaction with the lowest rate of pain recurrence.

2.6.3 Cluster headache
Pathophysiology

- The mechanism of the pain is similar to migraine, in that the trigeminovascular system is involved.

- The central disorder is likely to involve the pacemaker regions of the posterior hypothalamus.

Epidemiology

Migraine is 20 times more common. Cluster headache occurs predominantly in males (male to female ratio 6:1) over the age of 20 years.

Clinical presentation
Characteristic features

- Severe unilateral orbital, supraorbital and/or temporal headache described as an intense, constant and boring pain.

- Typically each attack lasts for 15–180 minutes, occurring one to three times daily for 4–8 weeks, with each cluster occurring once or twice a year. There is, however, considerable variation.

- Most (80–90%) patients will have recurrent attacks at the same time each day, particularly in the early hours of the morning ('alarm clock' headache).

- There are several important associated features (see below).

- During a bout, alcohol seems to be a potent trigger.

- A chronic form of cluster headache may develop from episodic cluster or may occur *de novo*, in which the patient experiences recurrent attacks for more than a year with little or no remissions.

Associated features

Patients should have one or more of these features in order to be diagnosed as having cluster headache:

> conjunctival injection

> lacrimation

> nasal congestion

> rhinorrhoea

> ptosis

> miosis

> eyelid oedema.

Physical signs

In chronic cluster headaches a permanent Horner's syndrome may develop, but examination is usually normal between attacks.

Differential diagnosis

> Episodic cluster headache is simple to diagnose, but the chronic form may be more difficult (see Section 1.1.2).

> Attacks with the features of cluster headache, but of shorter duration (3–45 minutes) and occurring more frequently (20–40 times per day) have been termed chronic paroxysmal hemicrania, and are almost invariably responsive to indomethacin.

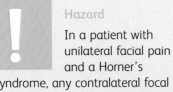

Hazard

In a patient with unilateral facial pain and a Horner's syndrome, any contralateral focal neurological signs should make you consider a carotid artery dissection (see Section 1.1.2).

Treatment

Acute

Try the following:

> Administering 100% oxygen via a close fitting mask at a rate of 15 L per minute relieves approximately 80% of attacks within 15 minutes.

> Sumatriptan 50–100 mg orally or 6 mg subcutaneously are as effective as oxygen.

> Ergotamine tablets or suppositories may be used the night before in anticipation of 'alarm clock' headaches.

> Verapamil 80 mg qds is effective in stopping a bout.

> Corticosteroids are also effective in stopping a bout, but recurrence is a problem.

Prophylaxis

The following agents may be helpful:

> Verapamil 240–600 mg daily has been used in the prevention of both episodic and chronic cluster headache, and is the drug of choice as a prophylactic agent. High doses need to be used. The starting dose should be 40 mg tds and an electrocardiogram (ECG) should be performed for every increment.

> Lithium carbonate is efficacious in the suppression of chronic, but less so of episodic, cluster headache in doses of 300–600 mg daily (maintaining serum levels at <1.2 mEq/L).

> Sodium valproate, topiramate and methysergide have also been used with some benefit.

2.6.4 Tension-type headache

Tension-type headache (TTH) is described as a constant tight or band-like sensation (non-pulsatile) around the head, which is usually bilateral (80–90%) and not aggravated by physical activity. It may be episodic (occurring on <15 days each month) or chronic (>15 days each month).

The term 'chronic daily headache' is often used for this type of headache, but is a descriptive, not diagnostic, term. Varieties of primary chronic daily headache are described below. Secondary causes are discussed in the differential diagnosis.

Varieties of primary chronic daily or near-daily headache include:

> chronic TTH

> transformed or chronic migraine (analgesic overuse)

> chronic cluster headache

> chronic paroxysmal hemicrania

> new persistent daily headache.

Pathophysiology

The pain of TTH is probably generated by the activation and sensitisation of second-order trigeminal neurones. The current phenotypic classification is likely to be reorganised once the underlying biological and genetic processes are better understood.

Epidemiology

Daily headache is common, with a lifetime prevalence of approximately 5% of the population.

Clinical presentation

Characteristic features include the following:

> The quality of the headache, as described above, may be of band-like, bifrontotemporal pressure, or a weight pressing down on top of the head.

> The pain is non-pulsatile.

> Occasional unilateral stabbing sensations may occur.

> Mild nausea (but not vomiting) and photophobia are common.

> Chronic forms are worsened by anxiety and stress, but pain is not limited to these occasions.

> Alcohol may relieve TTH, unlike migraine.

> There are no abnormal features on examination.

Investigations

Many patients are anxious to have a brain scan, but if there are no abnormal physical signs and the headache has the characteristic features as described above then a scan is not indicated, and reassurance is appropriate.

Differential diagnosis

If the headache is of more recent subacute onset, then the following can present with generalised non-specific headaches, and so must always be considered in the appropriate age group:

> expanding intracranial lesion (any age, but will produce symptoms more quickly in a young brain rather than atrophic one)

> progressive hydrocephalus (any age, but as for intracranial lesion)

> temporal arteritis (in those over 55 years old)

> idiopathic intracranial hypertension (in young females)

> primary angle-closure glaucoma (headache and eye pain associated with coloured haloes around lights, but may cause bilateral pain. Rare before middle age).

Key point

Over-diagnosed causes of chronic headache

Headache should not be attributed to:

> sinus disease, unless there are other symptoms supporting this

> disease of the ears, teeth or temporomandibular joint, unless there are other symptoms supporting this

> errors of refraction, as this only occasionally causes a very mild frontal headache not present on waking.

Treatment

Principles

Reassurance is a key component of treatment.

It is essential to identify contributory factors such as:

> functional or structural cervical or cranial musculoskeletal abnormalities

> depression

> analgesic overuse (see Section 2.6.1).

Non-pharmacological

These approaches are also useful:

> Encourage regular exercise in the sedentary.

> Suggest stress management if stress is prominent in the history.

> Physiotherapy may help to correct posture and to improve symptoms secondary to trauma such as whiplash, but it may be less successful in degenerative disease of the neck.

Pharmacological

Simple analgesia

Regular simple analgesia is inappropriate as it may be implicated in the genesis of the headache, although a single course of naproxen 500 mg bd for 3 weeks occasionally breaks the cycle of frequently occurring headaches.

Amitriptyline

This is the drug of choice. It is important to explain that this drug is not being used as an antidepressant, otherwise the patient may stop taking it when they find out. Start with 10 mg nocte and increase in 25 mg increments every 2 weeks to 75–100 mg. If tolerated, continue with this drug for 12 weeks before assessing efficacy, as it may take this long to work. If it has a beneficial effect then continue for a further 6–9 months before withdrawing the drug.

Other agents

Also consider the following:

> Other drugs such as prothiaden and sodium valproate.

> Selective serotonin reuptake inhibitors (SSRIs) seem to have little effect on chronic TTH, but may help if the patient is experiencing depression.

> Where chronic TTH and migraine coexist, in addition to the above measures the migraine may require symptomatic treatment (see Section 2.6.1), but on no more than 2 days per week.

Key point

Analgesic overuse, typically with paracetamol- or codeine-based compounds, requires that the appropriate drugs are withdrawn over 2–4 weeks if possible. It is wise to warn the patient that the headaches are likely to get worse before they get better, but unless the offending analgesics are withdrawn, the headache will not improve.

2.7 Epilepsy

Definition

Epilepsy is a condition characterised by recurrent (two or more) epileptic seizures, unprovoked by any immediate identified cause.

An epileptic seizure is a clinical manifestation presumed to result from an abnormal and excessive discharge from a set of neurones in the brain. The clinical manifestation consists of sudden and transitory abnormal phenomena which may include alterations in consciousness and motor, sensory, autonomic or psychic events perceived by the patient or an observer.

Pathophysiology

Pathological studies, increasingly from postoperative studies of resected foci, have shown a wide range of abnormalities, in particular the characteristic mesial temporal sclerosis seen in temporal lobe epilepsy, implying that these focal lesions may be epileptogenic. Diffuse cortical microdysgenesis may similarly play a part in the pathogenesis of idiopathic generalised epilepsy.

Aetiology

In childhood onset seizures, there is a strong association with congenital, developmental and genetic abnormalities.

In older patients, stroke is the commonest association (in 50% of first-time seizures in the over-sixties). At any age, head trauma, central nervous system infection and tumours have strong associations with epilepsy.

In general, there are likely to be multifactorial aetiologies. A genetic predisposition to epilepsy could lower the susceptibility to other aetiological factors.

Epidemiology

> Incidence: 40–70 per 100,000 people per year in developed countries.

> Prevalence: 0.5–1.0% of the general population have active epilepsy.

> Life-time prevalence: 2–5% of the general population.

Clinical presentation

Key point

A witness account is essential, and a hand-held video recording of an attack would be extremely useful, as the diagnosis of epilepsy is a clinical one.

Epilepsy may be most usefully classified according to seizure types (Table 45). The classification of epilepsy as syndromes is less useful clinically at present, partly because future classifications will change as more is learned about their underlying, possibly genetic, aetiologies.

Generalised seizures
Tonic–clonic
Features include:

> Sudden onset loss of consciousness often associated with an audible cry, followed by a fall to the ground.

> Tonic stiffening phase lasts 10–30 seconds, during which time respiration may be impaired, leading to cyanosis.

Table 45	Classification of epileptic seizures
Seizure type	**Characteristics**
Focal or partial seizures	*Simple* Motor – either limb or adversive head turning (frontal) Sensory or special sensory, eg visual – symptoms usually positive (pins and needles) rather than negative (numbness) Autonomic – rising epigastric sensation and changes in skin colour, BP, heart rate and pupil size may all indicate a temporal lobe origin Psychic – dysphasia/speech arrest, déjà vu, sensations of unreality or depersonalisation, fear, anger, elation, illusions or structured hallucinations may all originate from a temporal lobe focus
	Complex Simple partial onset followed by impairment of consciousness With impaired consciousness at onset Partial seizures evolving to secondary generalised seizures
Generalised seizures	Absence seizures: Typical Atypical
	Myoclonic seizures
	Clonic seizures
	Tonic seizures
	Atonic seizures
	Tonic–clonic seizures
Unclassifiable seizures	

> Followed by clonic phase, in which there is low-amplitude jerking of all four limbs. As the seizure progresses, its frequency slows and its amplitude increases. Lasts 30–60 seconds.

> Flaccidity of muscles with slow recovery of consciousness over 2–30 minutes.

> Associated with incontinence, tongue biting and autonomic features.

> May be more tonic or clonic.

> Does not imply pathological type, unless preceded by clear partial onset.

Typical absence

Features include:

> Sudden loss of consciousness and motor activity without warning, resulting in a blank stare.

> Attacks end suddenly and patients may continue with what they were doing, unaware of what has just happened.

> Short attacks lasting <30 seconds.

> Automatisms, slight clonic movements or eyelid fluttering may occur in longer attacks.

> These seizures occur as part of idiopathic generalised epilepsy.

Atypical absence

Features include:

> Blank stare.

> Onset and cessation are more gradual.

> Consciousness is only partially impaired.

> Focal signs are more prominent.

> Occurs in patients with diffuse cerebral damage.

Myoclonic

Features include:

> Brief jerk either in single muscle or generalised, which is of rapid onset and cessation.

> No loss of consciousness.

> Often part of idiopathic generalised epilepsies.

Focal or partial seizures

Simple

Features include:

> No alteration in consciousness and no amnesia.

> Sudden onset and cessation.

> Symptoms depend on site of underlying cortical lesion (Table 45).

> The seizure lasts for only seconds.

Complex

Features include:

> Often preceded by simple partial seizure (aura).

> Alteration in consciousness associated with blank staring, and often with motor signs such as unilateral dystonic posturing (temporal lobe).

> Automatism – this is a more or less coordinated involuntary motor activity occurring during a clouding of consciousness that occurs during or after an epileptic seizure, usually followed by amnesia. They may take many forms (Table 46).

> About 60% of complex partial seizures arise from the temporal lobes, and 30% from the frontal lobes.

Table 46	Clinical features of automatisms
Type	Feature
Oro-alimentary	Lip smacking
	Chewing
	Swallowing
Gestural	Fiddling with hands
	Picking at clothing
	Tidying
Ambulatory	Walking
	Running
	Circling
	Purposeless complex movement
Verbal	Humming
	Whistling
	Grunting
Mimicry	Displays of laughter, fear, anger and excitement

Automatisms may occur as part of a complex partial seizure from any location.

Key point

Juvenile myoclonic epilepsy (JME) is a syndromic diagnosis worth knowing about because:

> It is common, causing 5–10% of all cases of epilepsy.

> It has an extremely good prognosis if treated correctly.

Clinical features are:

> Myoclonic jerks, generalised tonic–clonic seizures, with or without absences and precipitated by sleep deprivation and alcohol.

> Clear diurnal variation, attacks frequently occurring within an hour of waking. Ask specifically about early morning twitching as this may not be reported.

> Of patients with JME, 90% become seizure-free when on sodium valproate, although high relapse rates occur off medication.

> Linked to chromosome 6.

Physical signs

> Uncommon unless seizures are due to an underlying cortical structural lesion.

> Epilepsy may occur as part of a wider phenotype in some neurodegenerative diseases.

> Consider the neurocutaneous syndromes.

Investigation

> Routine biochemical and haematological profiles.

> Electroencephalogram (EEG).

> MRI.

> A hand-held video recording is very useful, especially if the diagnosis is not clearly epilepsy.

Electroencephalogram

In practice, most patients require an EEG as part of their initial evaluation. However:

> A normal interictal EEG does not exclude epilepsy. An abnormal EEG may support a primary idiopathic process and provide evidence of photosensitivity.

> EEG is a poor guide to seizure control, with the exception of 3 Hz spike-and-wave changes which are sensitive to treatment (Fig 39).

> Minor asymmetries are not diagnostic.

Magnetic resonance imaging

Structural imaging is indicated as follows:

> partial seizures on history (Fig 40)

> deficit revealed on neurological or psychological examination

> difficult seizure control with antiepileptics

> generalised seizures, onset before 1 or after 20 years of age.

The last point is debated. The reason for suggesting it is that a generalised seizure with no suggestion of partial onset is extremely likely to be a primary idiopathic type of epilepsy in this age range. Some specialists will scan all new presentations.

Differential diagnosis

Half of new epilepsy referrals may have an alternative diagnosis.

The distinction between an epileptic attack and a non-epileptic attack is discussed in Table 47, but it should be remembered that they may coexist.

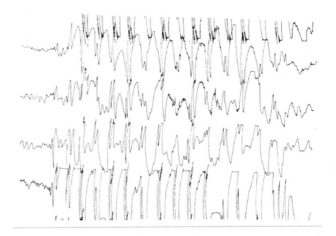

Fig 39 EEG showing 3 Hz spike-and-wave pattern.

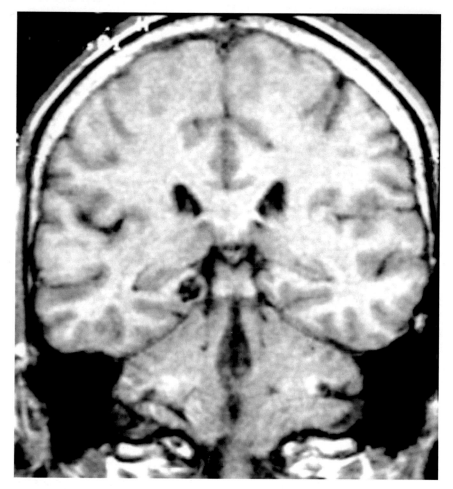

Fig 40 Right parahippocampal angioma in a patient with temporal lobe epilepsy seen on a coronal MRI scan.

Table 47 Differentiation between an epileptic attack and a non-epileptic attack

	Epileptic attack	Non-epileptic attack
Precipitant	Rare	Commonly stress related
Onset	Short	May be short or prolonged
Movement	Synchronous small amplitude jerks if clonic	Asynchronous flailing of limbs, pelvic thrusting and opisthotonus
Injury	Tongue biting (sides) and falls, but directed violence rare	May bite tongue (tip), cheeks, lip and hands, and may throw themselves to ground; also, directed violence occurs
Consciousness	Complete or incomplete depending on type	Variable, but may be inconsistent with seizure type
Response to stimuli	None unless it is complex partial seizure	May terminate the attack. Suggestible
Incontinence	Common	Sometimes
Duration	Minutes	May be prolonged
Recovery	Few minutes, but may be prolonged confusion	Rapid or very prolonged

Treatment

Emergency

For management of status epilepticus see Section 1.5.4.

Key point

When should antiepileptic medication be commenced?

To answer this, one needs an appreciation of the risks of seizure recurrence to balance against the risk of antiepileptic medication.

> The risk of recurrence is highest in the first few days and weeks, then falls with time.

> Thirty per cent of patients will have a recurrent seizure by 3 months, 67% by 12 months and 78% by 36 months. Antiepileptic medication reduces but does not abolish this risk.

> At 12 months the risk of recurrence in those with a focal seizure is 94%. In those with seizures precipitated by an acute illness it is much lower at 40%.

On the basis of these figures you can see that it might be desirable to treat some patients after one seizure rather than wait for the customary two seizures, as the risk of recurrence may be high (about 80% with time overall). If a patient presents having had a single seizure 12 months before, then the subsequent risk of recurrence may be lower and one may choose to wait.

The decision to initiate antiepileptic treatment is based on the risk of recurrent seizures versus the risks of the drug itself, not on arbitrarily waiting for two seizures to occur.

Natural history of epilepsy on treatment

> Reassure the patient that 70–80% of newly diagnosed patients treated with a single antiepileptic drug will eventually be seizure-free.

> If remission is defined as 5 years seizure-free, then about 40% of patients enter remission in the first year, 20% in the next 9 years and 10% in the next 10 years.

Once the decision to initiate treatment has been made, follow these general principles:

> Start the drug at a low dose, then titrate up slowly until the seizures are abolished or the maximum tolerated dose has been reached.

> For focal or partial seizures, or secondary generalised seizures, first-line drugs are usually carbamazepine or lamotrigine. Alternative treatments include levetiracetam, oxcarbazepine and sodium valproate.

> For most generalised or idiopathic epilepsies, sodium valproate is the treatment of choice. Lamotrigine is an alternative if sodium valproate is unsuitable.

> If seizures continue, reconsider the diagnosis, check compliance and review or obtain neuroimaging.

> If epilepsy is still thought to be the diagnosis, then introduce another first-line agent, for example carbamazepine, lamotrigine or sodium valproate. When a reasonable dose is achieved then the first drug can be withdrawn slowly.

> Adjust the dose of the second drug to optimum.

> If seizures continue, try both first-line drugs together. Thereafter add in a second-line drug at the expense of the least well-tolerated first-line drug. Consider other second-line drugs in a similar manner.

> Three drugs are rarely better than two.

Key point

'When can I come off my tablets, doctor?'

This question is likely to be asked by the patient when in some form of remission. The first two points that need to be highlighted are:

> No guarantees can be made that seizures will not recur.

> Think about driving: if the loss of a driving licence would be a devastating blow to the patient, they may decide to stay on medication.

The decision must be made by the patient, informed by the information you provide.

> In patients in remission for 2 years or more, the chance of a seizure in the next 2 years are 43% if the drug is withdrawn, compared with 10% in those maintaining therapy.

> This figure may alter with the presence or absence of certain risk factors (Table 48).

> Within 10–15 years after the onset of epilepsy at least 70% of patients are in 5 years remission and 50% are off all drugs.

Surgical treatment

Focal resections

Consider surgical options in patients with seizures of partial onset, which are refractory to intensive medical therapy over at least 2–3 years.

> Pre-surgical evaluation includes a detailed clinical assessment, EEG and video telemetry to obtain ictal EEG, high-resolution structural MRI (epilepsy protocol),

Table 48 Factors affecting risk of recurrent seizure following drug withdrawal

Risk	Factor
Increased risk	Age over 16
	Taking more than one antiepileptic drug
	A history of seizures after starting antiepileptic drugs
	A history of tonic–clonic seizures
	A history of myoclonic seizures
	An abnormal EEG in the previous year
Decreased risk	Risk of seizures declines the longer the seizure-free period

EEG, electroencephalogram.

a positron emission tomography scan if structural imaging is unclear, and neuropsychological and neuropsychiatric evaluation.

> One is looking for a convergence of data, implying one epileptogenic area. If this data are concordant then the chance of seizure freedom postoperatively is approximately 60–70%. Data suggesting multifocal foci indicates less chance of success.

> The commonest site of resection is the temporal lobe. The risk of serious morbidity or mortality during surgical resection is approximately 1%.

Other operations
Remember:

> Division of the corpus callosum is reserved for patients with severe intractable seizures and drop attacks. The operation is aimed at reducing the number and severity of attacks, especially the drop attacks.

> Hemispherectomy is reserved for children or adolescents with medically intractable seizures due to severe unilateral hemisphere damage.

Management of the pregnant patient with epilepsy
General information
Preconception counselling is very important.

> The background risk of major fetal malformations in developed countries is 1–2%, and this is thought to rise to 3% in mothers with epilepsy on no medication, 4–6% with one antiepileptic drug and up to 15% with two or more. There is some evidence that this risk is dose dependent.

> The background risk of neural-tube defects is 0.2–0.5%.

> Sodium valproate has the highest teratogenicity rate among antiepileptic medications. Carbamazepine and lamotrigine have the lowest recorded risks. More recently, it has been suggested that

levetiracetam has virtually no known teratogenic effects.

Principles of drug management
Remember:

> If possible, maintain the patient on as few drugs and at as low a dose as possible.

> Consider withdrawing drugs prior to pregnancy if the patient has been seizure-free for 2 years.

> Advise folic acid 5 mg daily for 12 weeks before and after conception, to reduce the risk of neural-tube defects.

> Serum alpha-fetoprotein measurement and high-resolution fetal ultrasound should be carried out at 16–18 weeks to screen for neural-tube defects, especially in those taking sodium valproate or carbamazepine.

> Oral vitamin K (20 mg/day) should be given to the mother if she is taking an enzyme-inducing drug (phenytoin, carbamazepine, phenobarbitone or mysoline) in the last month of pregnancy to protect the baby from haemorrhagic disease of the newborn. The risk lasts for a week or so postpartum and so some suggest that oral vitamin K be given to the baby for a further week to cover this period. However, vitamin K is still usually given by intramuscular injection to newborn babies. Fears still exist over the risk of childhood neoplasia with the injectable form, although more recent trials have failed to find this link.

Prognosis

Epilepsy carries an increased risk of death, mainly attributable to the underlying disease, accidents or suicide.

Hazard

Patients with epilepsy are at risk of SUDEP (sudden unexplained deaths in epilepsy) at a rate of 1 per 200–1,000 people per year. Young patients and those with frequent generalised seizures and learning disability have higher risk. The cause and strategies for prevention are not clear, although there is some evidence to suggest that either cerebrogenic cardiac arrhythmias or ictal apnoea may be responsible.

Occupational aspects

Key point

Driving

Patients may apply for a driving licence if they have been seizure-free for 1 year, or if they have an established pattern of seizures occurring only during sleep for the previous 3 years. Stricter rules apply to drivers of heavy goods vehicles (HGVs) and passenger-carrying vehicles (PCVs).

It is recommended, but not covered by legislation, that driving be suspended from the start of antiepileptic drug withdrawal until 6 months afterwards.

Employment

Recruitment is barred in the armed forces, the fire brigade, London Regional Transport, the merchant navy and diving. For many other occupations no specific legislation exists but employment is unlikely.

Leisure

To a large extent, this depends on the individual's particular seizure pattern, but in general adequate supervision for activities such as swimming, cycling and rock climbing is needed, together with an acceptance that risk is not something that can be eliminated from all activities.

2.8 Cerebrovascular disease

2.8.1 Stroke

The most widely accepted definition of a stroke is a clinical syndrome of presumed vascular origin characterised by rapidly developing clinical symptoms and signs of focal, and at times global (applied to patients with coma or subarachnoid haemorrhage), loss of cerebral function lasting for more than 24 hours or leading to death.

The classification of stroke is broadly into ischaemic and haemorrhagic (Table 49). Ischaemic stroke is dealt with in this section, and intracerebral haemorrhage and subarachnoid haemorrhage are discussed in Section 2.8.4.

Aetiology

An ischaemic stroke can be classified according to its mechanism using the Trial of Org 10172 in Acute Stroke Treatment (TOAST) classification. Strokes are divided into five categories:

> thromboembolism from the heart

> thromboembolism from major vessels

> occlusion of small penetrating vessels, found predominantly in the basal ganglia, internal capsule or pons (lacunar stroke) (Fig 41)

> other (ie not one of the above but a definite mechanism identified)

> cryptogenic.

Occlusion of vessels may occur as a result of thrombosis and local occlusion, or subsequent to embolisation and distal occlusion.

Thrombosis is attributable to any element of Virchow's triad:

> abnormality of the vessel wall (atherosclerosis (especially if ulcerated), dissection or vasculitis in large vessels and lipohyalinosis in the small perforating vessels)

> abnormality of the blood (eg polycythaemia)

> disturbances of blood flow (eg atrial fibrillation, turbulence of blood flow following dissection).

Table 49	Classification of stroke types
Pathology	**Mechanism**
Ischaemic (85%)	Cardioembolism – clot arising from the heart
	Large vessel atherosclerosis
	Small vessel thrombotic disease
	Embolic disease from cardiac source
	Other
	Cryptogenic (unknown cause)
Haemorrhagic (15%)	Primary intracerebral haemorrhage
	Secondary intracerebral haemorrhage
	Subarachnoid haemorrhage

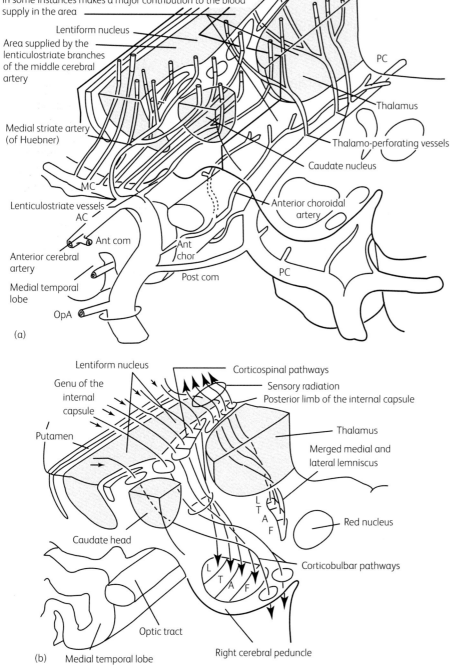

Area supplied by the thalamo-geniculate and thalamo-perforating branches of the posterior cerebral artery and the anterior choroidal artery which in some instances makes a major contribution to the blood supply in the area

Lentiform nucleus

Area supplied by the lenticulostriate branches of the middle cerebral artery

Medial striate artery (of Huebner)

Lenticulostriate vessels

PC

Thalamus

Thalamo-perforating vessels

Caudate nucleus

Anterior choroidal artery

MC

AC

Ant com

Ant chor

Anterior cerebral artery

Medial temporal lobe

Post com

PC

OpA

(a)

Lentiform nucleus

Genu of the internal capsule

Putamen

Corticospinal pathways

Sensory radiation

Posterior limb of the internal capsule

Thalamus

Merged medial and lateral lemniscus

L
T
A
F

Red nucleus

Caudate head

Corticobulbar pathways

L
T
A
F

Optic tract

(b)   Medial temporal lobe

Right cerebral peduncle

Fig 41 (a) Schematic representation of the blood supply to the region of the internal capsule. Note that the main motor pathways at capsular level are supplied by the middle cerebral branches, and the main sensory pathways are mainly supplied by the posterior cerebral-derived vessels. This explains why capsular strokes tend to be primarily motor or sensory. The blood supply of the sublenticular visual pathways, the optic tract and the lateral geniculate body is derived from anterior choroidal or posterior cerebral-derived vessels. **(b)** Key diagram of pathway anatomy in the internal capsule. The right internal capsule is shown from above and anteriorly to indicate the motor and sensory rotations between the internal capsule and upper midbrain. A, arm; F, face; L, leg; T, trunk.

The main modifiable risk factors for stroke are:

> hypertension

> atrial fibrillation

> cigarette smoking

> previous transient ischaemic attack (TIA)

> heart failure

> ischaemic heart disease

> diabetes mellitus

> excess alcohol

> hyperlipidaemia

> obesity

> inactivity

> elevated haematocrit

> recreational drug use (usually in the young).

Pathophysiology

Reduction in cerebral blood flow (CBF) below the normal (>50 mL/minute per 100 g of tissue) sets off a cascade of events which will ultimately lead to cell death if not reversed.

As CBF falls below about 20 mL/minute per 100 g, there is loss of electrical neuronal function, a potentially reversible stage. Below 10 mL/minute per 100 g irreversible damage starts to occur. The increased energy demands of the cell cannot be met and adenosine triphosphate becomes depleted. Consequently, energy-dependent ion homeostasis fails, leading to equilibration of all ions across the cell membrane (anoxic depolarisation) and the release of potentially toxic levels of glutamate and calcium influx. Several processes interact leading to an ischaemic cascade and, ultimately, cell death.

Epidemiology

> The annual incidence of stroke is 115–150 per 100,000 people.

> Stroke is the fourth single largest cause of death in the UK and second in the world.

> There are 1.2 million stroke survivors in the UK.

> One in eight strokes are fatal within the first 30 days.

> Stroke is the commonest cause of complex disability and half of all stroke survivors have a disability.

Physical signs

The neurological examination should enable one to identify the site of the lesion accurately, but in routine clinical practice this degree of accuracy has no value over and above a bedside system of classification, such as the Oxfordshire Community Stroke Study classification (see Table 18). In the case of evolving signs this simple analysis is more likely to be incorrect, but it is used in some units and is worth being aware of.

Investigations

The most important specific investigation is a CT scan to exclude haemorrhage, enable early treatment with interventional mechanical thrombectomy (in specialised vascular centres), intravenous thrombolysis and antiplatelet agents, and to exclude other possible diagnoses such as space-occupying lesions. In ischaemic stroke CT scans may initially appear normal, but remember that early signs of ischaemia are subtle and easily missed (see Fig 42).

At presentation patients should also have the following:

> an electrocardiogram (ECG)

> a chest X-ray

> blood tests (FBC, erythrocyte sedimentation rate, urea, electrolytes and glucose).

Differential diagnosis

Misdiagnosis of ischaemic stroke occurs in up to a quarter of cases, usually when a clear history is not available. Intracerebral haemorrhage is the most important differential diagnosis, and can only reliably be differentiated on CT scan. Other alternatives include brain tumour, subdural haematoma, cerebral venous thrombosis, focal cerebral infection, hemiplegic migraine, hypoglycaemia and postictal Todd's paresis. In a young person, consider multiple sclerosis.

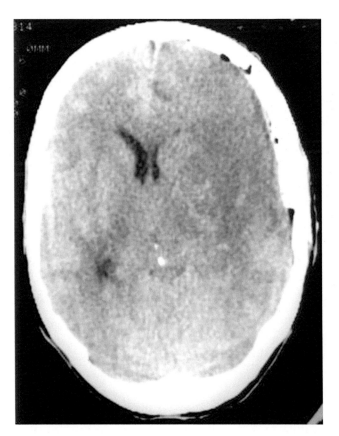

Fig 42 Acute changes of cerebral infarction due to occlusion of left middle cerebral artery shown on a CT scan.

Key point

Stroke is a clinical diagnosis, but the most important distinction – between ischaemia and haemorrhage – requires special investigation, ie a CT scan. This has an impact on subsequent management, and will become ever more important with the advent of acute therapies for ischaemic stroke.

Treatment

Short term

General care

Important points to consider in the investigation/management of an acute case are as follows:

> Early treatment is supportive in order to prevent complications.

> Careful monitoring of neurological status, blood pressure, oxygenation, glycaemic control, hydration, nutrition, swallowing function, temperature control and bladder function are all crucial, and proper management in these areas will have an enormous impact on the mortality and morbidity of stroke patients. Management of stroke patients in a designated stroke unit reduces mortality and long-term dependency. Much planning needs to go into the ongoing care of patients, often older patients, whose stroke has left them dependent.

Acute therapies designed to minimise the size of infarct

Specific early treatments designed to reduce the size of infarct include thrombolysis, interventional mechanical thrombectomy and neuroprotective agents.

> Thrombolysis: the National Institute of Neurological Disorders and Stroke (NINDS) trial demonstrated that compared with placebo, patients treated within 3 hours of onset of their stroke with intravenous recombinant

tissue plasminogen activator (rtPA) had a favourable outcome at 3 months. For every eight patients treated with rtPA within 3 hours, one additional patient will have minimal or no disability. There was a significant increase in the number of treated patients suffering from symptomatic intracranial haemorrhage (6.6%), but importantly there was no overall increase in mortality at 3 months. The time window for treatment with intravenous rtPA has been extended up to 4.5 hours from stroke onset following the results from the European Cooperative Acute Stroke Study III (ECASS III). For every 14 patients treated with intravenous rtPA, one additional patient will have minimal or no disability.

> Mechanical thrombectomy: recent randomised clinical trials have proven the benefit of endovascular mechanical thrombectomy in the management of acute stroke patients. This establishes a new standard of treatment in the management of acute ischaemic stroke patients. Mechanical thrombectomy is provided in addition to thrombolysis in ischaemic stroke patients presenting with major vessel occlusion confirmed on neuroimaging such as CT angiogram. The treatment should be provided within 6 hours of acute stroke onset with proximal intracranial anterior circulation occlusion (distal internal carotid artery, proximal middle cerebral artery occlusion).

> Neuroprotection: neuroprotective agents have been disappointing to date, but it is likely that they will need to be given in combination with thrombolysis so that cerebral tissue preserved in this manner will benefit from reperfusion.

Agents used to reduce stroke recurrence in the acute setting

These include antiplatelet therapy and anticoagulants.

> Antiplatelet therapy – aspirin prevents 10 deaths or recurrent strokes per 1,000 patients treated in the first 2 weeks following acute ischaemic stroke, and it should be commenced once haemorrhage has been excluded at a dose of 300 mg daily for 2 weeks. In patients who have received intravenous thrombolysis, aspirin at a dose of 300 mg once daily should be started 24 hours post-thrombolysis and continued for 2 weeks. It is then usual to switch to long-term prophylaxis at a dose of 75 mg daily.

> Anticoagulants – warfarin and heparin are not associated with any overall benefit in the treatment of stroke because of an increase in haemorrhagic complications, and so cannot be recommended for acute treatment. Heparin is used occasionally for 'stroke in evolution' and basilar artery thrombosis, and frequently for carotid or vertebral artery dissection (but without supportive evidence from randomised controlled trials).

Long term

The diagnosis has been made and treatment initiated. Subsequent management is directed at establishing the underlying cause of the stroke, initiating secondary preventative measures and managing the consequent impairment.

Further investigations

In appropriate circumstances the following are likely to be helpful in determining cause and identifying factors important in secondary preventative treatment.

> Electrocardiography should have been performed acutely but it is critical to ensure that it is reviewed. The diagnosis of atrial fibrillation will have a significant impact on further management.

> Carotid Doppler ultrasound scans and magnetic resonance angiography

should be performed to look for symptomatic internal carotid artery stenosis in a case of carotid territory ischaemia. If these two investigations are in agreement, they should avoid the need for intra-arterial angiography.

> Transthoracic echocardiography should be performed if an embolic source is suspected. In a young stroke patient in whom an embolic source is considered, transoesophageal echocardiography should be performed to rule out patent foramen ovale and the associated feature of interatrial septal aneurysm.

> Serum cholesterol.

> Thrombophilia screen – at present the significance of these tests is not clear, so reserve them for cases with no other clear aetiological risk factors, young patients and those with a strong family history. Similarly, a sickle cell screen is crucial when appropriate.

Secondary preventative treatment – risk factor reduction

Most of the evidence is from primary prevention studies, but removal of as many risk factors as possible is sensible.

Secondary preventative treatment – antiplatelet therapy

Consider:

> Aspirin is beneficial in secondary prevention of all vascular events, as demonstrated by the Antiplatelet Trialists' Collaboration, and it seems to reduce subsequent vascular events by about 23%. The time to commence it is established to be as soon as possible (ie after haemorrhage excluded), both by the International Stroke Trial (IST) and the Chinese Acute Stroke Trial (CAST).

> Dipyridamole modified release (MR) 200 mg bd – should be added if further events occur on aspirin monotherapy.

> If the patient is genuinely aspirin intolerant or the patient has a stroke while on aspirin, use clopidogrel 75 mg daily. Alternatively, dipyridamole MR monotherapy could be considered in patients with low vascular risk factors, but not in those with high vascular risk factors as dipyridamole MR alone seems to have no effect on non-stroke vascular events.

Secondary preventative treatment – anticoagulants

These should be prescribed for patients who have had an ischaemic stroke with atrial fibrillation. It is not clear exactly when to start this, but after major stroke wait at least 2 weeks (possibly less in minor strokes) to reduce the chances of haemorrhagic conversion. Atrial fibrillation carries a recurrent stroke risk of 12% per annum. Treatment for atrial fibrillation includes warfarin and newer anticoagulants such as dabigatran (direct thrombin inhibitor), rivaroxaban and apixaban (direct factor Xa inhibitor).

Secondary preventative treatment – carotid surgery

Two trials, the North American Symptomatic Carotid Endarterectomy Trial (NASCET) and the European Carotid Surgery Trial (ECST) studied patients with a recent TIA or minor stroke, and found a beneficial effect of carotid endarterectomy in those with ≥70% stenosis.

Secondary preventative treatment – carotid endovascular treatment

Endovascular treatment (angioplasty and stenting) is a less invasive alternative to surgery for internal carotid artery stenosis. The most obvious advantages are the avoidance of a surgical incision and the ability for it to be performed under local anaesthesia, thus avoiding the effects of

anaesthetic drugs and intubation. Because of this, the risk of potentially fatal complications such as myocardial infarction and pulmonary embolism is also reduced. The use of local anaesthesia also means a faster recovery for patients treated endovascularly, reducing the length of hospital stay and potentially reducing costs.

Carotid artery stenting is an alternative to carotid endarterectomy. Carotid artery stenting can be considered in patients with symptomatic carotid artery disease with 70–99% stenosis who are poor surgical candidates with increased associated comorbidity.

Secondary preventative treatment – cholesterol

Raised cholesterol is an important risk factor for ischaemic stroke. Elevated serum total cholesterol, triglycerides and low density lipoprotein (LDL) are risk factors for cardiovascular disease. Coronary artery disease is a major cause of death in stroke patients, and so it seems reasonable to treat a cholesterol level over 5 mmol/L (and some would say even lower) after a stroke or TIA with a statin. This is particularly important in patients with diabetes mellitus.

Complications

Complications of acute stroke include the following:

> cerebral oedema – the commonest cause of death, usually at 4–5 days

> haemorrhagic transformation

> seizures – complicate 10% of infarcts or haemorrhages, but do not influence mortality

> depression – occurs in 50% of those who suffer acute strokes, particularly with left anterior lesions

> deterioration in glycaemic control

- syndrome of inappropriate antidiuretic hormone secretion, peaking at 7–9 days
- pressure sores
- pulmonary embolism
- aspiration.

Prognosis

- Twenty per cent of cases result in death in the first month, 30% in the first year.
- In those alive at 1 year the annual death rate is 8.5%.
- The annual risk of recurrence is 13% in the first year, 5% thereafter.
- The risk of stroke or cardiac event by 5 years is 40%.
- It is very important to remember not only the risk of recurrent stroke but also of cardiac events.

Occupational aspects

Following stroke, patients often report reduced exercise tolerance and increased fatigue levels, which may continue beyond good functional recovery. This has implications for the timing of return to work when appropriate.

Driving is discouraged for 3 months.

2.8.2 Transient ischaemic attacks

A transient ischaemic attack (TIA) is an episode of acute loss of focal cerebral or monocular function with symptoms lasting <24 hours, which is thought to be due to inadequate cerebral or ocular blood supply as a result of an arterial, cardiac or haematological cause.

The definition of TIA has evolved and is tissue based rather than time based. With the development of neuroimaging (MRI diffusion-weighted imaging sequences) about one-third of TIA defined by the 24-hour criteria has abnormal diffusion-weighted MRI sequences in keeping with actual ischaemic infarct.

Investigation and secondary prevention is as detailed in Section 2.8.1. The distinct characteristics of TIAs are discussed below.

Clinical presentation

The diagnosis is made on a history of focal neurological symptoms (Table 50), as physical signs will almost certainly have disappeared by the time of assessment. The vascular territory involved, carotid or vertebrobasilar, is suspected on the same basis as for ischaemic strokes. Isolated dysarthria or homonymous hemianopia are more difficult to interpret, as they may be caused by TIAs in either territory.

Key point

- Non-focal symptoms such as loss of consciousness, dizziness, mental confusion, generalised weakness and incontinence are unacceptable as evidence of a TIA.
- Some focal symptoms occurring in isolation should also not be interpreted as TIAs (see below).

The following symptoms are not acceptable as evidence of a TIA if they occur in isolation:

- vertigo
- diplopia
- dysphagia
- loss of balance
- tinnitus
- scintillating scotomas
- amnesia
- drop attacks
- sensory symptoms confined to one part of limb or face.

Physical signs

Examine for the following:

- Cardiovascular abnormalities – the examination is usually normal but is necessary to exclude predisposing factors.
- Carotid bruits – not always present even if there is a very tight stenosis.
- Cholesterol embolus – if visualised on fundoscopy this may indicate that the aetiology is atheromatous plaque in the aortic arch or internal carotid artery in a case of amaurosis fugax.

Table 50 Symptoms raising the possibility of transient ischaemic attacks (TIAs)	
Carotid	Vertebrobasilar
Contralateral paresis, heaviness or clumsiness in the leg, arm/hand and face	Bilateral, unilateral or alternating paresis (may be contralateral and ipsilateral in face/limbs)
Contralateral and predominantly negative sensory symptoms in the leg, arm/hand and face	Sensory loss, unilateral or bilateral (may be contralateral and ipsilateral in face/limbs)
Contralateral homonymous hemianopia	Diplopia
Unilateral monocular visual loss	Bilateral visual loss
Aphasia	Dysphagia
Dysarthria	Dysarthria
Combination of the above	Combination of the above

Vertebrobasilar symptoms brought on by exercise of the ipsilateral arm may be the result of the stenosis of the proximal subclavian artery or aortic arch, leading to retrograde flow down the vertebral artery (Fig 43). On examination there may be a bruit in the supraclavicular fossa with reduced blood pressure and pulse pressure in the ipsilateral arm.

Differential diagnosis

Migraine and epilepsy are two of the commonest differential diagnoses encountered and the differential diagnosis of TIA include:

> partial epilepsy

> migraine with aura

> migraine equivalents

> multiple sclerosis

> intracranial space-occupying lesions

> intracranial vascular malformations

> cardiac dysrhythmia

> vestibular disorders

> peripheral nerve or root lesions

> anxiety and hyperventilation

> hypoglycaemia

> transient global amnesia.

Migraine

The difficulty arises when considering migraine equivalents, ie migraine without headache. The following points are helpful:

> Migrainous symptoms are usually positive (tingling and scintillating scotoma), whereas TIA symptoms are usually negative representing a loss of function (numbness, reduced vision and weakness).

> The spread of symptoms in migraine tends to be slow, ie over several minutes.

> After a migraine, patients often feel generally unwell for hours, which is not usually the case after a TIA.

Partial epilepsy

Features include:

> Symptoms are usually positive (jerking and tingling), and are brief compared with a TIA.

> Very frequent attacks are usually epileptic.

Note that occasionally focal lower limb shaking, occurring on standing, has been associated with severe contralateral carotid artery stenosis.

Prognosis

The risk of stroke following a TIA is increased:

> 13 times in the first year, and by seven times in each year subsequent to that one

> 4% in the first month

> 9% in the first 6 months

> 12% in the first 12 months

> 4% per annum thereafter.

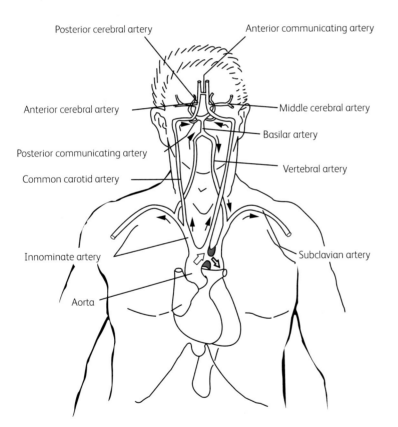

Posterior cerebral artery

Anterior communicating artery

Anterior cerebral artery

Middle cerebral artery

Posterior communicating artery

Basilar artery

Common carotid artery

Vertebral artery

Innominate artery

Subclavian artery

Aorta

Fig 43 Subclavian steal syndrome. The lesion is in the aortic arch between the take-off of the left common carotid artery and the left subclavian artery. The blood therefore tends to flow up both carotids and the right vertebral artery and then flows back down the left vertebral artery, ultimately rejoining the subclavian artery to supply the left arm.

Most strokes occur in the same territory as the previous TIA. Amaurosis fugax, possibly for this reason, has a much lower chance of leading to a stroke.

Key point

Patients with TIA have arterial disease, and as such have a higher risk of heart disease. In fact, the risk of myocardial infarct and sudden cardiac death is about 4% per annum, which emphasises the point that you must consider heart disease in TIA and stroke patients.

2.8.3 Intracerebral haemorrhage

Aetiology

Almost all cases of intracerebral haemorrhage (ICH) are caused by one of the following:

> Primary intracerebral bleed (80–85%)

> > hypertension

> > cerebral amyloid angiopathy.

> Secondary intracerebral bleed (15–20%)

> > oral anticoagulation, underlying bleeding disorder

> > tumours (primary versus metastatic)

> ruptured aneurysms and vascular malformations (arteriovenous malformations, cavernomas)

> cerebral venous sinus thrombosis

> cerebral vasculitis

> sympathomimetic drugs

> eclampsia.

> Rare causes

> > mycotic aneurysm (endocarditis)

> > haemorrhagic leucoencephalopathy

> > herpes simplex encephalitis.

Pathology

Chronic hypertension causes a vasculopathy in the small perforating arteries characterised by lipohyalinosis, fibrinoid necrosis and the formation of Charcot–Bouchard microaneurysms. Rupture of these results in haemorrhage in predominantly deep areas of the brain (Table 51).

Small haematomas dissect along white matter tracts, but large haematomas rupture into the parenchyma, causing destruction of tissue and elevation of intracranial pressure. Death occurs due to hemisphere and/or brainstem compression.

Epidemiology

> ICH occurs in 10–15% of all strokes.

> It is twice as common as subarachnoid haemorrhage.

Clinical presentation

An ICH is clinically indistinguishable from ischaemic stroke, but headache, vomiting and seizures at onset suggest ICH. A large haemorrhage will cause death or coma within hours, no matter its location. The onset may be rapid, but an ICH associated with anticoagulant therapy may evolve slowly.

Key point

An ICH cannot reliably be distinguished from ischaemia on clinical grounds, a CT scan *is essential to make the diagnosis.*

Physical signs

Smaller haematomas may have distinguishing physical signs depending on the site.

Supratentorial

Look for:

> Putamen – predominantly hemiplegia, and also aphasia, homonymous hemianopia, hemineglect and deviation of eyes away from the affected side.

> Thalamic – predominantly hemisensory deficit, and also hemiparesis, aphasia (dominant side) and neglect (non-dominant side). Ocular signs may be prominent with forced downward deviation of the eyes, skew deviation (vertical separation of gaze) and ipsilateral Horner's syndrome.

> Lobar – depends on the site of the lesion.

Infratentorial

Look for:

> Cerebellar – may be slow to develop, so the patient is unlikely to be comatose at onset. There will be deviation of the eyes away from the haemorrhage, ipsilateral fifth–seventh cranial nerve palsies and ipsilateral Horner's syndrome. Hemiplegia and aphasia are absent,

Table 51 Sites of hypertensive intracerebral haemorrhage (ICH)

Site	Percentage (%)
Putamen	35–50
Subcortical (lobar)	30
Cerebellum	16
Thalamus	10–15
Pons	5–12

as are cerebellar signs early on. Progresses to coma as a result of brainstem compression.

> Pontine – total paralysis, decerebrate rigidity (extension to pain), pinpoint reactive pupils and absent doll's eyes response.

Investigation

A CT scan will be diagnostic (Figs 44–46). If the patient is under 40 years old with no history of hypertension, it may be wise to enhance the scan to look for an underlying lesion.

An angiogram is warranted when there is significant suspicion of an underlying lesion. Factors that increase the likelihood of finding an abnormality are:

> The patient is under 45 years old.

> There is an absence of hypertension.

> There is lobar haemorrhage, unless the patient is over 65 years old as cerebral amyloid angiopathy (CAA) would then be a more likely aetiology.

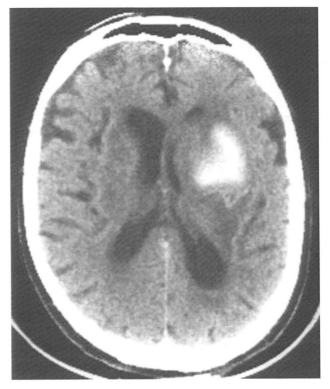

Fig 44 Putaminal haemorrhage on CT scan.

Key point

Consider cerebral amyloid angiopathy (CAA)

> It is a common cause of ICH in older people; it is sporadic, but there are a few autosomal dominant families.

> If there is subcortical, often multiple, haemorrhage, particularly in the occipital and parietal lobes.

> Pathological changes are found in 10% of septuagenarians and in 60% of those aged over 90.

> If there is any association between a CAA and an Alzheimer-type pathology.

> Of those with CAA, 10–30% will have progressive dementia.

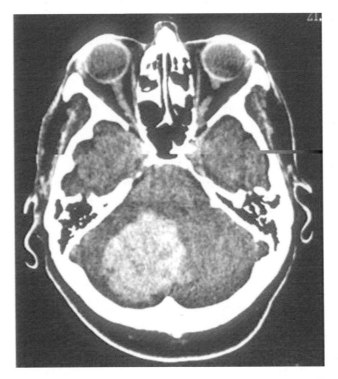

Fig 45 Cerebellar hemisphere haemorrhage on CT scan. (Courtesy of Professor M. Brown, Institute of Neurology, University of London.)

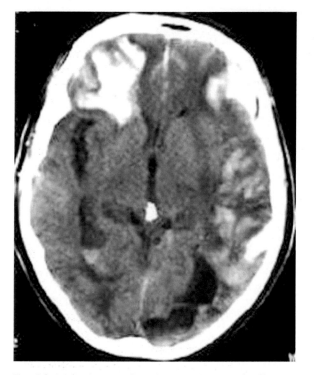

Fig 46 Multiple superficial haemorrhages of different ages seen on a CT head scan. This patient was presumed to have cerebral amyloid angiopathy (CAA). (Courtesy of Professor M. Brown, Institute of Neurology, University of London.)

Differential diagnosis

See Section 2.8.1.

Treatment

Medical management

See Table 52.

Surgical

Trials have not shown benefit for surgical intervention in ICH. However, selected patients may benefit from surgery.

Surgery is indicated in:

> Patients with a cerebellar haemorrhage over 3 cm, because of the risk of hydrocephalus and brainstem compression. Remember, these patients may deteriorate slowly. Do not wait for brainstem signs to occur as it will be too late to reverse any deficit.

> Young patients who were initially stable but subsequently deteriorate and may benefit from surgery, especially if there is superficial lobar haemorrhage.

Table 52	Principles of medical management of patients with intracerebral haemorrhage (ICH)
Priorities	**Action**
Immediate priorities (first few hours)	Protect and maintain airway
	Prevent hypoxia – give oxygen if saturation is <95% on pulse oximetry
	Regular monitoring and neurological observations – review if condition deteriorates
	Nursing – bed rest, elevate head of bed by 30° and protect pressure areas
Later priorities (first few days)	Maintain hydration – intravenous fluids if the patient cannot drink safely
	Consider nutrition – nasogastric (later via percutaneous endoscopic gastrostomy tube) if the patient cannot swallow safely
Other aspects	Hypertension – treat if blood pressure high and aim for systolic blood pressure <140 mmHg and diastolic pressure <80 mmHg within 1 hour of presentation
	Agitation – give the minimum sedation possible (often a difficult judgement)
	Pain – use paracetamol or codeine
	Bowels – use stool softeners etc to prevent straining

Surgery is not indicated if:

> The patient's Glasgow Coma Scale score is 4 or less (unless cerebellar) (see Section 1.5.5).

> There is only a small lesion or minimal deficit.

For other types of ICH, surgery is less likely to result in a beneficial outcome.

Complications

> Death.

> Hydrocephalus.

> Disability.

Prognosis

> 35–50% of patients will die by 1 month.

> 10% are independent at 1 month, 20% by 6 months.

2.8.4 Subarachnoid haemorrhage

Aetiology

Ruptured saccular (berry) aneurysms are the cause of 80% of non-traumatic subarachnoid haemorrhages (SAHs). These are usually found at bifurcations and branchings of the arteries of the circle of Willis or its major branches. The reason why some aneurysms rupture and others do not is not known, but the risk is greater for larger aneurysms than for smaller.

Epidemiology

The incidence of SAH is 8–12 per 100,000 people per year and is the diagnosis in 1–4% of patients presenting to emergency departments with headache. Risk factors include hypertension, cigarette smoking, heavy alcohol consumption (particularly binge drinking), adult polycystic kidney disease and some connective tissue disorders.

Clinical presentation

SAH can present with relatively minor symptoms, devastating neurological dysfunction or be a cause of sudden death.

The typical presentation is with the sudden onset of a severe headache: 'the worst headache I've ever had'; or 'like being hit on the back of the head with a hammer'. This usually occurs when the patient is active, rather than asleep, and often during exertion. There is frequently a transient loss of consciousness and also vomiting.

Between 20% and 50% of patients with documented SAH report a distinct and unusually severe 'warning headache' in the days or weeks prior to the episode of bleeding.

Physical signs

Many patients will have some or all of the following features:

> Impaired conscious level – their Glasgow Coma Scale (GCS) score can vary from 3 (minimum) to 15 (maximum).

> Focal neurological signs – in particular third nerve palsy (posterior communicating artery aneurysm), sixth nerve palsy (posterior fossa aneurysm, but also a false localising sign with raised intracranial pressure), bilateral leg weakness (anterior communicating aneurysm), nystagmus or ataxia (posterior fossa aneurysm) and aphasia, hemiparesis hemianopia (middle cerebral artery aneurysm).

> Neck rigidity.

> Retinal haemorrhages, which are thought to result from an acute increase in intracranial pressure that causes obstruction to the venous outflow from the eye.

Patients may be hypertensive, have cardiac dysrhythmias and have electrocardiogram (ECG) patterns mimicking myocardial infarction – all of which can lead to diagnostic confusion. Those whose SAH has led to syncope may have sustained a head injury, which can also make diagnosis difficult.

Investigation

Immediate

The investigation of choice in suspected SAH is an immediate CT scan without contrast, taking very thin cuts through the base of the brain to optimise the chances of seeing small collections of blood (see Fig 24). The sensitivity of modern scanners for detecting SAH is very high: 98–100% if scanning is performed within 12 hours of onset of symptoms, and 93% within the first 24 hours.

Lumbar puncture should be performed in suspected cases of SAH if the CT scan is negative, equivocal or technically unsatisfactory. 'Traumatic taps' occur in up to 20% of procedures and need to be distinguished from true haemorrhages: the 'three tube' method, which looks for decreasing numbers of erythrocytes in successively collected specimens, is not entirely reliable. The diagnosis of SAH is established by centrifuging the cerebrospinal fluid (CSF) specimen without delay and demonstrating the presence of xanthochromia (due to the presence of oxyhaemoglobin and bilirubin) by spectrophotometry (Fig 47). Note, however, that xanthochromia may not be present if the CSF is examined within 12 hours of haemorrhage occurring. Hence in the face of a normal CT scan, lumbar puncture should be delayed until 24 hours after the ictus.

Subsequent

In cases of proven SAH where intervention (radiological or surgical) is contemplated (see Treatment section), imaging of the cerebral vessels by four-vessel angiography is required.

Differential diagnosis

Many studies have shown that about 30% of patients with SAH are misdiagnosed at presentation. The differential diagnosis includes: infective causes of headache (meningitis, encephalitis and viral infection such as

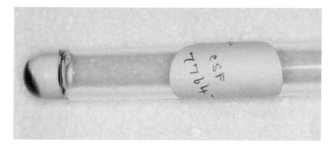

Fig 47 Test tube of blood-stained cerebrospinal fluid (CSF) after being spun down in a centrifuge to reveal xanthochromic supernatant in a case of subarachnoid haemorrhage (SAH).

influenza), other causes of headache (migraine, cluster or tension headache, and sinus-related headache), neck pain and psychiatric disorder.

Complications

The patient may present with neurological deficit, recover, but then develop hemiplegia or other focal signs 4–10 days after rupture because of delayed cerebral ischaemia.

The most feared immediate complication from aneurysmal SAH is rebleed from the symptomatic aneurysm. The risk of rebleed is between 4% and 15% within 24 hours of SAH and the case fatality can be up to 70%.

Treatment

Following the diagnosis of SAH, the patient should ideally be transferred to a tertiary neurovascular centre for further evaluation. Treatment options are considered after the diagnosis of an aneurysmal SAH is confirmed by angiography (computerised tomography angiogram and/or digital subtraction angiogram).

Medical management
General measures

In addition to appropriate management of airway, breathing and circulation, these include:

> Bed rest and monitoring for hypertension: high blood pressure does not need treatment unless there are signs of end-organ damage.

> Careful monitoring of fluid balance, aiming for euvolaemia with input and output charts.

> Analgesia (eg paracetamol, codeine or Oramorph) for headache.

> Deep vein thrombosis prophylaxis with anti-embolism stocking and/or sequential compression devices.

Specific measures

Prevention of vascular spasm – Nimodipine is used for the prevention and treatment of ischaemic neurological deficit due to vascular spasm after SAH; for prevention at a dose of 60 mg PO every 4 hours, and for treatment by intravenous infusion at a rate of 0.5–2 mg/hour. Once volume resuscitation (when necessary) has been completed, preventative treatment should be given to all patients with SAH who are not hypotensive. Intravenous nimodipine should only be administered in the setting of a neurological intensive care unit because hypotension is a common and serious problem.

Radiological (endovascular) or surgical intervention

The two methods of interventional treatment of ruptured aneurysmal SAH are endovascular intervention (coiling alone, or coiling and stenting) and surgical clipping of the ruptured aneurysm. Treatment should be offered as early as possible to avoid risk of rebleed. The randomised International Subarachnoid Aneurysmal Trial (ISAT)

showed coiling of ruptured aneurysms to be safer than clipping, and patients had a better functional outcome. The combined risk of mortality and morbidity was greater in the surgical than the coiling group (30.9% versus 23.5%).

Best practice is for patients with aneurysmal SAH to be discussed in a neurovascular multidisciplinary team meeting and a decision made whether to treat the aneurysm endovascularly or surgically. This decision is influenced by many factors, including local expertise. For younger patients, wide neck aneurysms and space-occupying intracerebral bleeds, surgical clipping is preferred over coiling. In patients with significant medical comorbidities, aneurysms with small necks and posterior circulation aneurysms, endovascular coiling is preferred. For aneurysms with wide necks, stent-assisted coiling should be considered. Age alone is not a contraindication to treatment.

Other issues

Patients should be treated for general vascular risk factors (hypertension, hypercholesterolaemia, diabetes, and they should stop smoking) and they must inform the Driver and Vehicle Licensing Agency (DVLA) regarding driving (if they make a full recovery their licence is usually returned after 3 months). There are no long-term lifestyle restrictions, except that they should not smoke.

Prognosis

With modern medical and surgical management, a poor outcome (death or severe disability) occurs in 20% of patients with SAH admitted to hospital. However, many of the worst affected do not ever reach hospital, meaning that the true mortality from SAH is nearer 50%. A good clinical outcome is expected in 90–95% of those admitted in good clinical condition (a GCS score of 14 or 15).

Prevention

Incidental aneurysms occur in up to 1% of the population. Any such patient should be referred for specialist advice, but most (aneurysms <7 mm in diameter) do not require treatment.

2.9 Brain tumours

Pathology

Brain tumours can arise within the brain parenchyma or adjoining structures (eg meninges), or invade by direct or haematological metastatic spread. Tumours can be benign or malignant, malignancy implying rapid growth, poor differentiation, high mitotic rate, necrosis and vascular proliferation. Metastasis to extracranial sites is rare. A benign tumour may be as devastating as a highly malignant tumour by virtue of its position, its ability to infiltrate locally or its propensity to transform to malignancy. The classification of brain tumours is shown in Table 53, and their age distribution in Table 54.

Epidemiology

Benign and malignant primary brain tumours are uncommon. Overall, the incidence is about 6–14 per 100,000 people annually. Malignant tumours of the brain are a rare occurrence accounting for approximately 2% of all cancers in adults. Approximately 4,400 people are newly diagnosed with a brain tumour each year in the UK compared with over 40,000 women with breast cancer and approximately 25,000 men with prostate cancer. The most common brain tumours in adults are benign meningioma and glioblastoma multiforme. Generally, the tumours that tend to occur in adults become more common with increasing age. Secondary ('metastatic') brain tumours are more common than primary brain tumours and are more likely to occur than primary tumours in older people.

Table 53 Classification of brain tumours

Type	Site	Diagnosis
Primary	Intraparenchymal	Gliomas
		Astrocytoma, many types
		Glioblastoma multiforme
		Oligodendroglioma
		Mixed glioma, eg oligoastrocytoma
		Ependymal tumours
		Neuronal tumours, eg gangliocytomas
		Primitive neuroectodermal tumours, eg medulloblastoma
	Extraparenchymal (extrinsic/extra axial)	Meninges: meningioma
		Cranial nerve sheath: schwannomas/neuromas
		Pituitary gland: microadenomas and macroadenomas
		Bone: osteomas
		Blood vessel: haemangioblastomas
Secondary	Direct extension	Nasopharyngeal
		Chordoma
		Glomus jugulare tumours
	Metastasis	
	Haematological	Primary central nervous system (CNS) lymphoma

Table 54 Age distribution of brain tumours by site

Location	Adult	Childhood
Supratentorial	(70% of adult brain tumours)	Craniopharyngioma
	Glioma	Pinealoma
	Meningioma	Gliomas (mainly astrocytomas of optic nerve and thalamus)
	Pituitary	
	Metastasis (commonest)	
Infratentorial	(Mainly cerebellar, and occurrence in the brainstem is rare)	Medulloblastoma (infancy)
	Metastasis	Cerebellar astrocytoma
	Acoustic neuroma	Ependymoma of fourth ventricle
	Cerebellar haemangioblastoma	

Clinical presentation

The nature of the clinical presentation will reflect the site of the tumour (Figs 48 and 49) and its rate of expansion.

General symptoms

Rapidly expanding tumours or those blocking the flow of cerebrospinal fluid and causing obstructive hydrocephalus will present with symptoms (postural headache, nausea and vomiting, and diplopia) and signs (papilloedema and sixth nerve palsy) of raised intracranial pressure. Headaches tend to be worse in the morning and coughing, sneezing and stooping may make the headaches worse. Seizures (partial or generalised) sometimes occur and are one of the most common presenting symptoms in patients with meningiomas. Impairment of consciousness may occur as the tumour enlarges. A stroke-like presentation with sudden onset symptoms usually reflects bleeding into a tumour.

Symptoms due to the location in the brain

As a tumour grows it can damage the nearby brain tissue. This may lead to:

> limb numbness or weakness

> cerebellar signs

> visual field defects (eg bitemporal hemianopia in pituitary tumours)

> hearing defects (acoustic neuromas)

> dysphasia

> dysphagia

> anosmia

> personality changes

> symptoms of hormone imbalance (pituitary tumours).

Common presentations are shown in Table 55. Rarely, patients may present with paraneoplastic syndromes (see Section 2.11.1).

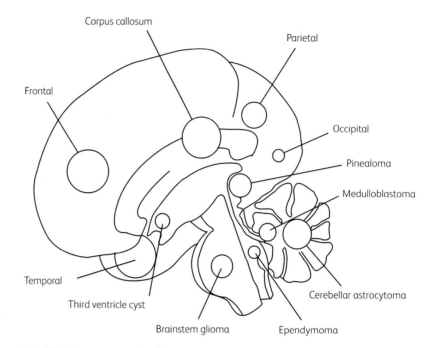

Fig 48 Main intracerebral tumour sites.

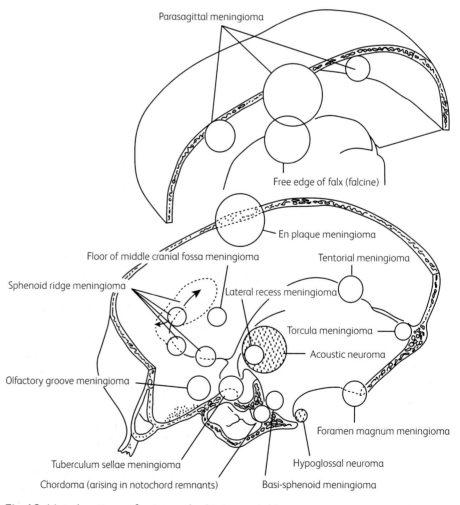

Fig 49 Main locations of extracerebral intracranial tumours.

Table 55	Brain tumours: common presentations
Site	**Common symptoms and signs**
Frontal	Personality change
	Contralateral motor signs
	Dysphasia (dominant hemisphere)
	(Note: Foster Kennedy syndrome – ipsilateral optic atrophy and contralateral papilloedema)
Parietal	Contralateral sensory change/cortical sensory loss
	Visual field defect (optic radiation)
	Neglect
	Apraxias
	(Note: Gerstmann's syndrome – agraphia, left/right disorientation, acalculia and finger agnosia)
Occipital	Homonymous hemianopia with or without macular sparing
Temporal	Memory and behavioural disturbance
Parasagittal	Gait abnormality (small steps)
	Spastic paraparesis (consider in the differential diagnosis of spinal cord compression)
Posterior fossa	Raised intracranial pressure
	Ataxia and nystagmus
	Cranial nerve lesions
Pituitary	Bitemporal hemianopia (pressure on optic chiasm)
	Endocrine disturbance
	Cranial nerve III, IV, Va, Vb and VI (lateral extension to cavernous sinus)
	(Note: pituitary apoplexy – sudden blindness and subarachnoid haemorrhage)

Investigation

The most important investigation is the CT or MRI scan. CT is particularly good if there is a stroke-like presentation in order to rule out haemorrhage. If a tumour is suspected it is important that contrast is used as some tumours may be isodense to brain tissue and therefore do not show up without it. An MRI is preferable for:

> posterior fossa tumours

> detecting multiple lesions, which are more suggestive of metastases.

The high incidence of metastases compared with primary brain tumours makes a chest X-ray and blood tests (FBC, erythrocyte sedimentation rate, urea and electrolytes, liver function tests, calcium and phosphates) essential. Further investigation of a patient with cerebral metastases will be guided by clinical symptoms and signs, eg anaemia may lead to oesophagogastroduodenoscopy and colonoscopy in search of a gastrointestinal malignancy.

Pituitary function tests are performed if a mass is seen in the pituitary fossa on a CT or MRI scan.

Lumbar puncture is unlikely to be safe and has a low positive yield.

Cerebral biopsy should be performed in most patients to exclude potentially treatable causes and also to classify and grade the tumour. Four malignancy grades are recognised by the World Health Organization system, with grade I tumours the biologically least aggressive and grade IV the biologically most aggressive tumours. The histological criteria for malignancy grading are not uniform for all tumour types and thus all tumours must be classified before the malignancy grade can be determined.

Differential diagnosis

The important conditions to consider in the differential diagnosis of a space-occupying lesion are as follows:

> Vascular causes such as haematoma with mass effect, giant aneurysm, arteriovenous malformation, cerebral infarct with oedema and venous thrombosis.

> Trauma resulting in haematoma/contusion.

> Infection of the central nervous system (CNS) including abscess, tuberculosis, herpes simplex encephalitis and hydatid cysts.

> Many inflammatory conditions that may cause focal signs, particularly multiple sclerosis and neurosarcoidosis.

Treatment

In some cases, treatment aims for a cure. If a benign tumour can be removed by surgery then a cure is likely. In other cases a cure is unrealistic and treatment aims to control the progression of the tumour by reducing the bulk or by limiting the growth or spread of the tumour so that it progresses less rapidly. The main treatments used for brain tumours are surgery, chemotherapy, radiotherapy and medication to control the symptoms. The treatment or combination of treatments used in each case depends on the following factors:

> the type of tumour (benign or malignant)
> the grade of the tumour if it is malignant
> the exact site of the tumour
> the patient's general health.

Symptomatic treatment
Consider steroids in the acute setting for the symptomatic treatment of oedema: dexamethasone 12 mg intravenously, followed by 4 mg qds orally or intravenously for no more than a week (it loses efficacy after this). The patient may require anticonvulsant medication for seizures (phenytoin or sodium valproate are the most often used). Analgesia is a very important part of symptomatic treatment and strong analgesics such as morphine may be required. Nausea and vomiting can be controlled with antiemetics such as cyclizine and prochlorperazine.

Surgery
Surgery is usually the main treatment option for benign tumours. Aggressive surgical resection for malignant lesions is impossible because the lesions are widely invasive beyond the macroscopic margins, and large-volume resections are associated with unacceptable morbidity. Surgery may be attempted if the lesion is situated in the frontal lobe or occipital pole.

Radiotherapy
Radiotherapy is not curative, but some tumours are sensitive. In the treatment of malignant cerebral glioma, radiotherapy offers a survival benefit of approximately 6 months. Radiotherapy is sometimes used instead of surgery

when an operation is not possible for a malignant brain tumour. It may be used as an adjunct to surgery if it is not possible to remove all the tumour with surgery, or to kill cancerous cells that may be left behind following surgery.

Chemotherapy
The benefits of chemotherapy in the treatment of primary malignant brain tumours are not clear but it is sometimes used as an adjunctive treatment to surgery and radiotherapy depending on various factors such as the type of tumour.

Prognosis
The length of survival following diagnosis of a brain tumour is dependent on the age of the patient, the histologic subtype and grade of the tumour, and the presenting symptoms. Survival chances have improved gradually but remain poor. Age-standardised net survival for patients diagnosed with malignant brain tumours during 2010–2011 in England and Wales show that only 41% of men survive for at least 1 year, falling to 18% for 5 years or more; 39% of women survive for 1 year or more, and 20% are predicted to survive for at least 5 years. A patient with a grade I–II glioma may survive for years, whereas a patient with a grade IV tumour will survive for a maximum of a few months if treated with surgery alone. The prognosis for metastatic disease is poor.

Disease associations
Neurocutaneous syndromes
The vast majority of brain tumours are sporadic. However, there are a number of familial syndromes that are well documented as being associated with an increased incidence of brain tumours. Even in the most common of these (neurofibromatosis type 1 and

neurofibromatosis type 2), the precise relative risk is difficult to define. The prevalence of neurocutaneous syndromes is higher in the medical examination (such as PACES) setting than in real life. Beware the patient with skin lesions and neurological signs! Table 56 summarises these syndromes.

2.10 Neurological complications of infection

2.10.1 Variant Creutzfeldt–Jakob disease

Aetiology

Variant Creutzfeldt–Jakob disease (vCJD) (formerly 'new variant CJD'), first described in 1996, is believed to be the human equivalent of bovine spongiform encephalopathy (BSE) or 'mad cow disease'. Although numerically a rare condition, it has major public health implications and a high media profile. Unlike the more common (yet still very rare) sporadic CJD, vCJD typically affects younger individuals. As for sporadic CJD, there is no curative treatment, all cases are progressive and fatal, and the mainstay of management is palliation.

Key point

> Glycosylation patterns of the disease-associated prion protein (PrP) in vCJD resembles that in BSE-infected cattle, but is not seen in sporadic CJD.

> In mice, the characteristics of the agents responsible for vCJD and BSE were identical, but different from those in sporadic CJD.

Table 56 Brain tumours as part of neurocutaneous disorders

Syndrome	Genetics	Features
Von Hippel–Lindau disease	Autosomal dominant, 3p26–25	Brain: haemangioblastoma (cerebellar, less common in cerebral hemispheres and brainstem)
		Eyes: retinal angioma Skin: hamartomas Visceral organs: tumours and cysts Phaeochromocytoma
Neurofibromatosis 1	Autosomal dominant, 17q11.2	CNS: optic and chiasmatic nerve glioma, neurofibroma and plexiform neurofibroma Eyes: Lisch nodules Skin: café-au-lait spots (numerous) and axillary and/or inguinal freckles
Neurofibromatosis 2	Autosomal dominant, 22q11–13.1	Brain: bilateral acoustic neuromas. Less commonly, meningioma, glioma and other neuromas. Schwannomas compress in cranial or spinal roots in their foramina Eye: presenile cataracts Skin: cutaneous neurofibroma and café-au-lait spots (less numerous)
Tuberous sclerosis	Autosomal dominant, 9q34.134.2 (some families)	Brain: cortical tubers, subependymal nodules and astrocytoma Eye: hamartomas Skin: shagreen plaques, ungual fibroma and facial angiofibromata (adenoma sebaceum) Other: widespread hamartomatosis

CNS, central nervous system.

Of the approximately 250 cases seen worldwide, the majority (>75%) have been diagnosed in the UK. All the initial cases were in individuals who had the prion protein gene (*PRNP*) codon 129 methionine homozygous (MM) genotype. The size of the potential public health impact of vCJD has been difficult to predict. The possibility of transmission to patients with the PRNP codon 129 methionine-valine heterozygous (MV) and valine homozygous (VV) genotype with longer incubation periods than seen in MM individuals remains (all possible genotypes are susceptible in animal models), as does transmission via contaminated blood transfusions. Continued surveillance will be necessary.

Clinical presentation

In vCJD, the mean age of onset is 29 years and the mean disease duration is 14 months, compared with the 60 years and 5 months, respectively, in sporadic CJD.

Psychiatric symptoms are often prominent, more so than in sporadic CJD. Sensory symptoms, often in the form of hyperpathia, are frequent.

Cerebellar signs are prominent early in the course of the disease. Up-gaze paresis, which is uncommon in sporadic CJD, often occurs in vCJD. Pyramidal signs, primitive reflexes (such as grasp and pout reflexes) and myoclonus may also be seen, although the latter is less prominent than in sporadic CJD.

Hazard

Psychiatric or sensory symptoms are prominent early features in vCJD compared with rapidly progressive dementia in sporadic CJD.

Investigation

The following may be helpful:

> An MRI brain scan often demonstrates the characteristic 'pulvinar sign' of high signal in the posterior thalamic pulvinar, sometimes likened in shape to a hockey stick.

> Cerebrospinal fluid may show elevated levels of the neuronal protein 14.3.3. This protein is a marker of acute neuronal damage, so elevated values are non-specific.

> Unlike sporadic CJD, electroencephalography does not show evolving periodic sharp wave complexes, but slow wave activity may be seen.

> Ultimately vCJD diagnosis requires pathological confirmation, usually post-mortem. Because of the proposed lymphoreticular spread of prions, tonsil biopsy undertaken in specialist centres may be used to establish ante-mortem diagnosis.

2.11 Neurological complications of systemic disease

2.11.1 Paraneoplastic conditions
Introduction

Key point

> Paraneoplastic syndromes can occur up to several years prior to detection of the underlying tumour. In some cases, the tumour is not identified until autopsy.

> The tumour is usually small, suggesting that it is being held at bay by the immune response.

> An immune response is directed against a tumour antigen is also expressed on neural tissue (onconeural antigen). Paraneoplastic disorders are therefore autoimmune in nature.

> The pathogenesis of certain paraneoplastic conditions is antibody mediated (Lambert–Eaton myasthenic syndrome, LEMS) whereas in others it may be cytokine- or T-cell-mediated.

> Identification of a particular associated antineuronal antibody will direct the hunt for the underlying tumour.

> None of the paraneoplastic syndromes is invariably associated with malignancy.

Non-neurological malignancies can affect the nervous system in many ways. This can be by infiltration or compression, either by direct spread of the primary tumour or by haematogenous metastatic spread. However, a wide range of non-metastatic remote complications are also described. Many of these can be attributed to cachexia, to competition between a tumour and body tissues for substances such as glucose and tryptophan, or to the adverse effects of chemotherapy such as vincristine and cisplatin. Others appear to have an immunological basis. It is this latter group that will be discussed as paraneoplastic conditions.

Clinical presentation

Numerous neurological paraneoplastic syndromes are described. Given the broad range of symptoms, what is it that makes the clinician consider a diagnosis of paraneoplastic syndrome?

> Conditions that progress rapidly over weeks to months before reaching a plateau.

> Patients are usually significantly disabled at the time of presentation, and mild waxing and waning symptoms are unlikely to be paraneoplastic in origin.

> Presentations are usually stereotyped as described below.

Paraneoplastic conditions involving the central nervous system

> Paraneoplastic encephalomyelitis (PEM) includes:

  > Limbic encephalitis – symptoms are anxiety, depression, impairment of recent memory and fluctuating confusion. More than 70% are associated with small-cell lung carcinoma (SCLC). This is also described in Hodgkin's disease (HD).

  > Brainstem encephalitis – there are variable brainstem signs and there may be corticospinal tract involvement. Mainly associated with SCLC.

  > Myelitis/anterior horn cell disease – this can mimic motor neurone disease. Any sensory signs are due to associated subacute sensory neuronopathy (SSN). Often associated with brainstem encephalitis.

> Paraneoplastic cerebellar degeneration (PCD) can occur causing ataxia, dysarthria and nystagmus. There may be associated PEM. This is also described with SCLC, gynaecological tumours and HD.

> In cases of paraneoplastic opsoclonus / myoclonus syndrome, 50% of the children affected have neuroblastoma, whereas in adults it is associated with cerebellar and brainstem signs and encephalopathy. Clonazepam may offer relief.

> Necrotising myelopathy mimics transverse myelitis or cord compression.

Paraneoplastic conditions involving the eye
Cancer-associated retinopathy is a triad of photosensitivity, ring scotomatous visual field loss and attenuated calibre of retinal arterioles.

Paraneoplastic conditions involving the neuromuscular junction
This can lead to:

> Stiff person syndrome – stiffness of proximal limbs and trunk. Described with breast cancer and HD. In association with breast cancer, antibodies to amphiphysin have been described.

Key point

Stiff person syndrome is also associated with organ-specific autoimmune diseases and insulin-dependent diabetes mellitus. Of those affected, 60% have antibodies to glutamic acid decarboxylase.

> LEMS – weakness of proximal muscles, mainly in the legs, and autonomic dysfunction. There is also post-tetanic stimulation of deep tendon reflexes and antibodies to the presynaptic voltage-gated calcium channel. Usually in association with SCLC.

> Myasthenia gravis – muscle fatigability, ptosis and ophthalmoplegia. Associated with anti-acetylcholine receptor (AChR) and thymoma.

Paraneoplastic conditions involving the nerve

This leads to:

> Subacute sensory neuronopathy – rapid progressive loss of all sensory modalities, especially proprioception, may result in pseudoathetosis. This may be associated with myelitis, but is usually in association with SCLC. The differential diagnosis of this striking neuropathy includes Sjögren's syndrome.

> Motor neuronopathy – affects legs more than arms, often in a patchy distribution, but spares bulbar musculature. Associated with HD and other lymphomas.

> Paraneoplastic vasculitic neuropathy – a mononeuritis multiplex associated with SCLC, endometrial cancer and others.

> Chronic gastrointestinal pseudo-obstruction (CGP) – involves the myenteric plexus causing subacute progressive nausea, vomiting, constipation, abdominal distention and pain. Associated with SCLC and thymoma.

> Brachial neuritis – asymmetric pain, weakness and wasting in the muscles of the shoulder girdle is usually idiopathic, but can occasionally be associated with malignancy.

> Autonomic neuropathy – may rarely be paraneoplastic.

Paraneoplastic conditions involving muscle

This includes:

> Dermatomyositis – associated with cancer in 10% of cases.

> Necrotising myopathy – necrosis without inflammation; this is rare.

Investigations

Cerebrospinal fluid (CSF) analysis may show an increased level of protein and a mild pleocytosis. Associated anti-neuronal antibodies may be identified in both serum and CSF, but this is an emerging field. Table 57 summarises our knowledge of onconeural antigens to date.

Treatment

This is a difficult issue. There is limited evidence that a complete cure of the malignancy driving the immune response leads to either partial or complete resolution of the paraneoplastic condition. Immune therapies such as corticosteroids, plasma exchange and intravenous immunoglobulin may improve the neurological symptoms and does not appear to prejudice the oncological outcome.

Table 57 Onconeural antigens

Antibody	Antigen	Associated cancer	Syndrome
Anti-Hu	All neuronal nuclei	SCLC	PEM, SSN, CGP, LEMS opsoclonus
Anti-Yo	Purkinje cell cytoplasm	Gynaecological, breast	PCD, opsoclonus
Anti-Ri	Neuronal nuclei	Breast, SCLC, non-SCLC	PCD, opsoclonus
Anti-amphiphysin	Synaptic vesicles	Breast and SCLC	PEM, stiff person syndrome
Anti-VGCC	Presynaptic VGCC	SCLC	LEMS, PCD
Anti-AChR	AChR	Thymoma	Myasthenia gravis
Anti-Tr	Neuronal cytoplasm, Purkinje cells and spiny dendrites	HD	PEM, PCD
Anti-Ma2	Testis-specific proteins	Testicular cancer, non-SCLC	PEM, PCD
Anti-CV2/CRMP5	Cytoplasm of oligodendrocytes	SCLC, thymoma	PEM, PCD, LEMS, CGP, opsoclonus, SSN
Anti-NMDA	NMDA receptor	Gynaecological	PEM, stiff person syndrome
Anti-VGKC	VGKC complex	SCLC, benign adenoma, thymoma, prostate adenocarcinoma	PEM, PCD, LEMS, stiff person syndrome

AChR, acetylcholine receptor; CGP, chronic gastrointestinal pseudo-obstruction; HD, Hodgkin's disease; LEMS, Lambert–Eaton myasthenic syndrome; NMDA, N-methyl-D-aspartate; PCD, paraneoplastic cerebellar degeneration; PEM, paraneoplastic encephalomyelitis; SCLC, small-cell lung carcinoma; SSN, subacute sensory neuronopathy; VGCC, voltage-gated calcium channel, VGKC, voltage-gated potassium channel.

3 Investigations and practical procedures

3.1 Neuropsychological assessment

An organised and thorough ('bedside') cognitive examination performed by the clinician is important in both initial assessment and diagnosis of a patient's condition and in subsequent follow-up. A number of cognitive screening instruments are available which can be administered in around 10–30 minutes. These are not diagnostic tests, and do not substitute for a formal cognitive assessment by a neuropsychologist, but are helpful adjuncts to the clinical evaluation which may indicate the need or otherwise for further investigation.

The most frequently used is the Mini-Mental State Examination (MMSE) (score range 0–30, impaired to normal), but this is heavily weighted towards verbal tasks, and although specific, lacks sensitivity for mild cognitive impairment. Other cognitive screening instruments, in order of increasing duration, include the Six-item Cognitive Impairment Test (6CIT, score range 0–28, normal to impaired, ie negatively scored), the Montreal Cognitive Assessment (MoCA, score range 0–30, impaired to normal) and the Addenbrooke's Cognitive Examination-III (ACE-III, score range 0–100, impaired to normal).

Orientation and attention

Is the patient orientated in place, person and time? Disorientation in person is seldom organic. Poor orientation should prompt examination of attention. This can be done by testing digit span, the immediate recall of a string of digits. The normal forward digit span is five to six digits, and backwards three to four. Patients who perform poorly on digit recall often perform poorly on subsequent tests that require concentration (eg serial subtraction of 7 from 100, reciting the months of the year backwards). These faculties are particularly impaired in acute confusional states.

Language

Listen carefully to the patient's general conversation. See Section 1.2.17 for assessment of language.

Memory

Memory functions may be divided into episodic memory (recollection of events) and semantic memory (working knowledge of the world). Episodic memory impairments may be further classified into anterograde or retrograde, depending on the relation to the onset of a disease.

Episodic memory

Ask the patient to relate his or her life history from early childhood to the present day and have this verified by a relative (retrograde episodic memory). Anterograde episodic memory can be tested by making the patient register new information, such as a name and address or a list of words, and then testing recall a few minutes later after other (distractor) tests. Impairment of anterograde episodic memory is the typical presenting feature of Alzheimer's disease.

Semantic memory

Tested by both naming and describing objects. Difficulty naming (anomia) alone may not necessarily imply semantic impairment.

Frontal lobe dysfunction

This includes executive function, our ability to plan and reason.

Verbal fluency

Ask the patient to give as many words (not proper nouns) beginning with a certain letter within 1 minute (letter or phonological fluency). Then ask them to name as many animals as possible, beginning with any letter, within a further minute (category or semantic fluency). Normal individuals will name approximately 20 words and slightly more animals. In frontal lobe dysfunction, there is generally a greater decrease in letter fluency than category fluency; this pattern of impairment is reversed in Alzheimer's disease.

Concrete thinking
Cognitive estimates

Ask the patient to estimate/guess the answers to the following questions:

> How high is the Post Office (British Telecom) tower?

> How far is it from London to New York?

> How tall is the average man?

> How long is the average woman's spine?

> How many camels are there in the Netherlands?

Patients' answers may be both fixed and wildly inaccurate.

Proverbs

Enquire as to the meaning of 'People in glass houses should not throw stones'. The patient may interpret such proverbs literally.

Visuoperceptual/visuospatial

Test the following:

> dot counting

> line bisection

> copying of geometric figures, eg intersecting pentagons, Necker cube

> draw a clock face, put in all the numbers, and set the hands at ten-to-two.

Look for signs of neglect. Impairment in the ability to perform these tasks usually reflects non-dominant parietal lobe dysfunction. Obviously the latter three tests also have a motor component.

Cortical and subcortical dementias

Dementias may be divided into those in which the pathology is predominantly subcortical or cortical. Good examples of subcortical dementia are progressive supranuclear palsy and Huntington's disease. Typically patients are lethargic and withdrawn with slow thought processing. Memory impairment reflects frontal dysfunction, with recollection aided by cues. Cortical dementia, as seen in Alzheimer's disease, is more rapid and the amnesia more severe. Aphasia, apraxia and agnosia may also be present. The lack of motivation and attention that characterise subcortical dementias are not usually seen. As neurodegenerative diseases progress there is often an overlap of symptoms between cortical and subcortical dementias.

3.2 Lumbar puncture

Principle

Analysis of the cerebrospinal fluid (CSF) can yield valuable diagnostic information in a wide range of clinical circumstances.

Indications

Suspected infection

> Meningitis – bacterial, viral, fungal.

> Encephalitis – eg herpes simplex.

Suspected bleeding

> Subarachnoid haemorrhage.

Suspected neoplasia

> Particularly malignant meningitis (diffuse meningeal infiltration) – at least 10 mL of fresh CSF should be sent for cytological evaluation. Liaise with laboratory before lumbar puncture as formalin fixative may need to be added to CSF sample on the ward before transport to maximise detection of malignant cells. Repeat sampling (two to three times) may be necessary.

Suspected inflammatory conditions

> Central nervous system – multiple sclerosis, acute demyelinating encephalomyelitis (ADEM), neurosarcoidosis.

> Peripheral nervous system – Guillain–Barré syndrome, chronic inflammatory demyelinating polyneuropathy (CIDP).

Other indications

> Idiopathic intracranial hypertension.

> Rapidly progressive dementia.

Contraindications

> Symptoms or signs of raised intracranial pressure (eg papilloedema) without brain imaging.

> Presence of focal neurological signs (eg hemiparesis, aphasia) without brain imaging.

> Local infection (skin, bone, pustular acne).

> Thrombocytopenia or a clotting disorder (eg therapeutic anticoagulation).

Practical details

Performed properly, lumbar puncture should not be a painful or terrifying experience. As in all invasive procedures, careful explanation before and during the procedure helps to allay patient anxieties.

Correct positioning of the patient is crucial to success; without it failure is more likely. Lumbar puncture is routinely performed with the patient lying on the left side (for a right-handed operator), knees drawn up to the chest, uppermost shoulder vertically over the other (Fig 50). Alternatively, the patients may sit on the bed leaning forward onto a chair or table; this position is often easier in obese subjects.

Ensure all equipment (eg manometer, sample bottles) and an assistant are to hand before commencing. Under strict aseptic conditions, a small amount of local anaesthetic is injected into the skin, and massaged with finger or thumb in order to disperse the 'bleb'. This enables you to remain confident about the 'feel' of the anatomical landmarks, which is crucial to success. Ensure adequate time is allowed for the local anaesthetic to work.

A vertical line from the anterior superior iliac spine crosses the spinal column at the desired L3/4 space. The needle should be angled slightly headwards, aiming in the direction of the navel (Fig 51).

If anatomical landmarks cannot be discerned (eg scoliosis, extreme obesity), lumbar puncture should be performed under radiological guidance.

CSF pressure reading should be obtained in the lateral position (not sitting) with the patient relaxed. If the patient starts in a sitting position it is possible, after needle insertion into the subarachnoid space, to move the patient carefully into a lying position to enable pressure recording.

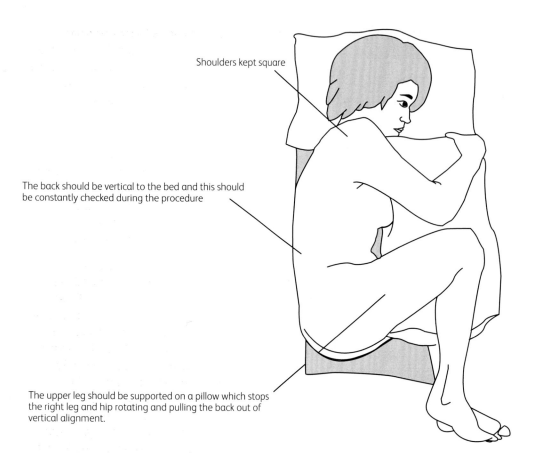

Shoulders kept square

The back should be vertical to the bed and this should be constantly checked during the procedure

The upper leg should be supported on a pillow which stops the right leg and hip rotating and pulling the back out of vertical alignment.

Fig 50 The correct position for lumbar puncture.

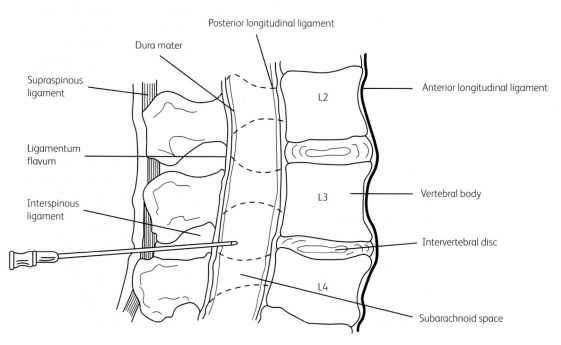

Posterior longitudinal ligament

Dura mater

Supraspinous ligament

Ligamentum flavum

Interspinous ligament

Anterior longitudinal ligament

L2

L3

Vertebral body

Intervertebral disc

L4

Subarachnoid space

Fig 51 Lumbar puncture needle shown *in situ* at L3/4 (often the easiest level). The needle is angled slightly headwards. If inserted at 90°, it tends to hit the upper surface of the arch of L4, producing a very characteristic grating sensation and an appropriate response from the patient.

Medical Masterclass Third edition

Post-procedure, the patient needs to rest for no more than 30 minutes. Enforced bed rest has not been shown to reduce the incidence of post-lumbar puncture headache (see below).

Hazard

A common mistake is to insert the needle too low. Remember that the L3/4 space is located between the iliac crests (Fig 51). Remember also that the spinal cord ends at approximately L1, so it is quite difficult to go too high.

Normal findings

> Opening pressure: 80–200 mm of water (CSF).

> Lymphocytes or mononuclear cells: no more than 5/μL.

> No red blood cells.

> Total protein 0.15–0.5 g/L.

> Glucose 60–80% of blood glucose concentration.

> No xanthochromia (see Section 2.8.4).

A 'bloody tap' is not uncommon – if the patient has a normal blood count, then the ratio of white cells to red cells is approximately 1:1,000. Hence, if the red cell count is 10,000/μL, the expected white cell count in the CSF sample will be 10/μL.

Complications
Post-lumbar puncture headache
This occurs in about 10% of procedures. It is not related to CSF volume taken but to continuous CSF leak from the hole made in the dura. Incidence is

therefore related to the size of the hole, and predictors include:

> gauge of the needle; atraumatic needles reduce risk

> angle the bevel is inserted (horizontal insertion parts the dural fibres whereas vertical insertion slices through them)

> number of attempts.

The headache is of typical low-pressure type: worse on standing and ameliorated by lying down. Patients should be reassured. Symptoms normally resolve in a matter of days with bed rest, adequate fluid intake (occasionally intravenous) and simple analgesia.

Cerebral herniation
This rare catastrophic event is largely avoidable with brain imaging to exclude mass lesions prior to undertaking lumbar puncture.

3.3 Neurophysiology

Neurophysiological investigation uses a variety of techniques to aid the diagnosis of disease processes affecting both the central and the peripheral nervous systems.

3.3.1 Electroencephalography
Principle
It is thought that the electroencephalography (EEG) signals reflect extracellular current flow from the summation of excitatory and inhibitory postsynaptic potentials.

Normal findings
The waking EEG pattern consists of mainly alpha (8–12 Hz) and beta (>12 Hz) activity, with minimal gamma (4–7 Hz) activity.

In sleep, there is increasing delta (1–3 Hz) activity as the depth of sleep becomes greater. In drowsiness, there is disappearance of alpha activity with increased beta and gamma activities.

Indications
To evaluate suspected epilepsy and altered consciousness (eg brain death), and to detect structural lesions (eg tumour) and certain diseases (eg herpes simplex encephalitis or Creutzfeldt–Jakob disease, CJD).

In epilepsy, the EEG is used to distinguish partial from generalised seizures, localise the epileptic focus in partial seizures and characterise epilepsy syndromes, eg 3-Hz spike-and-wave activity in absence attacks. Prolonged EEG monitoring or video telemetry improves diagnostic accuracy in epilepsy. The EEG is not useful in aiding the diagnosis of a patient presenting with 'funny turns'. Minor asymmetries should not be considered pathological.

The typical sign of a focal cerebral lesion is polymorphic focal activity. In herpes simplex encephalitis, the EEG shows slowing with periodic sharp-wave complexes over the temporal lobe. EEG changes in CJD are discussed in Section 2.10.1.

3.3.2 Evoked potentials
Principle

Evoked potentials measure electrical conduction through the nervous system in response to sensory stimulation.

Visual evoked potentials (VEPs) are elicited by monocular visual stimulation with a chequerboard pattern. Normally, a response is recorded from the visual cortex approximately 100 ms after eye stimulation – the P100 latency.

Brainstem auditory evoked potentials (BAEPs) are elicited by monaural stimulation with repetitive clicks, which generate waves in the eighth cranial nerve and the brainstem. Normally, five waveforms occur (I–V) within 10 ms of the stimulus, representing sequential activation of structures of the auditory pathway.

Somatosensory evoked potentials (SSEPs) are generated by electrical stimulation of a peripheral nerve, with recordings over the spine and scalp to assess central sensory processing. Responses depend on which nerves are stimulated.

Indications
Look for:

> VEPs – abnormal (delayed P100 latency) in optic neuritis in multiple sclerosis (MS), tumours compressing the optic nerve, ischaemic optic neuropathy, toxic amblyopias, glaucoma and Leber's hereditary optic atrophy.

> BAEPs – abnormal (as indicated by the presence, latency and interpeak intervals of waveforms I–V) in the eighth cranial nerve and brainstem lesions (eg MS), acoustic neuromas and brainstem gliomas.

> SSEPs – conduction delay or block arises in any disease affecting the central nervous system sensory pathways, eg MS. Abnormally large SSEPs may be seen in myoclonus of cortical origin.

3.3.3 Electromyography
Principle
An electromyogram (EMG) records electrical activity of motor units from resting and voluntary muscle activity. Relaxed muscle normally shows no spontaneous electrical activity, except in the end-plate area where neuromuscular junctions are found. All voluntary muscle activity is recorded as motor unit potentials. A motor unit potential is the sum of muscle fibre potentials innervated by a single anterior horn cell.

Indications
Look for:

> EMG is commonly used to evaluate anterior horn cell diseases, inflammatory muscle diseases, muscular dystrophies, myotonic disorders, neuromuscular junction disorders, axonal peripheral neuropathies and chronic radiculopathies.

> Single-fibre EMG is mainly used to diagnose myasthenia gravis and other neuromuscular junction transmission disorders by the detection of jitter (see Section 2.2.5).

3.3.4 Nerve conduction studies
Principle
Motor nerve conduction studies (NCS) are done by recording the compound muscle action potential (CMAP) of a muscle to stimulation of its motor nerve (Fig 52).

Sensory NCS are done by recording sensory action potentials in sensory fibres when these fibres are stimulated. Supramaximal stimulation is used. Conduction velocity and amplitude of responses are measured.

F-waves can also be recorded in the muscle after the CMAP. Its latency represents conduction retrogradely up the motor nerve to the anterior horn cell and back to the muscle. Increased latency with normal motor conduction may be seen in radiculopathies (ie proximal disease).

Indications
NCS are used to determine the presence and extent of peripheral nerve damage in entrapment neuropathies; whether the pathological process is axonal or demyelinating; or whether conduction block is present.

Key point
Demyelination slows conduction velocities markedly; axonal loss reduces the amplitude of response although conduction velocity remains relatively normal.
NCS are also used to evaluate neuromuscular junction disorders, eg myasthenia gravis where there is a decremental response to repetitive nerve stimulation.

3.4 Neuroimaging

3.4.1 Computerised tomography and computerised tomography angiography
Principle
Computerised tomography (CT) images are produced by detecting X-rays that have been directed through tissue. The images depend on how much of the original beam has managed to pass through the tissue, known as X-ray attenuation. Contrast agents improve the sensitivity and specificity of CT. Enhancement occurs when the blood–brain barrier is compromised, eg in inflammatory lesions or tumours.

Computerised tomography angiography (CTA) is based on detecting enhancement of arterial vessels after the injection of contrast using fast helical CT scanners.

Indications
Non-contrast CT is used for diagnosing early stroke and in trauma. Non-contrast CT can detect parenchymal haemorrhagic stroke, subdural haematoma, subarachnoid haemorrhage (SAH), epidural haematoma and early cytotoxic changes seen in ischaemic stroke. In the early stages of ischaemic stroke there is loss of grey and white matter differentiation with effacement of

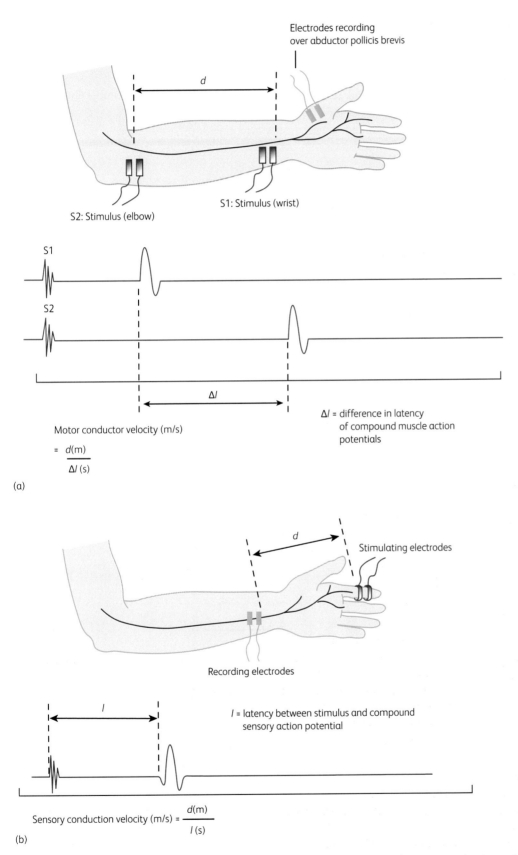

Fig 52 Principles of nerve conduction studies (NCS). **(a)** Measurement of motor conduction velocity in the median nerve. **(b)** Measurement of sensory conduction velocity in the median nerve.

cortical sulci. A CT head scan is preferred as it is readily accessible in most hospitals compared with a magnetic resonance imaging (MRI) scan. A non-contrast CT head scan can detect thrombus within the proximal middle cerebral artery (MCA) (hyperdense MCA sign) and within the basilar artery. It is also used to assess bony pathology, eg bony erosion from tumours, and when MRI is contraindicated. In head trauma, CT is indicated because it detects bony injuries, and traumatic intracerebral or subarachnoid haemorrhage.

CTA uses intravenous contrast to define intra and extracranial arteries. This is used to diagnose arterial stenosis or occlusion, intracranial aneurysms, intracranial vascular malformations such as arteriovenous malformation dural fistula etc and plan treatment where necessary.

Computerised tomography venography uses contrast to study the venous drainage of intracranial structures and is used to diagnose cerebral venous sinus thrombosis, cortical and deep vein thrombosis and stenosis.

Computerised tomography perfusion uses contrast to study cerebral blood flow (CBF), cerebral blood volume (CBV) and the mean transit time (MTT) in stroke patients. This helps to recognise areas of the brain that are infarcted and that are at risk of infarction.

Hazard
If SAH is strongly suspected a lumbar puncture must be performed, even if a CT scan is normal.

CTA may be used in patients who decline catheter angiography and have contraindications for magnetic resonance angiography (MRA) to detect carotid artery stenosis, carotid dissection, arteriovenous malformations and cerebral aneurysms. However, CTA is inferior to angiography or MRA.

Contraindications

Contrast agents are contraindicated in patients with asthma or who are allergic to the contrast itself. Renal failure is a relative contraindication. In pregnancy, the fetus must be shielded from the harmful radiation. Iodine-based contrast may induce thyrotoxic crisis in patients with hyperthyroidism and may cause hypertensive crisis in patients with phaeochromocytoma.

3.4.2 Magnetic resonance imaging and magnetic resonance angiography

Principle

A magnetic resonance image is obtained when a radiofrequency pulse excites the protons in the tissue, producing radio wave emissions. The signal intensity depends on the mobile hydrogen nuclei concentration of tissues. T1 (spin-lattice) and T2 (spin-spin) relaxation time constants depend on the physical properties of the tissue. As in computerised tomography (CT), contrast enhancement is due to disruption of the blood–brain barrier.

Magnetic resonance angiography (MRA) is performed using the time-of-flight (TOF) or phase-contrast (PC) techniques. In TOF MRA vessels are detected because of the inflow of unsaturated spins into the imaging plane. In PC MRA vessels are detected because moving protons within them accumulate phase shifts proportional to their velocity as they cross a magnetic gradient (Fig 53).

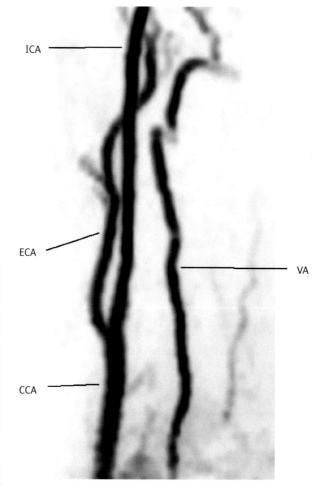

Fig 53 Normal magnetic resonance angiography (MRA) of right-sided carotid and vertebral artery systems. CCA, common carotid artery; ECA, external carotid artery; ICA, internal carotid artery; VA, vertebral artery.

Indications

Magnetic resonance imagining (MRI) is best for soft tissue and vascular abnormalities, and is superior to CT in detecting posterior fossa or spinal cord (eg syrinx and epidural abscess) lesions. Indications for MRI include stroke, tumour, degenerative diseases, multiple sclerosis, vascular lesions (eg aneurysm and vascular malformation), epilepsy, myelopathy and cerebral infections (eg abscess), herpes simplex encephalitis and meningitis.

In stroke, after taking into account the advantages of CT, note that haematomas of more than 2–3 days old are better seen with MRI. MRI can detect vasogenic oedema (subacute phase of stroke) better than cytotoxic oedema (hyperacute and acute phase of stroke).

Diffusion-weighted MRI (DWI) is used to detect early ischaemic stroke and is useful in diagnosing acute stroke (Fig 54) and perfusion-weighted MRI (PWI) detects cerebral tissue that is underperfused in the setting of acute stroke. If the defect in PWI is greater than that seen on DWI it may be that this tissue is under threat from ischaemia, but is not infarcted. Therefore it would survive if perfusion could be reinstated, for example using thrombolytic therapy (see Section 2.8).

On DWI sequence acute ischaemic stroke looks bright and the corresponding apparent diffusion coefficient (ADC) sequence appears dark.

Indications for MRA are similar to CT angiography, but the former provides better quality images. In the investigation of carotid artery stenosis, arterial angiography (which carries a risk of stroke) should not be required if MRA and carotid Dopplers are concurrent.

Axial fat-suppressed T1-weighted imaging is useful in diagnosing cervical artery dissection. This shows an intramural clot within the arterial wall which appears as a high signal also called the crescent sign.

Contraindications

Metallic objects, eg shrapnel in eyes, intracranial clips and pacemakers are contraindications for an MRI.

3.4.3 Angiography

Principle

Angiography (also called digital subtraction angiography) is an invasive procedure and is performed by introducing a catheter via the femoral or brachial artery, up the aorta, into the carotid or vertebral arteries and injecting radio-opaque contrast to enable detailed visualisation of vessels.

Indications

Angiography is used to diagnose aneurysms, arterial stenosis (eg thromboembolism, dissection, vasculitis and atherosclerosis), arteriovenous malformations and cerebral venous sinus thrombosis. Therapeutic interventional procedures can also be carried out, eg embolisation of aneurysms,

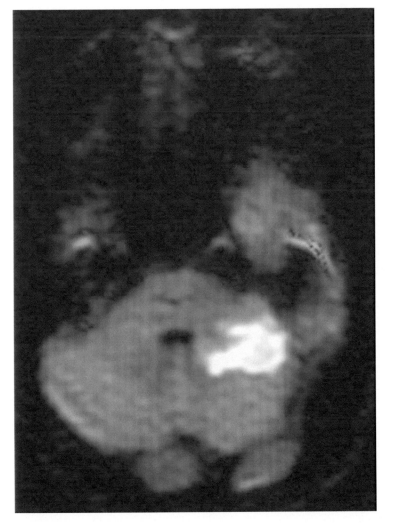

Fig 54 Diffusion-weighted MRI (DWI) scan demonstrating acute infarction in the right cerebellar hemisphere. (Courtesy of Professor M. Brown, Institute of Neurology, University of London.)

arteriovenous malformations or blood supply to tumours, arterial thrombolysis, angioplasty and stenting.

Complications

These include local haematoma or bleeding, infection, pseudoaneurysm formation, vessel damage, renal failure, contrast reaction, stroke or transient ischaemic attack and death. In experienced hands, diagnostic angiography carries a risk of stroke of <1%. However, interventional procedures carry a risk of major complications of up to 10%, including vessel perforation.

3.5 Single-photon emission computed tomography and positron emission tomography

Single-photon emission computed tomography (SPECT) and positron emission tomography (PET) are two methods by which functional, rather than conventional structural, neuroimaging can be performed. Functional neuroimaging can be divided into techniques that demonstrate synaptic activity or regional activation (called functional mapping) based on the close association between blood flow and neuronal activation/synaptic activity, and techniques that enable the detection of particular neurotransmitter or neurochemical substances.
Tracer design is therefore based on physiological molecules involved in metabolic turn over (such as oxygen, glucose and amino acids) and enzyme activation, or on neurotransmitters and their receptors. The specific tracers are labelled with gamma-emitting radioisotopes for SPECT and positron-emitting radionucleotides for PET.

Single photon emission computed tomography (SPECT)

Gamma-emitting radionucleotides are commercially available and images are taken with a routine nuclear medicine camera. This makes SPECT less expensive and more widely available compared with PET. The disadvantages are inferior spatial resolution and less quantification than are possible with PET.

Positron emission tomography (PET)

PET depends on positron (positively charged electrons)-labelled radionucleotides, which have a short half-life and are generated by a cyclotron. PET can only be performed, therefore, in a centre with a cyclotron. Commonly used positrons are oxygen (^{15}O), carbon (^{11}C) and nitrogen (^{13}N). Fluorine (^{18}F) is used to replace hydrogen. The image gathered represents the distribution of the emitted positrons. The increased sensitivity of PET over SPECT enables patients to undergo less radioactive exposure.

Functional imaging

Functional imaging techniques are concerned with describing activity of neurones in the brain associated with a given physiological, cognitive or pathological state, ie function of the brain as opposed to structure. Studies using PET may be steady-state or activation studies, in which a physical or cognitive task is associated with changes in cerebral blood flow in discrete brain regions.

Steady-state studies

These can show:

> a characteristic pattern of impaired metabolism in parietal and posterior temporal regions, as seen in early Alzheimer's disease

> patchy abnormalities, particularly in the distribution of the middle cerebral artery in vascular dementia

> reduced uptake of ^{18}F-DOPA in the basal ganglia in Parkinson's disease

> hypometabolism in the striatum in Huntington's disease.

Activation studies

These can be used for:

> localisation of cerebral function in normal volunteers, eg language, memory, attention and motor control

> studies of the reorganisation of the brain in the recovery of function following brain injury, eg after stroke (Fig 55).

3.6 Carotid Dopplers

Principle

The is a non-invasive technique which utilises the fact that sound waves reflected off red blood cells give an indication of the flow velocity within the vessel (Fig 56). A stenosed vessel gives a high-flow velocity. The accuracy of the test compared with angiography (the gold standard) is operator-dependent, but should approach at least 90% in good centres.

Key point

Carotid Dopplers cannot distinguish between an absence of flow (complete occlusion) and very low flow (tight stenosis with a patent vessel).

Indications

This is used to screen for carotid artery stenosis (atherosclerotic disease or dissection) when clinically suspected. The results from ultrasound should be compared and confirmed with alternate vascular imaging such as that produced by magnetic resonance angiography (MRA) or computerised tomography angiography (CTA) before planning on treatment.

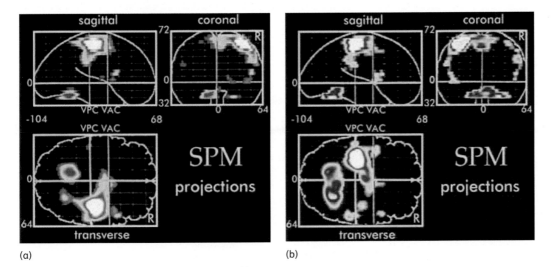

(a)   (b)

Fig 55 Statistical parametric maps (SPM) of brain areas activated (in comparison with rest) by a paced, sequential, finger-to-thumb opposition task in patients with lesions of the left internal capsule **(a)** using the left hand, and **(b)** recovered right hand. The SPMs are presented as projections through the brain seen from side (sagittal), back (coronal) and top (transverse) views. The frontal pole is on the right side of the transverse section. Highly significant changes of activity between active and resting states are shown in colour, coded to represent levels of significance (white being the greatest significance). In comparing **(b)** with **(a)** it can be seen that the same task has led to activations that are not only bilateral but are more extensive, reflecting recruitment of other motor areas not normally activated by simple motor tasks. (Reproduced from Chollet *et al. Ann Neurol* 1991; 29: 63–71 with permission of Lippincott, Williams and Wilkins Inc.)

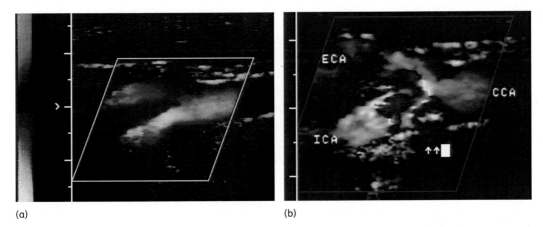

(a)   (b)

Fig 56 Colour flow Doppler ultrasound scans. **(a)** Normal carotid bifurcation; **(b)** internal carotid artery stenosis causing turbulent blood flow (seen in blue). CCA, common carotid artery; ECA, external carotid artery; ICA, internal carotid artery. (Courtesy of Professor M. Brown, Institute of Neurology, University of London.)

4 Self-assessment

4.1 Self-assessment questions

MRCP(UK) Part 1 examination questions

Question 1

Clinical scenario

A 62-year-old man presented with a 2-month history of intermittent double vision and ptosis. His symptoms were worse in the evenings or when he was tired. On examination he had mild bilateral ptosis and fatigable weakness of his upper limbs, which was worse proximally.

Question

Which antibody is most likely to be positive in this patient?

Answer

A anti-acetylcholine receptor antibody

B anti-glutamic acid decarboxylase antibody

C anti-muscle specific tyrosine kinase antibody

D anti-voltage-gated calcium channel antibody

E anti-voltage-gated potassium channel antibody

Question 2

Clinical scenario

An 18-year-old man presented to clinic with a 1-year history of progressive difficulty in walking and climbing stairs. There was no family history of muscle weakness. On examination, he had wasting of his quadriceps and hamstrings in his lower limbs bilaterally, with increased muscle bulk in his lower legs. There was mild weakness of flexion and extension in his hips and knees bilaterally. Deep tendon reflexes and sensory examination were normal.

Investigation:

serum creatine kinase	18,000 U/L (normal range 24–195)

Question

Which investigation is most likely to confirm the diagnosis?

Answer

A anti-glutamic acid decarboxylase antibody

B anti-Jo-1 antibody

C dystrophin gene analysis

D mitochondrial DNA analysis

E single-fibre electromyography

Question 3

Clinical scenario

A 59-year-old man presented with an 8-month history of gradually progressive unsteadiness. On examination, he had full range of eye movements, with two beats of nystagmus on left-horizontal gaze. Hearing was mildly reduced in both ears and Weber's test did not lateralise. Rinne's test revealed that bone conduction was better than air conduction bilaterally. Otoscopy revealed wax in both ear canals. When he stood with his eyes shut, he was unsteady.

Question

What part of the nervous system is most likely to be affected?

Answer

A cerebellum

B cochlear

C dorsal columns of the spinal cord

D midbrain

E vestibulocochlear nerve

Question 4

Clinical scenario

A 27-year-old man presented with a 3-day history of weakness of the left side of his face, which he first noticed when he woke up. On examination, he had difficulty raising his left eyebrow, closing his left eye and blowing out his left cheek.

Question

What is the most likely diagnosis?

Answer

A Bell's palsy

B carotid cavernous fistula

C cerebrovascular accident

D myasthenia gravis

E parotid gland tumour

Question 5

Clinical scenario

A 25-year-old woman presented with a 3-week history of pins and needles on her right outer thigh. She was 32 weeks pregnant and had type 1 diabetes. Two years ago, she had an episode of optic neuritis in her left eye that had resolved without treatment. On examination there was a patch of hypersensitivity on the right outer thigh, which did not go past the midline or below the right knee. There was no weakness and all lower limb reflexes were present.

Question

What is the most likely diagnosis?

Answer

A diabetic amyotrophy

B femoral nerve palsy

C lumbar radiculopathy

D meralgia paraesthetica

E multiple sclerosis

Question 6

Clinical scenario

A 30-year-old man was admitted after a motorcycle accident. He had sustained excessive bruising of his upper limb, chest and shoulder regions on the left. On examination, he was unable to abduct or externally rotate his left upper arm at the shoulder joint.

Question
Which nerve is most likely to be injured?

Answer
A axillary
B dorsal scapular
C long thoracic
D musculocutaneous
E suprascapular

Question 7

Clinical scenario
A 17-year-old woman was admitted to the emergency department with recurrent seizures. She had received three doses of 10 mg diazepam intravenously. After each dose her seizures stopped for about 10 minutes, but then returned. She was currently on levetiracetam 1,000 mg twice a day, having previously been on Lamotrigine without benefit. She had been investigated with an electroencephalogram (EEG) and magnetic resonance imaging (MRI) of the brain a week ago: both were normal.

Question
What is the most likely diagnosis?

Answer
A cryptogenic generalised epilepsy
B frontal lobe epilepsy
C juvenile myoclonic epilepsy
D non-epileptic attack disorder
E syncope

Question 8

Clinical scenario
A 34-year-old woman presented with a 2-week history of left upper limb weakness. Two years ago she had optic neuritis in her left eye, which had resolved without treatment.

On examination, she had mild left facial weakness and left upper limb weakness, increased deep tendon reflexes in the knees bilaterally, and an extensor left plantar response. An MRI of the brain was performed.

Question
Lesions in which area of the brain are most suggestive of multiple sclerosis?

Answer
A corpus callosum
B frontal lobe
C occipital lobe
D red nucleus
E thalamus

Question 9

Clinical scenario
A 30-year-old woman was seen in the clinic complaining of visual disturbance. On examination she had an absent right corneal reflex.

Question
Which cranial nerve provides the efferent (motor) pathway for the corneal reflex?

Answer
A third cranial nerve
B fourth cranial nerve
C fifth cranial nerve
D sixth cranial nerve
E seventh cranial nerve

Question 10

Clinical scenario
A 68-year-old woman presented with a 7-month history of daily headaches. The headaches started on waking, were dull and generalised, and fluctuated in intensity. At its peak there was associated mild nausea and slight blurring of vision. When she was younger she used to get headaches during her menstrual cycle. She took co-codamol, two tablets every 6 hours to control her headaches. Neurological examination was normal.

Question
What is the most likely diagnosis?

Answer
A medication overuse headache
B migraine
C raised intracranial pressure
D temporal arteritis
E tension-type headache

Question 11

Clinical scenario
A 34-year-old woman presented to the neurology clinic with a 1-week history of gradually worsening difficulty with speech and swallowing, with dragging of her right leg. On examination, there were fasciculations on the left side of her tongue, which deviated to the left on protrusion. Her right leg was weak with increased tone and brisk deep tendon reflexes. Her left leg was normal.

Question
Where is the likely site of the neurological lesion?

Answer
A left medulla
B left midbrain
C left pons
D right medulla
E right midbrain

Question 12

Clinical scenario
A 45-year-old woman was referred after her optician noticed that she had nystagmus. On examination, she had rhythmic oscillations of the eyes of maximal intensity when the eyes were looking inferiorly, with the fast phase beating in a downward direction.

Question
Which area is most likely affected to cause this nystagmus?

Answer
A cerebellum
B craniocervical junction
C hypothalamus
D medial geniculate nucleus
E ventral midbrain

Question 13

Clinical scenario

A 55-year-old man presented to clinic complaining of right arm weakness. On examination, he had weakness of the right elbow and wrist extension and sensory loss over the middle finger.

Question

Which nerve root is likely to be affected?

Answer

A C5

B C6

C C7

D C8

E T1

Question 14

Clinical scenario

A 19-year-old woman reported that she had first noted unequal pupils when looking in the mirror a couple of weeks earlier, and this had persisted. She thought her left pupil was larger than the right. Vision was not affected, and she was otherwise in good health. On examination she had an enlarged left pupil that did not obviously constrict with illumination or on accommodation, and absent knee and ankle deep tendon reflexes.

Question

What is the most likely diagnosis?

Answer

A Argyll Robertson pupil

B Holmes–Adie pupil

C Horner's syndrome

D simple (physiological) anisocoria

E third cranial nerve palsy

Question 15

Clinical scenario

A 25-year-old man presented to the outpatient clinic with a 2-week history of a right foot drop. He denied any history of trauma or back pain.

Question

Which feature is more suggestive of a right L5 lumbar radiculopathy rather than a right common peroneal nerve palsy?

Answer

A absent right ankle jerk

B numbness over the web of the first and second toes of the right foot

C weakness of ankle dorsiflexion

D weakness of ankle eversion

E weakness of ankle inversion

Question 16

Clinical scenario

A 66-year-old woman complained of drooping of her right eyelid towards the end of the day over the past 3 months. She had a past medical history of hypothyroidism and diabetes. Seen in a morning clinic, no obvious neurological abnormality was seen, but on prolonged upgaze some drooping of the right eyelid was noted.

Question

What is the most likely diagnosis?

Answer

A age-related ptosis

B Horner's syndrome

C myasthenia gravis

D third cranial nerve palsy

E thyroid eye disease

Question 17

Clinical scenario

A 60-year-old man presented with a 2-week history of back pain. He denied any history of trauma. On examination, he had weakness of dorsiflexion of the right big toe.

Question

Which nerve root would you expect to be affected in this case?

Answer

A L2

B L3

C L4

D L5

E S1

Question 18

Clinical scenario

A 35-year-old man presented with a 3-week history of headaches in his left temple and left periorbital region. He described at least two severe attacks a day, each lasting around an hour. The pain used to wake him up around 4am every morning. The pain was associated with right-sided nasal congestion and excessive tear production in the right eye.

Question

What is the most likely cause of the headache?

Answer

A cluster headache

B episodic migraine

C hypnic headache

D paroxysmal hemicrania

E trigeminal neuralgia

Question 19

Clinical scenario

A 71-year-old woman presented with progressive instability of stance and gait that developed over a month. Four months previously she had been diagnosed with metastatic ovarian carcinoma and had been receiving chemotherapy since then. Examination was notable for bilateral gaze-evoked nystagmus and scanning speech. A CT brain scan and brain MRI examination were unremarkable.

Question

What is the most likely cause of her new presentation?

Answer

A chemotherapy-induced peripheral neuropathy

B malignancy-associated polymyositis

C malnutrition-associated vitamin B_{12} deficiency

D multiple intracranial metastases

E paraneoplastic cerebellar degeneration

Question 20

Clinical scenario

A 29-year-old man presented with a 2-day history of headache, nausea and vomiting. Examination revealed high fever, global confusion and neck stiffness. He had mild right-sided weakness with a right extensor plantar reflex. Intravenous antibiotics were started.

Question
What is the most important investigation to do next?

Answer
A blood culture
B brain CT scan
C brain MRI
D full blood count
E lumbar puncture

MRCP(UK) Part 2 examination questions

Question 21

Clinical scenario
A 70-year-old woman was referred for forgetfulness and failure to look after herself at home. When she attended clinic with her daughter she denied any memory problems other than what she thought might be expected for old age, but her daughter told of her mother's repetitive questioning, repeatedly misplacing household items and she reported finding food items in the fridge which were well past their eat-by dates. Symptoms had gradually worsened over approximately 8 months since the death of her husband. She was a smoker and was treated for hypertension.

On examination, there were no focal neurological signs. On the Mini-Mental State Examination she scored 21/30, losing marks for orientation in time and place, 5-minute recall and drawing intersecting pentagons.

Question
What is the most likely diagnosis?

Answer
A Alzheimer's disease
B Creutzfeldt–Jakob disease
C depression
D frontotemporal dementia
E vascular dementia

Question 22

Clinical scenario
A 28-year-old man presented with a 3-year history of muscle pain and weakness which developed after prolonged exercise. He said that he was not able to exercise gently through the initial pain barrier. He also complained of having intermittent episodes of dark urine after exercise.
On examination, there were no focal neurological signs.

Question
What is the most likely diagnosis?

Answer
A acid maltase deficiency
B carnitine palmitoyltransferase deficiency
C McArdle's disease
D necrotising myopathy
E polymyositis

Question 23

Clinical scenario
A 75-year-old man presented to the clinic with his daughter who complained that over the past few months her father was seeing things that were not there, such as children in the garden, or insects in the bath, or that people on TV were actually in the room with him. These caused him no particular concern or anxiety. He was otherwise in good health, with no history of hypertension, diabetes, alcohol misuse or previous psychiatric disease.

On examination, he had no focal neurological signs except for reduced arm swing when he walked.

Question
What is the most likely diagnosis?

Answer
A Charles Bonnet syndrome
B delirium
C dementia with Lewy bodies
D epilepsy
E psychotic depression

Question 24

Clinical scenario
A 70-year-old man with a progressive amnesic syndrome of 8 months' duration was diagnosed with Alzheimer's disease on the basis of poor performance on cognitive screening tests (Mini-Mental State Examination score 20/30) and global brain atrophy on CT scan. His daughter reported that he repeatedly complained of things being stolen from his house, where he lived alone, and seeing someone he did not know in the house when he looked in the mirror. He sometimes phoned her in the middle of the night, apparently very agitated, to tell her of these happenings.

Question
What is the most appropriate treatment?

Answer
A benzodiazepine receptor modulator
B cholinesterase inhibitor
C dopamine receptor antagonist
D N-methyl-D-aspartate (NMDA) receptor antagonist
E selective serotonin reuptake inhibitor

Question 25

Clinical scenario
A 30-year-old woman attended the neurology clinic after being diagnosed with multiple sclerosis. She had suffered an episode of optic neuritis 5 years previously, which had resolved after 3 months. About 4 weeks ago, she presented with an episode of paraesthesiae of her upper limbs that had lasted for 3 weeks. She did not have any limb weakness. Her MRI of the brain and cerebrospinal fluid investigations were compatible with a diagnosis of multiple sclerosis. She was keen to discuss her prognosis.

Question
Which is associated with a worse prognosis?

Answer

A female, rather than male, gender

B later, rather than earlier, age of onset

C longer, rather than shorter, first remission

D optic neuritis or sensory symptoms at onset, rather than motor weakness

E relapsing-remitting, rather than primary progressive, disease course

Question 26

Clinical scenario

A 19-year-old man was referred to clinic with difficult-to-control epileptic seizures. He was getting two to three tonic–clonic seizures a week. He was also noted to have almost daily brief jerks of his upper limbs in the mornings.

Neurological examination was normal.

Question

What is the most appropriate antiepileptic medication to prevent further seizures?

Answer

A carbamazepine

B clobazam

C phenytoin

D pregabalin

E valproate

Question 27

Clinical scenario

A 65-year-old man was referred with a 6-month history of muscle weakness and mild dysphagia. He complained of difficulty opening jars, gripping objects and difficulty walking.

On examination he had disproportionate weakness in his finger flexors compared with the corresponding extensors, and disproportionate knee extensors compared with hip flexors. Reflexes were symmetrical. There were no cranial nerve signs.

Question

What is the most likely diagnosis?

Answer

A inclusion body myositis

B limb girdle muscular dystrophy

C motor neurone disease

D myotonic dystrophy

E polymyositis

Question 28

Clinical scenario

A 28-year-old man was referred to the outpatient clinic with a 5-year history of cramps and twitching of muscles affecting mainly his calf muscles, but also the upper arms occasionally. The symptoms were more noticeable when he exercised or was under stress.

On examination, he had intermittent fasciculations of his calf muscles and biceps. The rest of the neurological examination was normal.

Question

What is the most likely diagnosis?

Answer

A amyotrophic lateral sclerosis

B mononeuritis multiplex

C multiple sclerosis

D myotonic dystrophy

E peripheral nerve hyperexcitability

Question 29

Clinical scenario

A 59-year-old man presented with an 8-month history of progressive weakness of the upper and lower limbs. Over the last 2 months he complained of increasing dysphagia affecting liquids more than solids, and worsening shortness of breath at rest.

On examination, he had a brisk jaw jerk, tongue fasciculations and weakness of elbow flexion and hip flexion of Medical Research Council (MRC) grade 4/5 bilaterally.

Question

Which treatment would be expected to increase his life expectancy the most?

Answer

A gastrostomy

B immunoglobulin

C non-invasive ventilation

D physiotherapy

E riluzole

Question 30

Clinical scenario

A 47-year-old man presented with a 1-year history of tremor affecting both hands. The tremor was worse with anxiety and on movement, and it was not affected by alcohol intake. He had a history of severe asthma. There was no family history of tremor.

On examination, he had a postural tremor in his upper limbs bilaterally.

Investigations:

serum copper	26 μmol/L (normal range 12–26)
serum caeruloplasmin	230 mg/L (normal range 200–350)
serum thyroid-stimulating hormone	4.8 mU/L (normal range 0.4–5.0)
24-hour urinary copper	0.3 μmol (normal range 0.2–0.6)

Question

What is the most appropriate treatment?

Answer

A citalopram

B levetiracetam

C primidone

D propranolol

E topiramate

Question 31

Clinical scenario

A 58-year-old man was referred to the outpatient clinic with an 8-month history of increasing difficulty walking, associated with several falls. He felt faint when he stood up quickly. He had a history of depression, for which he had been on citalopram 20 mg daily for 10 years.

On examination, his blood pressure was 148/84 mmHg supine and 130/74 mmHg after standing for 3 minutes. He had bilateral gaze-evoked nystagmus and his speech was quiet and slow. There was coarse bilateral tremor of his hands and he had marked rigidity of his upper limbs and trunk. His gait was broad-based and he had difficulty walking heel-to-toe.

Question
What is the most likely diagnosis?

Answer
A citalopram-induced extrapyramidal syndrome
B corticobasal degeneration
C idiopathic Parkinson's disease
D multiple system atrophy
E progressive supranuclear palsy

Question 32

Clinical scenario
A 68-year-old man was referred with a 2-month history of cognitive decline, especially of short-term memory loss. He had become withdrawn and agitated over the previous 1 month. He drank 30 units of alcohol per week.

On examination, his Mini-Mental State Examination score was 10/30. He had involuntary jerking movements of his upper limbs. He was easily startled by abrupt noise.

Question
What is the most likely diagnosis?

Answer
A Alzheimer's disease
B Creutzfeldt–Jakob disease
C dementia with Lewy bodies
D Huntington's disease
E Korsakoff's syndrome

Question 33

Clinical scenario
A 68-year-old woman presented with a 3-week history of pain in the right foot and a right foot drop that developed over 2 days. Two months previously she had developed a right wrist drop that had come on over 1 week and recovered after 3 weeks. Her past medical history included asthma of recent onset and an 8-year history of type 2 diabetes mellitus.

On examination, she had weakness of right ankle dorsiflexion and eversion.

The rest of the neurological examination was normal.

Question
What is the most likely diagnosis?

Answer
A chronic inflammatory demyelinating polyneuropathy
B mononeuritis multiplex
C motor neurone disease
D multifocal motor neuropathy with conduction block
E multiple sclerosis

Question 34

Clinical scenario
A 54-year-old woman was admitted with a 3-day history of headache and confusion. While in the emergency department she had a tonic–clonic seizure. Her past medical history included a liver transplant, performed 5 years previously for hepatitis C-induced liver failure. She was on tacrolimus and corticosteroids for post-transplantation immunosuppression.

On examination, her temperature was 39.6°C, her pulse was 128 beats per minute and her blood pressure was 110/70 mmHg. She was lethargic and not rousable. She had bilateral upgoing plantar responses.

Investigations:

haemoglobin	100 g/L (normal range 115–165)
white cell count	14.6 × 10⁹/L (normal range 4.0–11.0)
platelet count	175 × 10⁹/L (normal range 150–400)
erythrocyte sedimentation rate	68 mm/1st h (normal range <30)
serum alanine aminotransferase	77 U/L (normal range 5–35)
serum aspartate aminotransferase	50 U/L (normal range 1–31)
serum alkaline phosphatase	105 U/L (normal range 45–105)
serum C-reactive protein	100 mg/L (normal range <10)
MRI of the brain	haemorrhage and enhancement in the right parietal and temporal lobes

Question
What is the most appropriate management?

Answer
A aciclovir
B ceftriaxone
C methylprednisolone
D plasmapheresis
E stop tacrolimus

Question 35

Clinical scenario
A 40-year-old woman presented to the emergency department with an occipital headache of sudden onset, followed by confusion and decreased consciousness. On examination, her Glasgow Coma Scale score was 12/15. She had neck stiffness and Kernig's sign was positive.

Investigations:

MRI of the brain	blood in subarachnoid space and intraventricular space
CT angiogram of brain	no aneurysm detected

She made good progress on conservative management initially, but 13 days after admission her level of consciousness started to deteriorate significantly and she became confused again.

Question
What is the most likely cause of her clinical deterioration?

Answer
A aneurysm rebleed
B cerebral abscess
C communicating hydrocephalus
D meningitis
E venous sinus thrombosis

Question 36

Clinical scenario
A 26-year-old woman presented with a 4-week history of headaches. The headaches were worse when she woke up in the mornings and were

occasionally associated with nausea and vomiting. Her only medical history was of acne, for which she took doxycycline. She was also taking vitamin B complex supplements, vitamin C, selenium and zinc because she had heard that they were beneficial from a health point of view.

On examination, she had enlarged blind spots and bilateral papilloedema. Visual acuity was 6/12 in both eyes. Investigations:

MRI of the brain	normal
magnetic resonance venogram (MRV)	normal

Question
What is the most likely cause of her neurological presentation?

Answer
A doxycycline
B selenium
C vitamin B
D vitamin C
E zinc

Question 37
Clinical scenario
A 34-year-old woman was admitted with a severe headache. The headache had started while she was running in the gym: initially it was mild then it progressively got worse and she began vomiting. She noticed tingling in her left hand, which spread up the arm, eventually affecting the left side of her face over a period of 3 minutes. She noticed difficulty getting words out when the headache was severe. The severe headache lasted for 24 hours.

On examination, her blood pressure was 120/84 mmHg. She had some mild neck discomfort but no focal neurological deficit.

Question
What is the most likely cause of her neurological presentation?

Answer
A internal carotid artery dissection
B migraine

C partial seizure
D subarachnoid haemorrhage
E transient ischaemic attack

Question 38
Clinical scenario
A 60-year-old man presented with a troublesome tremor. Six months previously he had undergone emergency laparotomy for peritonitis. He needed a further two operations and spent 6 weeks in intensive care. Since discharge from intensive care he had noticed uncontrollable shaking of his upper and lower limbs for most of the day. He was taking paroxetine 40 mg daily for depression.

On examination, his cognition was normal. He had a resting tremor of his left arm and jerky movements of his upper limbs, worse on movement. He also had rigidity of both upper and lower limbs.

Question
Which treatment is most likely to improve his abnormal movements?

Answer
A carbamazepine
B clonazepam
C levodopa
D propranolol
E valproate

Question 39
Clinical scenario
A 46-year-old woman presented with a 3-day history of double vision. Ten days previously she had become unsteady when walking and had fallen twice. Two weeks before the onset of these symptoms she had taken a course of antibiotics for a urinary tract infection. She had been treated for cervical cancer 3 years previously.

On examination, she had a left-sided internuclear ophthalmoplegia with truncal and limb ataxia. She was areflexic.

Question
What is the most likely diagnosis?

Answer
A brainstem infarct
B Lambert–Eaton syndrome
C Miller Fisher syndrome
D multiple sclerosis
E paraneoplastic cerebellar degeneration

Question 40
Clinical scenario
A 25-year-old man was referred to the neurology clinic with a 3-year history of involuntary jerking of his arms and legs. He was currently on clozapine for a major depressive illness, and he had been on several other neuroleptics in the past. He never knew his father, who died in a psychiatric hospital when he was only 2 years old, and his paternal grandfather was also said to be 'twitchy', although he died of a heart attack in his sixties.

On examination, he had mild rigidity of his upper limbs and jerky movements of his hands.

Question
What is the most likely diagnosis?

Answer
A Creutzfeldt–Jakob disease
B Huntington's disease
C Sydenham's chorea
D tardive dyskinesia
E Wilson's disease

4.2 Self-assessment answers

Answer to Question 1
A: anti-acetylcholine receptor antibody

Anti-acetylcholine receptor antibody is present in approximately 85% of patients with generalised myasthenia gravis and 50% of patients with ocular myasthenia gravis.

Answer to Question 2

C: dystrophin gene analysis

Becker muscular dystrophy is caused by a deficiency or defect in, rather than absence of, dystrophin. It is X-linked and milder than Duchenne muscular dystrophy.

Answer to Question 3

C: dorsal columns of the spinal cord

A patient who has difficulty with proprioception can still maintain balance by using vestibular function and vision. In the Romberg's test (the standing patient is asked to close his or her eyes), a loss of balance is interpreted as a positive test. A positive Romberg's test suggests that the ataxia is sensory in nature, ie depending on loss of proprioception, which is carried in the dorsal columns of the spinal cord.

Answer to Question 4

A: Bell's palsy

Bell's palsy is a condition that usually causes a temporary seventh cranial nerve lower motor neurone weakness. It is usually unilateral and approximately 70% of affected patients make a complete recovery.

Answer to Question 5

D: meralgia paraesthetica

Meralgia paraesthetica is a painful mononeuropathy of the lateral cutaneous nerve, commonly due to focal entrapment as it passes through the inguinal ligament, eg in pregnancy. The lateral cutaneous nerve is responsible for the sensation of the anterolateral thigh and is a purely sensory nerve.

Answer to Question 6

E: suprascapular

The suprascapular nerve innervates the supraspinatus and infraspinatus muscles. The supraspinatus muscle (in addition to the deltoid muscle) is responsible for shoulder abduction. The infraspinatus muscle (in addition to the teres minor muscle) is responsible for external rotation of the shoulder.

Answer to Question 7

D: non-epileptic attack disorder

The lack of response to treatment and normal investigations make a non-epileptic attack disorder the most likely diagnosis.

Answer to Question 8

A: corpus callosum

Lesions of the corpus callosum are highly suggestive of multiple sclerosis.

Answer to Question 9

E: seventh cranial nerve

The fifth cranial nerve provides the afferent (sensory) pathway for the corneal reflex.

Answer to Question 10

A: medication overuse headache

Medication overuse headache is caused by taking painkillers or triptan medications too regularly.

Answer to Question 11

A: left medulla

Lesions of the medulla result in loss of function of the cranial nerve on the side of the lesion and contralateral hemiplegia.

Answer to Question 12

B: craniocervical junction

A lesion of the craniocervical junction causes a downbeat nystagmus.

Answer to Question 13

C: C7

C7 supplies triceps and wrist extensors (motor function) and middle finger (sensory function).

Answer to Question 14

B: Holmes–Adie pupil

This is the typical clinical picture of Holmes–Adie pupil.

Answer to Question 15

E: weakness of ankle inversion

An L5 nerve root lesion, but not a common peroneal nerve palsy, causes weakness of ankle inversion. The ankle jerk is supplied by the S1 nerve root. Numbness over the web of the first and second toes of the foot is indicative of a common peroneal nerve palsy.

Answer to Question 16

C: myasthenia gravis

Muscle weakness that is worse at the end of the day and/or made evident by repetitive muscle contraction (ie fatiguable weakness) is typical of myasthenia gravis, which has a predilection for the eyelids, extraocular and bulbar muscles, as well as proximal limb muscles.

Answer to Question 17

D: L5

An L5 nerve root lesion causes weakness of ankle dorsiflexion, inversion and eversion, and dorsiflexion of the big toe. L2 weakness affects hip flexion and thigh adduction; L3 weakness affects thigh adduction and knee extension; L4 weakness affects knee extension and ankle inversion; and S1 weakness affects plantar flexion, eversion and knee flexion.

Answer to Question 18

A: cluster headache

The description is typical of cluster headache.

Answer to Question 19

E: paraneoplastic cerebellar degeneration

The constellation of ataxia, nystagmus and scanning speech (dysarthria) points towards cerebellar dysfunction. The normal brain imaging rules out gross lesions. Paraneoplastic cerebellar degeneration fits this scenario.

This syndrome has been associated with anti-Yo antibodies and affects 1–3% of all cancers; ovarian cancer, uterine cancer, small-cell lung cancer, breast cancer and Hodgkin's lymphoma.

Answer to Question 20
B: brain CT scan

The overall clinical picture is suggestive of a meningitic process. Although focal and lateralising neurological signs might be seen in complicated pyogenic meningitis (eg due to cortical venous thrombosis, subdural collection), their presence should always call for initial brain imaging looking for a brain abscess that might have ruptured and produced this picture. If the CT scan is not indicative of a space-occupying lesion, one can proceed with lumbar puncture. In all cases of suspected pyogenic meningitis, intravenous antibiotics should not await diagnostic confirmation. Brain MRI is not a suitable choice in an unstable confused patient. Blood counts may show leucocytosis or leukopenia (or could be normal), and blood culture can be positive (depending on the culprit organism).

Answer to Question 21
A: Alzheimer's disease

The insidious onset of symptoms indicative of an amnesic syndrome in late life is typical of Alzheimer's disease.

Answer to Question 22
B: carnitine palmitoyltransferase deficiency

In carnitine palmitoyltransferase (CPT) deficiency, patients typically develop symptoms after prolonged exercise, whereas in McArdle's disease patients develop symptoms within minutes of starting exercise and may also describe a 'second wind' phenomenon. Myoglobinuria secondary to rhabdomyolysis is more common in CPT deficiency than in McArdle's disease.

Answer to Question 23
C: dementia with Lewy bodies

New onset visual hallucinations in late life with subtle parkinsonian features suggests dementia with Lewy bodies, particularly in the absence of risk factors for other causes (visual impairment, depression, drug use).

Answer to Question 24
B: cholinesterase inhibitor

Cholinesterase inhibitors are licensed for the treatment of mild-to-moderate Alzheimer's disease, and can sometimes help neuropsychiatric as well as mnemonic problems.

Answer to Question 25
B: later, rather than earlier, age of onset

Earlier age of onset is associated with a better prognosis in multiple sclerosis.

Answer to Question 26
E: valproate

Valproate is the most effective treatment for juvenile myoclonic epilepsy.

Answer to Question 27
A: inclusion body myositis

The pattern of weakness described is characteristic of inclusion body myositis.

Answer to Question 28
E: peripheral nerve hyperexcitability

Peripheral nerve hyperexcitability or benign fasciculation syndrome is associated with voltage-gated potassium channel antibodies. It causes muscle fasciculations and cramps, but no muscle wasting or weakness.

Answer to Question 29
C: non-invasive ventilation

Non-invasive ventilation increases life expectancy by up to 6 months in motor neurone disease.

Answer to Question 30
C: primidone

Essential tremor is best treated by propranolol (which is contraindicated in this patient because of his asthma) and primidone.

Answer to Question 31
D: multiple system atrophy

Multiple system atrophy is parkinsonism associated with cerebellar and autonomic features.

Answer to Question 32
B: Creutzfeldt–Jakob disease

The rapid cognitive decline associated with personality changes, myoclonic jerks and startle response is very suggestive of Creutzfeldt–Jakob disease.

Answer to Question 33
B: mononeuritis multiplex

Mononeuritis multiplex is a painful, asymmetrical, asynchronous sensory and motor peripheral neuropathy involving isolated damage to at least two separate nerve areas. It is associated with diabetes mellitus and Churg–Strauss syndrome.

Answer to Question 34
A: aciclovir

The clinical picture is that of viral encephalitis which is treated with aciclovir.

Answer to Question 35
C: communicating hydrocephalus

This is the classical picture of the delayed complication of communicating hydrocephalus, which develops 10 or more days after a subarachnoid haemorrhage. It is characterised by the unexpected deterioration of a patient's condition when they are expected to be recovering.

Answer to Question 36
A: doxycycline

Tetracycline antibiotics can cause intracranial hypertension.

Answer to Question 37
B: migraine

The spreading of symptoms is classically associated with migraine.

Answer to Question 38
B: clonazepam

The clinical presentation is post-hypoxic myoclonus, which is best treated with clonazepam.

Answer to Question 39
C: Miller Fisher syndrome

Miller Fisher syndrome is a post-infectious, immune-mediated condition characterised by the clinical triad of ophthalmoplegia, ataxia and areflexia.

Answer to Question 40
B: Huntington's disease

The family history, suggestive of an autosomal dominant disease with anticipation, and clinical presentation of involuntary choreiform movements and parkinsonian features such as rigidity, would be compatible with Huntington's disease.

Medical ophthalmology

Author

Dr G Heath

Editor-in-Chief

Dr JD Firth

The ophthalmology section of the second edition of Medical Masterclass was written by Dr P Frith, Dr H Towler and Dr JD Firth (editor). This third edition of Medical Masterclass contains entirely new material, but many sections from the first edition have been retained and updated, and we gratefully acknowledge the contribution of these authors.

Medical ophthalmology: Section 1

1 PACES stations and acute scenarios

1.1 Clinical examinations

1.1.1 Examination of the eye

Examination of the eye may be required during examination of the cranial nerves in the neurology station of PACES (Station 3) or as part of examination of the eye in Station 5 (brief clinical consultation). Eye examination by the non-specialist requires the following assessments:

> visual acuity

> visual fields

> pupil responses

> ocular media and fundus using the ophthalmoscope

> ocular movements.

The necessary techniques are described in *Clinical Skills for PACES*. The following short notes emphasise important aspects about use of the ophthalmoscope and pharmacological methods of dilating the pupil.

How to use the direct ophthalmoscope

The direct ophthalmoscope provides an image that is magnified and upright but of a very limited area, so that the retina has to be 'scanned' to provide the observer with a composite view. It also lacks depth perception, and examination of the peripheral retina is restricted. Its advantages are its ease of use, relatively simple construction and maintenance, and ability to examine the retina through an undilated pupil. When

using the direct ophthalmoscope, remember:

> First, check that the batteries and bulb are satisfactory.

> It is always preferable to examine the eye through dilated pupils, although this may not always be possible (see below). Select the larger aperture if the pupil is dilated; the smaller if not.

> Stand about 1 metre from the patient and rotate the lens dial to provide the sharpest image. You should remove spectacles if normally worn by you or the patient, unless either of you has a high error of focus.

> Shine the ophthalmoscope light at the patient's pupils and look for the normal red reflex from the retina (the same as the 'red eye' from flash photography). Any opacity within the media of the eye such as a cataract (Fig 1) or vitreous haemorrhage (Fig 2) will darken the red reflex. A subluxed (partially dislocated) lens may be evident, especially if the pupil is dilated (Fig 3).

> Examine each eye in turn, using your right hand and eye for the patient's right eye and vice versa (if you can do so). Try to remain as upright as possible because this enables the

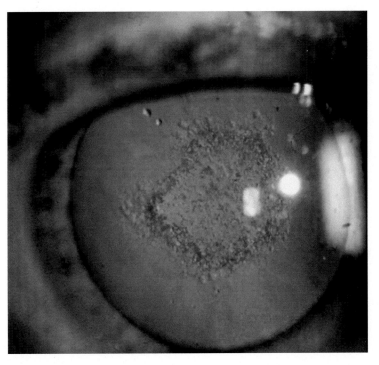

Fig 1 Early cataract seen against the red reflex. The granular appearance in the centre of the pupil is typical of a posterior subcapsular cataract due to use of systemic corticosteroids.

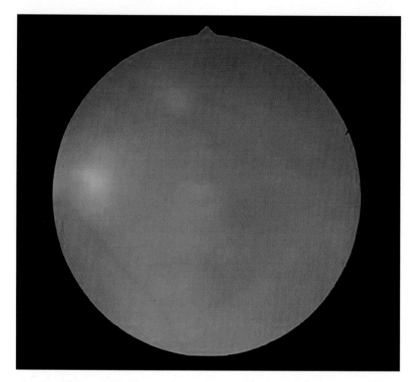

Fig 2 Vitreous haemorrhage: the optic disc can just be seen through a diffuse vitreous haze caused by red cells. With a dense haemorrhage the red reflex may be entirely obscured.

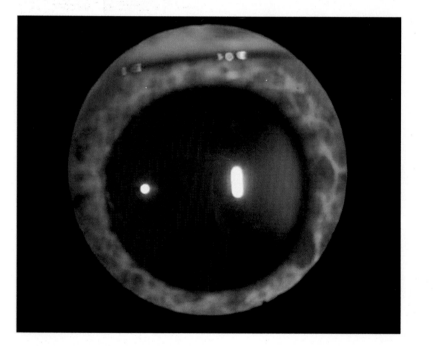

Fig 3 A horizontally subluxed lens, which can be seen following blunt trauma, or in Marfan syndrome (where the lens normally subluxes upwards) or homocystinuria (where it normally goes downwards).

patient to look beyond you and maintain fixation on a distant object. It is also important to approach from a slightly temporal direction, which means that the optic disc is easily identified and sharp focus on it is possible. If you approach the eye straight on, the pupil will constrict and the rather featureless retina at the macula may be difficult to identify.

> Once the optic disc is identified it should be systematically assessed for colour, swelling, cupping, haemorrhage, venous pulsation (often present, so try to count the pulse), neovascularisation and pigmentation (Figs 4 and 5).

> Next follow the four main vascular arcades peripherally (temporal and nasal, above and below) assessing vessel calibre and regularity, and arteriovenous (AV) crossing changes for AV nipping, while also looking for neovascularisation or vascular occlusion. Cotton-wool spots are most frequently seen between vascular branches along the major arcades or close to the optic disc (Fig 6).

> Next, examine the macula looking for the normal bright light reflex from the fovea, while also assessing any pigmentary change (Fig 7), haemorrhage or hard exudates. Subtle macular changes may not be readily seen with the direct ophthalmoscope.

> Finally, examine the more peripheral retina in all quadrants by asking the patient to look up and down, and right and left.

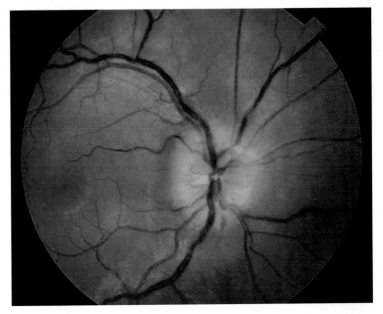

Fig 4 Optic disc swelling. If vision is normal, this may be papilloedema secondary to raised intracranial pressure; if vision is reduced, an acute optic neuropathy is likely.

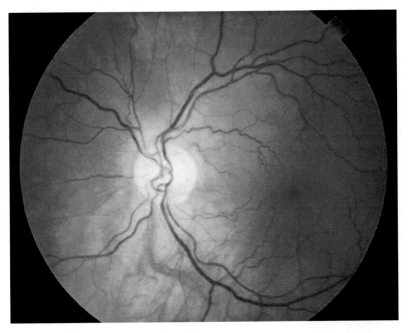

Fig 5 Optic disc atrophy. This may follow a course of optic nerve swelling secondary to either a compressive lesion, papilloedema (swelling secondary to raised intracranial pressure), inflammation (eg optic neuritis) or ischaemia. Hereditary optic neuropathies may result in atrophy in addition to ischaemic insults to the retina such as central retinal artery occlusion.

Key point

Use the green filter ('red-free') on the ophthalmoscope to give better contrast, especially when examining for diabetic retinopathy or vascular changes – it will mean fine red structures are more clearly defined.

Dilatation of pupils

Key point

Indications for dilatation of the pupils

Examination of the fundus of the eye is complete only if the pupil is dilated. It is possible to examine the optic disc through an undilated pupil, particularly if the room is dark, but the macula or more peripheral retina will not be seen adequately.

Hazard

Contraindications to pupil dilatation for fundoscopy:

> patients with acute head injury or those in a coma, in whom it is important to observe serial neurological signs that include pupil size and reactivity

> patients at risk of acute angle-closure glaucoma, if an inappropriate dilating agent is used (see below).

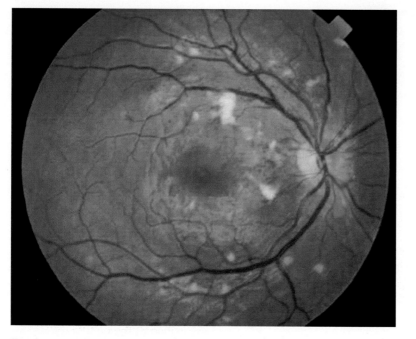

Fig 6 Cotton-wool spots. These represent retinal microinfarcts, scattered between branches of major retinal vessels.

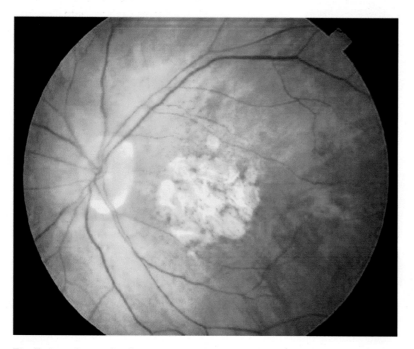

Fig 7 Atrophy at the fovea in age-related macular degeneration. Pigmentation may also be found.

Before dilatation

Before dilating the pupils, assess and record the pupil reactions – including the relative afferent responses. Patients should be warned of the following:

> Near vision especially will be blurred for about 2 hours.

> Bright lights may be uncomfortable.

> Driving is not advisable.

> If they develop eye pain or discomfort, they should phone back immediately or attend an eye emergency department.

Choice of dilating agent

The various dilating agents that can be used are shown in Table 1. For diagnostic purposes, tropicamide drops are ideal: 1% for adults and 0.5% for children. They block the parasympathetic terminals in the pupillary constrictor muscle. A brown iris dilates more slowly than a blue one, and its dilatation is more prolonged; in very dark eyes cyclopentolate 1% drops can be used, but the patient should be warned to expect a more sustained blurring of vision. Phenylephrine 2.5% drops stimulate the sympathetic system and act synergistically with tropicamide to enable maximum pupil dilatation. However, phenylephrine should be used with caution both in children and in adults with ischaemic heart disease, because it may induce hypertension, exacerbate angina or cause arrhythmias as a result of its sympathomimetic action when absorbed.

The procedure

One or two drops are placed in the lower conjunctival fornix of each eye and 15–20 minutes allowed for the

Table 1	Dilating drops		
Agent	**Mode of action**	**Duration (hours)**	**When to use**
Tropicamide 1%	Parasympathetic block	2–4	Adult
Tropicamide 0.5%	Parasympathetic block	2–4	Child
Cyclopentolate 1%	Parasympathetic block	6–8	Very dark iris
Phenylephrine 2.5%	Sympathomimetic	2–4	Full examination of peripheral retina, or photography
Phenylephrine 10%	Sympathomimetic	2–4	Very dark iris

pupils to dilate. Tropicamide drops sting: if children are reluctant to allow drops to be put directly into their eyes, lie the child down, place a drop at the inner corner of each closed eye and wait. The child will always open the eye and so the drop rolls in with minimum fuss.

Complications

Dilatation of the pupil can precipitate acute (angle-closure) glaucoma in susceptible eyes, but this is rare, occurring in less than one in 1,000 patients and lower with tropicamide than cyclopentolate. The onset of acute glaucoma is during the recovery phase of pupil dilatation, usually several hours after the drops have been instilled. Eyes at risk are typically long-sighted (hypermetropic), with spectacle lenses that are convex and magnifying. These eyes have shallow anterior chambers and are predisposed to obstruction of the drainage angle between the iris and cornea when the pupil is mid-dilated hence the alternative term – angle-closure glaucoma. Shallowing of the anterior chamber can also occur as a result of the progressive enlargement of the lens with age, particularly if there are any coexisting cataracts. Short-sighted (myopic) eyes are not predisposed to acute glaucoma. Patients with known chronic or primary open-angle glaucoma may be safely dilated.

1.2 Brief clinical consultations

1.2.1 Gradual loss of vision: age-related macular degeneration

Scenario

Mr Smith, a 73-year-old man, has been admitted to the medical assessment unit after he fell without an apparent cause. He has complained of poor vision, which he says had been getting worse for some time. What is the likely cause of this visual problem?

Introduction

Gradual painless loss of vision often implies a degenerative rather than a pure inflammatory or vascular aetiology. That said, visual loss secondary to vascular retinopathies such as those associated with diabetes may appear to be gradual as a result of slowly increasing macular oedema.

It is important to establish whether the visual loss is central, peripheral or involves the entire visual field. The commonest cause of central, gradual, visual loss in older people is age-related macular degeneration (AMD) However, patients with diabetic retinopathy may also experience gradual central visual

loss if they develop progressive macular oedema. Peripheral visual loss may be suggestive of a rare retinal dystrophy such as retinitis pigmentosa. However, retinitis pigmentosa typically occurs in younger individuals with symptoms suggestive of night blindness (nyctalopia) as a result of degeneration of the rod photoreceptors. Patients suffering from macular dystrophies, by contrast, may also experience symptoms similar to those with AMD, but the onset typically occurs in a much younger age group. A further distinction between dystrophic conditions and AMD is that the former are often hereditary, which may be identified in the history.

Glaucoma may also present with gradual visual loss. Unlike macular degeneration, the visual loss tends to affect the mid-peripheral visual field before affecting central vision. Moreover, ophthalmoscopy would reveal bilateral cupped optic discs (see Fig 8). However, it is noteworthy that glaucoma may exist alongside AMD since the incidence of both of these conditions increases with age.

Beginning the encounter

Doctor: hello my name is Dr A. I understand that your vision has been getting worse for some time, is that right?

Patient: *yes*

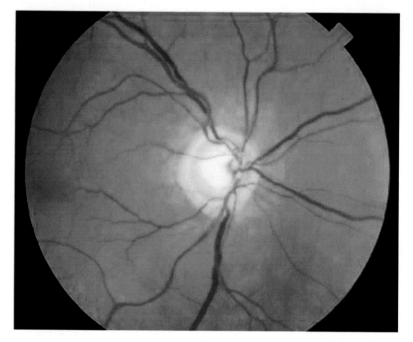

Fig 8 A cupped optic disc in a patient with glaucoma: the peripheral rim of the disc is narrow and pale and the central cup is wide.

Doctor: before we get onto the details of that, can you tell me if you have any major medical problems? Any problems with diabetes?

Patient: [gives list (with doctor politely but firmly discouraging lengthy detail).]

Doctor: are you on any tablets or medications?

Patient: [gives details (and will probably have been asked to produce a written list).]

These introductory questions will provide useful clinical context and may immediately give a clue to the likely diagnosis eg are there any medical conditions (such as diabetes) or drugs (such as hydroxychloroquine) that may be contributing to the patient's visual symptoms.

Focused history

Doctor: please tell me what you mean by 'poor vision'? Did the problem come on suddenly or gradually? [The scenario suggests that it was gradual in this case, but it's important to check information.]

Doctor: do you have spectacles, and does your vision improve if you wear them? Does the problem affect your central vision, peripheral vision or both? Are both of your eyes affected and, if so, are they affected to the same extent?

Doctor: have you had any pain in your eyes?

Doctor: have you ever had a problem with your eyes in the past?

Doctor: is there a family history of eye disease?

Doctor: do you smoke? Do you drive?

> It is important to establish what the patient means by 'poor vision' and whether this improves when they wear spectacles (if they have them). Failure to improve implies a structural cause to account for their symptoms. Distorted vision is suggestive of a maculopathy. Quite often, affected patients will comment on the fact that objects with straight edges appear kinked or wavy. This is secondary to disruption of the regular arrangement of the photoreceptors within the macular area.

Key point

Painless, gradual, central visual loss in the absence of any anterior segment problems in older patients is highly suggestive of a maculopathy. Generalised visual loss, by contrast, suggests involvement of the whole retina or severe optic nerve disease.

> The patient's previous ocular history may be relevant, such as previous trauma, inflammation (choroiditis resulting in retinochoroidal scars) or treatment (such as laser photocoagulation for diabetic retinopathy).

> It is important to acquire a smoking history since this has a deleterious effect on the retinal vasculature and can exacerbate known retinal diseases such as AMD.

Key point

It is always important to establish whether or not the patient drives since they may not meet the standard to perform this task, necessitating notification to the regulatory authorities (Driver and Vehicle Licensing Agency (DVLA) in the UK).

Focused examination
Ophthalmic examination
Check the following:

> Visual acuity – assess using the Snellen chart provided, or with the most appropriate written material available. The patient should wear their distance (not reading) glasses. If they do not have these with them, then vision should be tested using a pinhole occluder, which should be provided and would simulate the vision achieved with glasses. The Snellen chart used will be scaled to be

tested at a reduced distance, but will equate to a 6-metre standard. It is important to establish the distance that the chart is scaled to (usually 3 metres). For example, if the patient is able to read the top letter designed to be read at 3 metres, this would equate to 6/60, which implies that what the patient can read at 6 metres, another person with normal vision would be able to read at 60 metres. If the patient is unable to read the letters at the distance required, then bring the chart closer (1 metre) and reassess. If the patient is still unable to discern the letters at this new distance then the next approach is to assess the patient's ability to count fingers, recognise hand movements or perceive light in order of severity of visual loss.

> Visual fields – via confrontation (see *Clinical Skills for PACES*).

> Pupil assessment (see *Clinical Skills for PACES*) – if the pupils are fixed and dilated then the examiners have instilled a mydriatic to enable you to examine the ocular fundus. If the pupils are not dilated and the visual loss is monocular, it important to assess for a relative afferent pupillary defect (RAPD).

> Ocular fundoscopy – Use a direct ophthalmoscope as described earlier. Look at the appearance of the optic disc before systematically examining the retinal vasculature and maculae.

Mr Smith's left ocular fundus finding is illustrated in Fig 7. The right ocular fundus displayed a similar appearance.

Questions from the patient

[On the assumption that Mr Smith's left ocular fundus was as illustrated in Fig 7, and the right ocular fundus displayed a similar appearance:]

Patient: why is my vision poor?

Doctor: when I shone a light to examine the back of your eyes, there appeared to be some age-related changes affecting a region known as the macular area. The macula contains many complex cells that are vital in allowing us to see fine detail and colour. The condition is known as macular degeneration.

Patient: is there any treatment?

Doctor: I'm not sure, and we need to get specialist help to find out. There are two forms of macular degeneration – a wet and a dry type. Although the wet form of the disease is potentially more aggressive, there is a treatment available which involves injections delivered locally into the eye by an eye specialist. At the moment there is no treatment to reverse the changes related to the dry form of the disease.

Patient: what's the next step to find out what's wrong?

Doctor: it is important that I refer you to see an eye specialist to investigate this further, and I will refer you to them now, during this admission. They will be able to perform more sophisticated tests to examine your eyes and work out which type of macular degeneration you have.

Questions from the examiner

Examiner: can you tell me more about macular degeneration?

Doctor: macular degeneration is the commonest cause of sight impairment in the Western world. There are two forms – dry (atrophic) and wet (exudative). The dry form is more common and results in slow deterioration of central vision. The wet form can result in a rapid visual loss as result of leakage of fluid or blood from choroidal neovascularisation. These are abnormal blood vessels that invade the retina through degenerative layers underlying the retina.

Examiner: why did you suggest that this patient be reviewed during his admission? Wouldn't a routine *ophthalmological outpatient appointment suffice?*

Doctor: although Mr Smith has signs that are highly suggestive of dry macular degeneration, further investigation sometimes reveals that the patient's condition is transforming into the wet form of the disease, making them eligible for intravitreal treatment [the ophthalmologist may employ rapid sophisticated techniques such as optical coherence tomography, see Section 3.1, to establish the true nature of the condition].

Further discussion

Choroidal neovascularisation consists of a blood vessel complex that extends through a membrane underneath the retina known as Bruch's membrane into the space underneath either the retinal pigment epithelium or the retina itself. Macular degeneration is the commonest association. Other conditions that can lead to choroidal neovascularisation include myopic degeneration (retinal degeneration associated with high degrees of short-sightedness) and inflammation. The neovascular complex may result in haemorrhage, leakage of fluid or exudates resulting in irreversible fibrosis and loss of vision.

Treatment consists of injecting a vascular endothelial growth factor (VEGF) antagonist into the vitreous cavity in an attempt to shrink the neovascular complex and reverse some of its sequelae. The treatment has a short-lived effect, necessitating either monthly or bi-monthly injections in most patients. Unsurprisingly, the prognosis is better for those patients treated early, hence the importance of detecting cases as soon as is practicable. The same injections are employed in the treatment of macular oedema secondary to other vascular aetiologies such as diabetes and retinal vein occlusion.

1.2.2 Reduced vision in a diabetic

Scenario

Ms Kennedy, a 35-year-old woman with type 1 diabetes, has been admitted to a general medical ward for treatment for cellulitis affecting her left foot. Her left vision has been poor since she was a child, but she has become concerned during her admission that the vision in her right eye has reduced. What is the likely cause of the problem with her right eye?

Introduction

Diabetes mellitus may cause a plethora of ophthalmic manifestations. These are listed in Table 2.

Diabetic retinopathy is the commonest and most serious ocular complication associated with diabetes. Duration of diabetes is positively correlated with the incidence and prevalence of diabetic retinopathy and is the most important risk factor. Poor diabetic control is positively correlated with the severity of retinopathy, especially in patients with type 1 diabetes. Pregnancy, in particular, may be associated with a rapid progression in diabetic retinopathy. The risk appears to be increased in those women whose condition was poorly controlled pre-pregnancy, whose control was exerted too rapidly during the early stages of pregnancy, and if there is coexisting pre-eclampsia. Hypertension and diabetic nephropathy are also associated with a greater risk of developing severe retinopathy.

Beginning the encounter

Doctor: hello my name is Dr A. I understand that the vision in your right eye has deteriorated, is that right?

Patient: yes

Table 2 Ophthalmic complications of diabetes

Common	Uncommon	Rare
Retinopathy	Accelerated age-related cataract	Diabetic papillopathy (swelling of optic nerve)
Unstable refraction	Neovascular glaucoma	Pupillary light near dissociation
	Recurrent styes	Acute onset cataract
	Ocular motor nerve palsies	
	Reduced corneal sensitivity	

Doctor: before we get onto the details of that, can you tell me how long you have been diagnosed with diabetes and tell me more about it? And do you have any other medical problems?

Patient: [gives list (with doctor politely but firmly discouraging lengthy detail).]

Doctor: are you on any tablets or medications?

Patient: [gives details (and will probably have been asked to produce a written list).]

These introductory questions will provide useful clinical context and may immediately give a clue to the likely diagnosis (eg if her diabetes is poorly controlled this may lead to worsening retinopathy or refractive changes as a result of osmotic changes relating to her crystalline lens).

Focused history

Doctor: I understand that the vision in your left eye has been poor for a long time. Please tell me more about that – when were you first aware of it? [The scenario says since childhood.] Did you receive any surgery or patching of your good eye to try and improve the vision in your bad eye?

Doctor: now tell me about the right eye – how is the vision affected? Does it fluctuate? Is it affected at all distances? [Ms Kennedy reports that distance vision is affected more than near vision.]

Doctor: have you attended your retinal screening appointment lately, or are you under the care of an eye specialist at the hospital already? [If the answer to the latter is yes:] have you received any laser treatment to your eyes?

Doctor: do you drive? [see Section 1.2.1]

Focused examination

Ophthalmic examination
Check the following:

> visual acuity – as in Section 1.2.1

> visual fields – via confrontation (see *Clinical Skills for PACES*)

> pupil assessment (see *Clinical Skills for PACES*) – as in Section 1.2.1

> ocular fundoscopy – as in Section 1.2.1. Look in particular for signs of diabetic retinopathy.

Questions from the patient

[On the assumption that findings in Ms Kennedy were that vision in her right eye was 6/36, but improved to 6/6 with a pinhole; that she was able to read small print at 30 cm; and that ophthalmoscopy revealed some microaneurysms within the macular area and occasional haemorrhages and hard exudates. She could perceive hand movements in the left eye. She had never received laser treatment.]

Patient: what is the problem?

Doctor: after looking at the back of your eyes, I can see some changes relating to diabetes, but this does not explain the reason why your vision is reduced for long distances since you saw much better when I asked you to view the letters through the small pinholes. I therefore suspect that, as a result of your current diabetic control, your lens has altered, making you short-sighted, especially as you were able to read the small print close to you.

Patient: am I going to go blind?

Doctor: no, I don't think so … I think you have become temporarily short-sighted owing to the fact that your diabetic control is not very good – the sugar levels in the blood affect the lens of the eye. As your diabetic control improves, I am confident that your distance vision will improve, but since I can also see some changes at the back of your right eye relating to your diabetes, which is your only seeing eye, I will arrange for you to see an eye specialist soon.

Patient: can I carry on driving?

Doctor: no, at the moment I don't think that would be sensible, for your own safety and that of others. You should cease driving until you have seen the eye specialist.

Questions from the examiner

Examiner: does she need to be seen by an ophthalmologist as she is able to see 6/6 with a pinhole?

Doctor: although her vision improves with a pinhole suggesting a refractive change, the fact that I could observe haemorrhages and hard exudates within the right macular area makes

me suspicious of early diabetic maculopathy. Since she has only one seeing eye as a result of left amblyopia, and that my view of her macula is only two-dimensional, I would prefer that she is reviewed by an ophthalmologist. The ophthalmologist would be able to visualise her macula in a three-dimensional fashion (and hence identify subtle macular oedema) and perform specialised tests such as an optical coherence tomography [see Section 3.1] to categorise further. In addition, the ophthalmologist could arrange for her to undergo formal refraction to confirm my suspicions and put the patient's mind at rest.

Examiner: assuming that the vision in her right eye is corrected to 6/6, is she able to drive with one eye?

Doctor: I'd want to get specialist advice on this, but I think the answer is yes. As long as she can read a car number plate at 20 metres or have a visual standard of at least 6/12 in her best eye, with a normal visual field, then she is eligible to drive from an ophthalmological perspective.

Further discussion

Patients with diabetes are invited to attend a retinopathy screening examination on an annual basis as part of the NHS Diabetic Eye Screening programme. During this assessment, the patient's visual acuities are measured and they have digital ocular fundus photographs which are subsequently graded by trained healthcare professionals such as optometrists or medical photographers, supervised by a consultant ophthalmologist. Patients with mild, non-proliferative diabetic retinopathy are suitable for screening, including patients with haemorrhages within the macula as long as the visual standard is greater than 6/12.

Key point

Refractive changes are not uncommon in patients with unstable diabetes. This is often attributed to osmotic imbalances affecting the crystalline lens or the patient's cornea. The most common scenario is that the patient becomes temporarily myopic (short-sighted). As a result, patients may comment on the fact that their vision is blurred for the distance only, which often improves following improvement in glucose control.

1.2.3 Sudden loss of vision: giant cell arteritis

Scenario

Mr Davis, a 75-year-old man, has attended the emergency department after he lost vision in his left eye suddenly for approximately 20 minutes. He has been diagnosed with polymyalgia rheumatica 2 months previously by his general practitioner (GP). He has been told that he has suffered a stroke. What is your diagnosis?

Introduction

Patients with acute loss of vision need to be talked through the event in order to unearth those exact details that will provide the diagnosis. The following are important differentials:

> Amaurosis fugax – this represents a transient loss of vision that is usually complete and affects one eye. The period of visual loss rarely lasts more than 30 minutes and is sudden in onset. It is often referred to as a

retinal transient ischaemic attack (TIA) and involves the ipsilateral carotid vasculature or one of its branches. Although the cause is often embolic, it is important to recognise that vasculitides may present in a similar fashion. Other causes of transient, unilateral loss of vision include retinal vasospasm, which may or may not be accompanied by a migraine attack. These patients are often younger than those suffering from a TIA and the diagnosis is one of exclusion.

> Arterial occlusion – patients present with sudden, painless visual loss. The visual loss is complete if the central retinal artery is involved or partial if it involves a branch of one of the arterioles. Although emboli are the commonest cause, vasculitides may also cause such devastating visual loss. The condition is often referred to as a retinal stroke.

> Retinal vein occlusion – this may result in a relatively acute loss of vision, but not as abrupt as the loss experienced with its arterial counterpart. Patients often notice visual loss on waking up.

> Vitreous haemorrhage – this should always be considered in a patient with diabetes who presents with acute, painless visual loss associated with floaters.

> Retinal detachment – patients who are myopic (short-sighted), have previously undergone intraocular surgery (eg cataract surgery), or have a collagen vascular disorder such as Marfan or Stickler's syndromes, are at risk of developing this condition in which the visual loss is often preceded by flashes and floaters.

> Migraine equivalent – possible homonymous loss, a geometric pattern, persistence with the eyes closed, and scintillation all suggest a migraine equivalent, even if a headache is not a feature (acephalgic migraine). The visual disturbance tends to migrate in keeping with cortical depression experienced in migraine.

Beginning the encounter

Doctor: hello my name is Dr A. I understand that you suddenly lost the vision in your left eye, is that right?

Patient: yes

Doctor: before we get onto the details of that, can you tell me more about the polymyalgia rheumatica and if you have any other major medical problems?

Patient: [gives list (with doctor politely but firmly discouraging lengthy detail).]

Doctor: are you on any tablets or medications?

Patient: [gives details (and will probably have been asked to produce a written list).]

These introductory questions will provide useful clinical context and may immediately give a clue to the likely diagnosis (eg are there any cardiovascular risk factors that may predispose to the patient's symptoms).

Focused history

Key point

Sudden monocular visual loss in an older patient is due to giant cell arteritis until proved otherwise.

Doctor: tell me about the problem with your left eye – what happened? Was the visual loss sudden and complete? Did you have any pain?

Doctor: have you been suffering from headaches? [If the answer is yes, take a focused headache history ascertaining character, location, relieving and exacerbating factors.] Have you had any problems chewing your food, and if so, in what way? [There is a need to differentiate symptoms suggestive of claudication, when pain develops over time, from those indicating structural problems such as temporomandibular joint disease, when there is pain on initiating movement.]

Doctor: have you had any similar episodes before? Any problems with your speech? Any associated weakness in either your arms or legs?

Doctor: do you drive?

Focused examination

Ophthalmic examination

Check the following:

> visual acuity – as in Section 1.2.1

> visual fields – via confrontation (see *Clinical Skills for PACES*)

> pupil assessment (see *Clinical Skills for PACES*) – as in Section 1.2.1

> ocular fundoscopy – as in Section 1.2.1. Look in particular for emboli (suggestive of atherosclerotic disease) and signs of optic disc swelling (its presence may be suggestive of giant cell arteritis).

Hazard

The ocular fundi of patients presenting with amaurosis are often normal in appearance.

Cardiovascular assessment

> Check temporal artery pulses for tenderness and pulsatility.

> Check blood pressure in each arm (ask the examiner for a result).

> Auscultate the carotids (is there a bruit?) and heart (murmurs and pulse – is it irregularly irregular?).

Questions from the patient

[On the assumption that Mr Davis gave a history of recent headaches in addition to that of polymyalgia:]

Patient: have I suffered from a stroke doctor?

Doctor: no, I don't think so, but losing your vision temporarily suggests that you may have a problem with the blood supply to your eye. We often describe this as a transient ischaemic attack or TIA for short, but in your case I need to perform some other tests as you also complained of headaches and have a history of polymyalgia, which is also likely to be relevant. I think you may have a condition known as giant cell arteritis, which causes inflammation of the blood vessels.

Patient: is that serious?

Doctor: yes, it is a serious problem. I intend to keep you in hospital and perform some blood tests urgently. Depending on the results of these I can commence you on the correct treatment, which is steroids, while you are in hospital. Starting treatment will significantly reduce the risk of losing your sight, which is one of the risks of this condition. I will also arrange for you to undergo a biopsy of one of your arteries, but I can commence treatment before you have a biopsy.

Patient: am I going to be blind?

Doctor: I hope not, but that is the main risk of giant cell arteritis and why I want to get the relevant tests done straight away, and start you on treatment without delay if they support my suspicion of the diagnosis.

Questions from the examiner

Examiner: when do you investigate patients for giant cell arteritis?

Doctor: giant cell arteritis is rare in patients under the age of 50. Patients over this age who have new onset headaches associated with scalp tenderness, and particularly with tenderness over one of the branches of the cranial arteries, would make me suspicious. Other symptoms that are suggestive include jaw and tongue claudication, general malaise with or without unintentional weight loss and symptoms suggestive of polymyalgia rheumatica. There are numerous ocular symptoms associated with giant cell arteritis including sudden loss of vision due to either involvement of the optic nerve or the central retinal artery [as in this case], double vision or transient loss of vision. Some of these symptoms can occur in the absence of systemic symptoms, so it is important to investigate such patients in the same manner as those who do have systemic symptoms.

Examiner: what investigations would you choose?

Doctor: I would request urgent blood tests in the first instance – the most important of which would be a full blood count (FBC) [looking for a normocytic anaemia and thrombocytosis], C-reactive protein (CRP) and erythrocyte sedimentation rate (ESR) [both of which would be expected to be raised – especially the CRP]. I would also request a temporal artery biopsy.

Examiner: how would you manage a patient in whom you suspect the diagnosis of giant cell arteritis?

Doctor: if the blood tests are supportive in a patient with visual symptoms, jaw or tongue claudication, I would commence the patient on intravenous methylprednisolone straight away. I would continue this for 3 days before switching to oral prednisolone. In patients who have other symptoms,

I would prescribe oral prednisolone (1 mg/kg). I would also arrange a referral to a rheumatologist.

Examiner: would you wait for the temporal artery biopsy before starting treatment?

Doctor: no, not if the patient had visual symptoms, jaw or tongue claudication.

Further discussion

Symptoms suggestive of complicated giant cell arteritis include evolving visual loss, jaw and tongue claudication. Symptoms of uncomplicated giant cell arteritis include headaches, scalp tenderness, symptoms of polymyalgia rheumatica, scalp tenderness and constitutional symptoms (weight loss, loss of appetite, fatigue and fevers). Although not evidence based, the British Society for Rheumatology and British Health Professionals in Rheumatology guidelines suggest treating complicated giant cell arteritis with intravenous methylprednisolone at the outset before switching to oral prednisolone.

 Key point

Eye manifestations of giant cell arteritis include the following:

> anterior ischaemic optic neuropathy

> posterior ischaemic optic neuropathy

> arterial occlusion (central retinal, cilioretinal or, rarely, branch retinal)

> amaurosis fugax

> diplopia (secondary to involvement of the cranial nerves or brainstem)

> ocular ischaemic syndrome (low eye pressure, ischaemic uveitis, retinal haemorrhages).

Temporal artery biopsy remains the gold standard test and should ideally be performed within a week of commencing corticosteroids to reduce the risk of acquiring a false negative result. The use of temporal artery ultrasound appears to be a promising alternative if employed within a few days of commencing corticosteroids.

> **Hazard**
> A trial of corticosteroids is not sufficient for diagnosis of giant cell arteritis: it doesn't discriminate between other inflammatory causes and is associated with significant toxicity when administered for a protracted time period (patients with giant cell arteritis require treatment for at least 18 months, and often longer).

1.2.4 Headaches and swollen optic discs

> **Scenario**
> Ms Rogers, a 30-year-old woman, has been referred to the emergency department for urgent assessment. She has been complaining of headaches and intermittent blurred vision, and her GP thought that her optic discs looked abnormal. What is the likely diagnosis and what management would you recommend?

Introduction

Ophthalmoscopy can identify that a person's optic disc/s is/are swollen, but the cause cannot be established via the appearance alone. The term papilloedema is reserved for optic disc swelling secondary to raised intracranial pressure.

Raised intracranial pressure (ICP) may be identified radiologically (space-occupying lesion or cerebral venous thrombosis) or, in the absence

of such radiological features, measurement of the cerebrospinal fluid (CSF) pressure via a lumbar puncture (LP) in the lateral decubitus position, with a reading of ≥ 25 cm H_2O confirming the diagnosis. In the absence of these features, the term optic disc swelling should be used. Patients with swollen optic discs always require investigation.

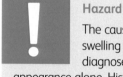

> **Hazard**
> The cause of optic disc swelling cannot be diagnosed by the appearance alone. History, serological, radiological and (where appropriate) CSF investigations are required.

Some of the common causes of apparent optic disc swelling are listed in Table 3.

Other causes of optic disc swelling include optic nerve tumours, infiltration (eg lymphoma), infections (eg syphilis), drugs (eg ethambutol) and hereditary optic neuropathies (eg mitochondrial disorders such as Leber's optic neuropathy).

Establishing whether or not the optic disc is truly swollen often requires further investigations performed by an ophthalmologist, such as optical coherence tomography and ultrasonography of the nerves.

Beginning the encounter

Doctor: hello my name is Dr A. I understand that you've had headaches and a problem with your vision, is that right?

Patient: yes

Doctor: before we get onto the details of that, can you tell me if you have any major medical problems? Any problems with blood pressure or neurological problems like multiple sclerosis?

Patient: [gives list (with doctor politely but firmly discouraging lengthy detail).]

Doctor: are you on any regular tablets or medications? Have you had any courses of medication prescribed recently, such as antibiotics?

Patient: [gives details (and will probably have been asked to produce a written list).]

These introductory questions will provide useful clinical context and may immediately give a clue to the likely diagnosis (eg the oral contraceptive pill and tetracyclines can be associated with raised ICP).

Focused history

Doctor: tell me more about your headaches [ascertain location, character, exacerbating and relieving factors]. Do you ever feel that you can hear your heart beat in your ears or a whooshing sound when you lie down [symptoms suggestive of pulsatile tinnitus]?

Doctor: tell me more about the problem with your eyes. Does it affect one eye or both eyes (and which is worst)? When does it cause you the most difficulty? Have you had to stop doing anything that you used to do? Does your vision ever change? [Patients with papilloedema often notice fluctuations in their vision lasting seconds, termed visual obscurations, with changes in posture or with Valsalva manoeuvres such as coughing.] Have you experienced double vision? [Sometimes the abducens nerve is affected in patients with raised ICP.]

Doctor: have you had any other problems with your nerves – funny feelings, numbness, weakness? Any problems with your arms or legs?

Doctor: tell me more about your weight? Has it increased or decreased lately?

Table 3	Common causes of optic disc swelling
Cause	**Typical features**
Papilloedema	Normal central vision, colour vision and pupil function May have enlarged blind spots on formal visual field examination Symptoms of raised ICP
Optic disc drusen	Common cause of pseudo disc swelling Lumpy appearance. Normal optic nerve function and no symptoms of raised ICP. Often identified by optometrists when patients attend for a routine eye examination
Typical optic neuritis	Reduced central vision (can be severe) associated with pain on eye movements. Reaches a visual nadir over a 2-week period. Defective colour vision (especially red – appears washed out). RAPD is present. The optic disc may be swollen in one-third of typical cases. The vision tends to improve gradually over several weeks in the absence of treatment
Atypical optic neuritis	As above, except no spontaneous visual recovery, may be bilateral, presence of autoimmune disease or recent infection, history of recent vaccination, optic discs invariably appear swollen
Anterior ischaemic optic neuropathy	Sudden loss of vision usually affecting one eye. Pain is not a feature unless there are symptoms of giant cell arteritis. Often affects older individuals with vasculopathic risk factors. Central vision is often affected and a typical visual field defect is altitudinal, affecting either the inferior or superior half of the visual field. Colour vision to reds is often affected (less severe compared with optic neuritis) and a RAPD is present in the affected eye

ICP, intracranial pressure; RAPD, relative afferent pupillary defect.

Focused examination

Ophthalmic examination

Check the following:

> visual acuity – as in Section 1.2.1

> visual fields – via confrontation (see *Clinical Skills for PACES*)

> colour perception – assess in each eye using a red neuro-tip

> pupil assessment (see *Clinical Skills for PACES*) – as in Section 1.2.1

> ocular fundoscopy – as in Section 1.2.1. Note the appearance of the optic disc:

> > do the margins appear clear and well delineated?

> > are the vessels emanating from the disc tortuous and dilated?

> > is there any evidence of haemorrhages or cotton-wool spots?

Neurological assessment

> perform a cranial nerve examination – in particular assess ocular motility

> rapid screening examination of arms and legs.

Cardiovascular assessment

> ask for blood pressure.

Questions from the patient

[On the assumption that the patient has bilateral papilloedema and the most likely diagnosis is idiopathic intracranial hypertension:]

Patient: what is causing my headaches?

Doctor: your symptoms and the fact that the optic nerves at the back of your eyes look swollen make me suspicious that the pressure in your head may be raised. It is impossible to say what is causing this until we have performed some tests, but the most likely diagnosis is a condition known as idiopathic intracranial hypertension. This is something that tends to affect women, especially those who have gained weight.

Patient: what causes it?

Doctor: the honest answer is that we don't know why some people develop raised pressure.

Patient: do I have to stay in hospital? My husband has to go to work and

will find it difficult to look after my son, who's 2 years old.

Doctor: I understand your concern, but I think that you should stay in hospital until we've worked out what's going on. We need to do some blood tests and a brain scan in the first instance, to rule out some important but unlikely causes, and then to perform a procedure known as a lumbar puncture, which involves inserting a needle in your back to measure the pressure in the fluid around your spine. All of these tests can be performed within 24 hours and the results processed very quickly. The sooner we know what the diagnosis is, the sooner we will be able to advise you about what to do. I do not think your hospital stay will need to be very long.

Questions from the examiner

Examiner: what investigations would you request in a patient who presents with headaches and optic disc swelling?

Doctor: headaches in the presence of optic disc swelling is suggestive of raised intracranial pressure until proven otherwise. The most important investigation would be a computerised tomography (CT) brain scan and venogram to look for a space-occupying lesion and cerebral venous thrombosis. I would perform a full blood count and clotting screen to ensure there were no relative contraindications to performing a lumbar puncture, and if the results of neuroimaging were normal, I would proceed with a lumbar puncture to measure the CSF pressure and analyse the constituents (cell count and protein).

Examiner: *assuming that this woman is diagnosed with idiopathic intracranial hypertension, how would you treat her?*

Doctor: I would want specialist advice from a neurologist and an ophthalmologist, but if there isn't an immediate threat to her vision, treatment would include lifestyle advice to promote weight loss, together with medical management such as acetazolamide. Acute visual loss is an indication for performing surgery urgently, either in the form of a shunting procedure or surgery to the optic nerve sheath.

Further discussion

Idiopathic intracranial hypertension
Idiopathic intracranial hypertension or pseudotumour cerebri describes a syndrome characterised by the following:

> raised ICP ($\geq$25 cm H_2O)

> no hydrocephalus on neuroimaging

> no evidence of an intracranial mass lesion or cerebral venous thrombosis

> normal CSF composition.

Cause and differential diagnosis
Although the cause is unknown, it primarily affects young, obese women; hence a patient who presents with headaches and bilateral optic disc swelling who is not obese should be considered to harbour sinister intracranial pathology until proven

Cause	Condition
Mass lesion	Tumour Subdural haematoma Abscess
Obstruction of venous flow	Venous sinus thrombosis Jugular vein compression
Obstructive hydrocephalus	Tumour
Exogenous substances	Antibiotics (tetracyclines) Corticosteroids (particularly withdrawal) Growth hormone Levonorgestrel implants Retinoids (vitamin A, isotretinoin)
Systemic conditions	Anaemia Polycystic ovarian syndrome Obstructive sleep apnoea Malignant (accelerated phase) hypertension
Increased CSF production	Choroid plexus papilloma
Decreased CSF absorption	Arachnoid granulation adhesions after, eg meningitis, subarachnoid haemorrhage
Idiopathic intracranial hypertension	

Table 4 Causes of chronic raised ICP

CSF, cerebrospinal fluid; ICP, intracranial pressure.

otherwise. Other causes of chronic raised ICP are shown in Table 4.

Treatment
The primary goals of treatment are twofold: first, to prevent visual loss, and second, to alleviate headache. If papilloedema remains untreated, the patient will lose vision and the optic disc will become atrophic and appear pale in appearance (Fig 5).

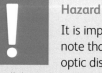

Hazard

It is important to note that atrophic optic discs cannot swell; hence papilloedema will not develop in a patient with previous optic atrophy who develops raised ICP.

Life style – weight loss is advised for obese patients, and may alone result in symptomatic improvement. In those

who struggle to lose weight despite lifestyle changes, bariatric surgery is an alternative.

Medical – carbonic anhydrase inhibitors such as acetazolamide decrease the production of CSF, which leads to a fall in CSF pressure with a concomitant improvement and resolution of papilloedema. If headaches are the predominant symptom, topiramate may be combined with acetazolamide. Topiramate has the added advantage of promoting weight loss in addition to a mild carbonic anhydrase inhibitory affect.

Surgical – in cases where there is acute visual loss or persistent papilloedema refractory to medical management, surgery may be considered. This may include a shunting procedure (ventriculo-peritoneal or lumbo-peritoneal), optic nerve sheath fenestration (a surgical window made in the optic nerve sheath to allow drainage) or intracerebral venous stenting (performed by an interventional radiologist). The rationale behind the latter is that patients with idiopathic intracranial hypertension often harbour at least one narrow cerebral, venous sinus. Stenting the stenosis promotes drainage of CSF which, in turn, leads to a reduction in ICP.

1.2.5 An acutely painful red eye

Scenario

Mr Read, a 25-year-old man, has attended the emergency department because his right eye has become red and increasingly painful over the past 3 days. The eye aches badly, bright light makes the pain worse and his vision has become slightly blurred. What is your diagnosis and what management would you recommend?

Introduction

Photophobia is the term used to describe a painful aversion to bright light. In the context of a patient presenting with a red eye, this usually implies inflammation of the iris musculature as it moves when exposed to different levels of illumination. The iris is under involuntary, autonomic control. When a bright light source is directed at the eye, the sphincter pupillae muscles contract leading to a constriction of the pupil. In the case of a patient presenting with a unilateral red eye, this will also occur when the light is directed to the uninvolved eye (as a result of the consensual response). The pupil may also constrict when focusing on a near object as part of the accommodative reflex.

Key point
Assessing for photophobia

To assess for photophobia in a patient presenting with a unilateral, red eye, shine the light into the uninvolved eye or ask the patient to focus on your finger at a distance of approximately 15 cm. Pain elicited via these two methods suggest photophobia. Photophobia is highly suggestive of significant pathology such as anterior uveitis or corneal ulceration.

Hazard

Danger signals
In the patient with a red eye:

> Pain, photophobia and visual blurring – these are *not* features of a benign condition: the patient requires urgent ophthalmological assessment, including slit-lamp examination.

> Pupil involvement – a semi-dilated pupil is acute glaucoma until proven otherwise and a small (miosed) pupil is acute anterior uveitis until proven otherwise. Both of these conditions require urgent ophthalmological management.

There are many causes of a red eye, some of which are listed in Table 5.

Beginning the encounter

Doctor: hello my name is Dr A. I understand that your right eye has become red and painful, is that right?

Patient: *yes*

Doctor: before we get onto the details of that, can you tell me if you have

any major medical problems? Do you have any problems with arthritis?

Patient: [gives list (with doctor politely but firmly discouraging lengthy detail).]

Doctor: are you on any regular tablets or medications?

Patient: [gives details (and will probably have been asked to produce a written list).]

These introductory questions will provide useful clinical context and may immediately give a clue to the likely diagnosis (eg a history of autoimmune rheumatic or vasculitic disorder).

Focused history

Doctor: have you had any change in vision? [A distinct impairment of vision (the scenario states that in this case the vision is 'slightly blurred') suggests a serious problem and must never be ignored; see Table 5.]

Doctor: has there been any discharge from the eye? [A purulent discharge suggests bacterial conjunctivitis.]

Doctor: tell me more about the pain: what is it like? [Patients with conjunctivitis may complain of grittiness, but they do not have pain. Photophobia is common in corneal diseases and with intraocular inflammation. Pain made worse by reading, which requires accommodation, suggests acute anterior uveitis. Severe pain that radiates to the forehead and often wakes patients from their sleep suggests scleritis.]

Doctor: have you had any problems with your other eye? [Bilateral inflammation suggests a systemic cause.]

Specific questions about symptoms that would be helpful in this case are:

> previous similar episodes – anterior uveitis is often recurrent

> features to suggest a systemic disease – note particularly the presence of erythema nodosum, dysuria or urethral

Table 5   Differential diagnosis of a red eye

	Disease	Discriminating clinical features
Common	Bacterial conjunctivitis	Mucopurulent (yellow and sticky) discharge with normal vision
	Viral conjunctivitis	Watery discharge, preauricular lymphadenopathy, upper respiratory tract infection and discomfort
	Chlamydial conjunctivitis	Conjunctival follicles and recurrent stickiness. Often presents as a chronic, unilateral conjunctivitis that is refractory to topical antibiotics
	Allergic conjunctivitis	Itchy with mucoid discharge (white and stringy). Patient may have an atopic history
	Episcleritis	Discomfort (bruised feeling), sectoral and self-limiting
	Anterior uveitis	Pain, photophobia, visual blurring, irregular pupil and keratic precipitates
Unusual	Scleritis	Pain (may be worse at night) and systemic associations
	Corneal abscess	Soft contact-lens wear or trauma, white corneal infiltrate, pain and blurred vision
Rare	Endophthalmitis	Trauma or eye surgery, IV drug use and poor vision
	Acute glaucoma	Hazy cornea, mid-dilated, unreactive pupil and hard eye

IV, intravenous.

discharge, oral or genital ulceration, joint or back pain, shortness of breath or diarrhoea, and any signs of abnormality in immune status (eg HIV) or intravenous drug use. It is important to enquire about the use of contact lens wear (particularly soft lenses which are worn overnight) in any patient presenting with an acutely painful, red eye owing to the attendant risk of developing bacterial corneal ulceration.

Focused examination

Ophthalmic examination

Check the eye for the following:

> Where is it red? In conjunctivitis or diffuse scleritis the redness may involve the whole of the visible portion of the eye. Redness that is localised around the corneal limbus is suggestive of intraocular inflammation, and sectoral redness is commonly seen in sub-conjunctival haemorrhage, nodular scleritis and episcleritis (see Section 2.2). The conjunctiva may show prominent follicles in chlamydial and viral conjunctivitis.

> Is it sticky? This would suggest conjunctivitis.

> Size and shape of the pupil – in cases of acute anterior uveitis this may be irregular due to the formation of adhesions or the pupil may be small (miosed). In acute (angle-closure) glaucoma it is characteristically mid-dilated and unreactive. A relative afferent pupillary defect always indicates serious retinal or optic nerve disease.

> visual acuity – as in Section 1.2.1

> visual fields – via confrontation (see *Clinical Skills for PACES*)

> colour perception – assess in each eye using a red neuro-tip

> pupil assessment (see *Clinical Skills for PACES*) – as in Section 1.2.1

> ocular fundoscopy – as in Section 1.2.1.

In the absence of systemic symptoms, general examination of the patient is unlikely to give valuable clues.

Key point

In assessing the patient with a red eye, always check the contralateral eye carefully – a systemic cause is more likely if there is simultaneous bilateral inflammation.

Questions from the patient

[On the assumption that the patient seems most likely to have anterior uveitis and they have evidence of bilateral ocular inflammation:]

Patient: *what is causing the problem with my eye?*

Doctor: it looks as though you have got inflammation of the front part of your eye

Patient: *why has it happened?*

Doctor: I'm not sure. Sometimes it can happen for no reason that we can find, but sometimes it can be triggered by infection or by an autoimmune condition, which are conditions where the body seems to react against itself. As well as giving you treatment to cut down the inflammation in the eyes, it will be appropriate to do some tests to find out if there is some underlying cause.

Patient: *what is the treatment?*

Doctor: two sorts of eye drops: steroids to cut down the inflammation, and something to dilate the pupil, which helps relieve the pain and reduces the chances of the inflammation causing the pupil to get stuck to the lens of the eye.

Questions from the examiner

Examiner: *what investigations would you request in a patient who presents with anterior uveitis?*

Doctor: I would want specialist advice from an ophthalmologist, but a patient with a first uncomplicated attack does not need investigation. However, if attacks are recurrent or bilateral – as in this case – then I'd want to look for evidence of a systemic inflammatory process with a test for C-reactive protein (CRP), look for sarcoidosis with a chest X-ray and serum angiotensin-converting enzyme (ACE), look for renal inflammation with a urinary dipstick, check for evidence of tuberculosis (TB) or syphilis if clinically indicated, and check human leukocyte antigen (HLA) type.

Examiner: *why would you check the HLA type?*

Doctor: patients with HLA-B27 are much more likely to get recurrent attacks.

Examiner: *what is likely to happen to the patient's vision?*

Doctor: anterior uveitis normally settles and vision is expected to return to normal.

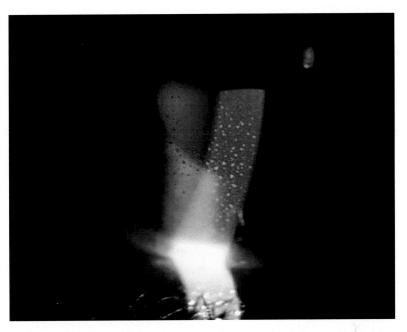

Fig 9 Slit-lamp view shows multiple white keratic precipitates (inflammatory cells) characteristic of iritis. These are deposited in the front chamber from the aqueous, as a sediment on to the inner surface of the cornea.

Further discussion

Specialist assessment of the patient with an acute red eye

This will involve:

> fluorescein staining – to reveal a corneal ulcer

> slit-lamp examination – to look for keratic precipitates (Fig 9), although larger precipitates on the corneal surface can sometimes be seen with a direct ophthalmoscope

> measurement of intraocular pressure – it is mandatory to exclude secondary glaucoma in those with inflammatory disorders of the eye.

Management of the patient with an acute red eye

This depends on the cause. Viral conjunctivitis is most commonly due to RNA viruses and is self-limiting. Herpes simplex corneal disease is treated with topical aciclovir. Episcleritis may be treated with oral non-steroidal anti-inflammatory agents or simply topical lubricants if the symptoms are mild: this is often a self-limiting disease. See Sections 2.1 and 2.2 for discussion of the management of anterior uveitis and scleritis, respectively.

2 Diseases and treatments

2.1 Acute anterior uveitis

Aetiology

Most cases of anterior uveitis are of unknown aetiology: some recognised causes are shown in Table 6.

Clinical presentation

The patient has a red, aching eye with photophobia, which tends to worsen over hours to a few days. Although the vision may be blurred, it is usually not severely affected. The pupil tends to be small (miosed) and may be irregular because the iris has adhered to the anterior lens (posterior synechiae), in which case it festoons on dilatation. There may be symptoms or signs to suggest an underlying cause (Table 6), but this would be unusual. Diagnosis is made by slit-lamp examination (Fig 9), which is essential whenever anterior uveitis is suspected.

Key point

Features of anterior uveitis on slit-lamp examination:

> 'Flare' – leak of protein from inflamed vessels into the anterior chamber makes the fluid in the aqueous look hazy.

> Keratic precipitates – inflammatory cells in the anterior chamber sometimes deposit on the inner surface of the cornea, forming keratic precipitates (Fig 9). Large precipitates are characteristic of granulomatous iritis such as that caused by sarcoid.

> Hypopyon – if the anterior uveitis is severe then inflammatory cells may sediment at the bottom of the anterior chamber, which is characteristic of Behçet's disease or endophthalmitis.

Hazard

Uveitis may only be described as anterior once the posterior segment of the eye (ie all structures behind the crystalline lens) have been examined and deemed to be devoid of inflammation. As a result, all cases of suspected uveitis should undergo a dilated ocular fundus examination by an ophthalmologist.

In the absence of systemic symptoms, general examination of the patient is unlikely to give valuable clues.

Investigation

A first uncomplicated attack of unilateral, acute, anterior uveitis does not require investigation in an otherwise well individual. Investigations are guided by the patient's history, uveitis phenotype and any other systemic features identified on examination. Possible causes are listed in Table 6. Appropriate investigations might include:

> Chest radiograph – looking in particular for evidence of sarcoidosis or tuberculosis.

> Serum C-reactive protein – suggests a systemic inflammatory process if raised.

> Urine dipstick (for haematuria and proteinuria, quantitating proteinuria by urinary albumin:creatinine ratio if present) and renal function – urinary beta-2 microglobulin is often raised in patients presenting with tubulo-interstitial nephritis and uveitis (TINU).

Table 6	Causes of anterior uveitis	
Autoimmune	**Drug induced**	**Infectious**
Ankylosing spondylitis	Rifabutin	Herpes zoster
Sarcoidosis	Cidofovir	Herpes simplex
Behçet's disease		Leptospirosis (uncommon)
Inflammatory bowel disease		Lyme disease
Juvenile chronic arthritis		Syphilis
Psoriatic arthropathy		Tuberculosis
TINU		Leprosy

There is a clear association of anterior uveitis with human leukocyte antigen (HLA)-B27 positivity. The most likely causes of acute anterior uveitis with systemic associations are HLA-B27/spondylitis/sacroiliitis and sarcoidosis.
TINU, tubulo-interstitial nephritis and uveitis.

> Full blood count (FBC), liver and bone profiles – serum calcium may be raised and the lymphocyte count low in sarcoidosis.

> Serum angiotensin-converting enzyme – may be raised in sarcoidosis.

> *Treponema pallidum* serology – uveitis may be the only feature of syphilis.

> Interferon-γ tests for *Mycobacterium tuberculosis* (also a Mantoux test) – indicated in patients suspected of suffering from this infection.

> Test for human leukocyte antigen (HLA)-B27 positivity – this does not influence immediate management, but patients with HLA-B27 are much more likely to experience recurrent attacks.

Treatment

Acute anterior uveitis responds promptly to topical treatment with corticosteroids and mydriatics in the vast majority of cases: drops are preferable by day and ointment by night. A typical regimen would include dexamethasone 0.1% every hour for the first week, together with atropine 1% or cyclopentolate 1% three times daily until review a week later. Although the latter mydriatic agents may blur the patient's vision for reading, they are important in preventing the formation of adhesions between iris and lens (posterior synechiae) while the inflammation is active.

Prognosis

Anterior uveitis often settles without sequelae provided that treatment is not delayed. Vision is expected to return to normal. Repeated attacks are more likely if uveitis is associated with a persistent systemic disease or if the patient is HLA-B27 positive, which carries a 10-fold increased risk of recurrence.

2.2 Scleritis

Aetiology

Scleritis is an inflammatory disease of the vessels supplying the sclera that may be associated with rheumatoid arthritis, systemic vasculitis (especially granulomatosis with polyangiitis) or other autoimmune rheumatic diseases such as relapsing polychondritis.

Clinical presentation

Scleritis may be anterior or posterior. Anterior scleritis may be nodular, diffuse or necrotising. Posterior scleritis may be associated with anterior disease, but can also occur in isolation unassociated with systemic disease.

Pain is the most common symptom of scleritis and is typically severe, worse at night and on eye movement. It typically wakes the patient from his/her sleep. Extreme redness and tearing are other common signs, and photophobia may also be a symptom of anterior scleritis. Such signs and symptoms notwithstanding,

severe necrotising scleritis in patients with vasculitis associated with polyarticular rheumatoid arthritis may occur without preceding pain or redness. Uncommonly, posterior scleritis may present with ocular pain, reduced visual acuity, proptosis, and limitation of extraocular movements despite the eye appearing white.

Key point

When a patient presents with pain in the eye, remember that:

> Severe eye pain that is worse at night is highly suggestive of scleritis.

> Severe, necrotising scleritis associated with rheumatoid arthritis may be painless.

Physical signs

The sclera is usually red and thickened, with dilatation of episcleral vessels (Fig 10). The redness may be localised, as in nodular scleritis, or diffuse.

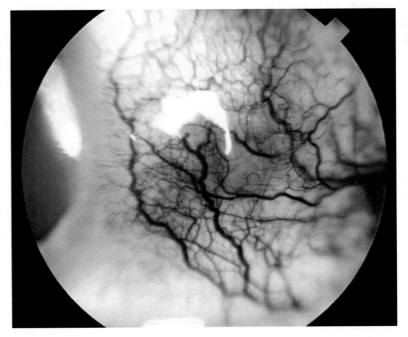

Fig 10 Anterior nodular scleritis before treatment. The episcleral vessels are markedly dilated and the underlying sclera swollen. There is scleral translucency with the underlying darker choroid visible in the centre of the nodule.

There may also be swelling or thinning (Fig 11). Scleral thinning and increased scleral transparency allow the underlying bluish choroid to show through, either after scleritis has healed (Fig 11) or in acutely necrotising scleritis (Fig 12). Full-thickness loss of sclera, called scleromalacia perforans, is usually associated with rheumatoid arthritis and is sight threatening: thankfully this is now rare owing to the early initiation of immunosuppressive treatment.

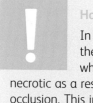

Hazard

In very severe scleritis, the sclera may appear white because it is necrotic as a result of vascular occlusion. This important sign, which can easily be overlooked, is an indication for urgent treatment with systemic corticosteroids.

General examination of the patient will clearly be directed by the history, but should particularly focus on the nose (discharge/bleeding and septal perforation – suggestive of polyangiitis with granulomatosis), ears (deafness or redness/pain – suggestive of relapsing polychondritis), upper respiratory tract (stridor), lungs (any abnormal signs – may be a manifestation of vasculitis, sarcoidosis or rheumatoid arthritis) and joints (in particular for signs suggestive of rheumatoid arthritis).

Investigation

Any associated systemic disease should be identified by:

> urine dipstick – for haematuria and proteinuria (quantitating proteinuria, if present, by urinary albumin creatinine ratio) and renal function

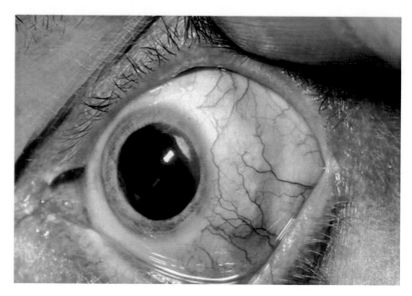

Fig 11 Healed anterior scleritis. After treatment with prednisolone and cyclosporin, the sclera has returned to normal thickness but is more translucent, allowing the darker choroid to show through.

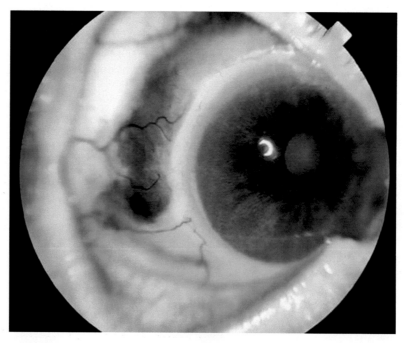

Fig 12 Necrotising scleritis in rheumatoid arthritis (scleromalacia perforans) with full-thickness scleral loss. Only thin conjunctiva and episclera cover the choroid.

> full blood count (FBC), electrolytes, and renal and liver function tests – looking in particular for anaemia of chronic disorders, neutrophilia and impaired renal function

> inflammatory markers – erythrocyte sedimentation rate and C-reactive protein

> serology for autoimmune rheumatic or vasculitic disorders – rheumatoid factor, anti-cyclic citrullinated peptide, antineutrophil cytoplasmic antibody, antinuclear antibody, anti-DNA antibodies, complement (C3 and C4) and immunoglobulin levels

> serology for infectious disorders where appropriate, such as *Treponema pallidum*

> chest radiograph.

Ocular ultrasonography is essential to diagnose posterior scleritis, showing thickening of the posterior eye coat which may also be evident on a CT or magnetic resonance imaging (MRI) of the eye and orbit. Scleral biopsy may be required in the rare event that lymphoma or infection is suspected.

Differential diagnosis

Episcleritis is a mild, non-sight-threatening disease that resolves spontaneously over 6–8 weeks. In contrast to scleritis, pain is not a feature and the redness will usually blanch with phenylephrine drops. Anterior uveitis is usually less painful and the redness is more marked around the cornea. Slit-lamp examination will distinguish these conditions. Rarely, lymphoma may present with scleral inflammation.

Treatment

Key point

Severe or necrotising scleritis requires immediate treatment.

Non-steroidal anti-inflammatory drugs, especially flurbiprofen, may be effective for milder cases, but systemic corticosteroids are frequently required to control the disease and immunosuppressive therapy is immediately essential for severe or necrotising causes of it. Remember:

> Flurbiprofen 100 mg three times daily will produce symptomatic improvement within 48 hours if effective.

> For necrotising or severe disease, prescribe oral prednisolone, 1 mg/kg per day initially, or intravenous pulse methylprednisolone, 500–1,000 mg. Unresponsive disease may require additional immunosuppressive therapy with cyclophosphamide.

> Corticosteroid-sparing treatment may be required if long-term therapy is necessary and the steroid dose cannot be reduced to acceptable maintenance levels. Agents used include methotrexate, mycophenolate mofetil, ciclosporin and azathioprine.

Complications

Complications include keratitis, uveitis, cataract, glaucoma and exudative retinal detachment in posterior scleritis. In rare cases, the globe may perforate.

Prognosis

Of patients with scleritis, 25% lose two or more lines of vision over 3 years, usually as a result of cataract or corneal involvement. Less than 5% of eyes lose useful vision in the longer term.

2.3 Retinal artery occlusion

Aetiology

Retinal arterial occlusion is caused by acute obstruction of the central retinal artery or one of its branches as a result of embolism, or less commonly of thrombosis. It occurs most commonly in the fifth or sixth decade. Associated conditions include carotid vascular disease, diabetes, hypertension, valvular heart disease, arrhythmias (especially atrial fibrillation with left atrial thrombus) and vasculitides (particularly giant cell arteritis). Uncommon causes which need to be considered in younger patients include atrial myxoma, coagulopathies and haemoglobinopathies. Intravenous drug abuse is also an associated factor.

Clinical presentation

Patients present with sudden, painless loss of vision. The visual loss may be transient (amaurosis fugax) or sustained, depending on whether or not arterial blood flow is re-established. Central retinal artery occlusion results in total visual loss and branch occlusion in altitudinal (upper or lower) visual field loss. It is important to realise that involvement of the inferior retina will result in a superior visual field defect and vice versa.

Uncommonly, visual loss may primarily affect the peripheral field with preservation of central vision if the macula is supplied by a cilioretinal artery arising from the short posterior ciliary vessels. Cilioretinal arteries are present in 25–30% of the population. Rarely, the converse situation of cilioretinal artery occlusion with sparing of the central retinal artery can occur.

Physical signs

> Visual acuity is usually profoundly reduced – such as to hand movements, or even to no light perception.

> A relative afferent pupillary defect is present.

> Retinal pallor may be sectoral or generalised; the retinal arteries are attenuated; and a 'cherry-red spot' may be seen at the macula as a result of the underlying choroidal circulation visible through the fovea (Fig 13). Sometimes an embolus may be visible within the arterial lumen, a Hollenhorst plaque (see Fig 14), and/or 'cattle-trucking' of the blood column in the arteries may be seen. In patients harbouring a cilioretinal artery, it may appear patent (Fig 15) or occluded (Fig 16).

A complete cardiovascular examination of the patient is required, looking in particular for arrhythmia (especially atrial fibrillation), hypertension, carotid bruit(s) and cardiac murmurs.

Investigation

> full blood count (FBC), glucose and renal/liver/bone profile

> inflammatory markers – erythrocyte sedimentation rate and C-reactive protein

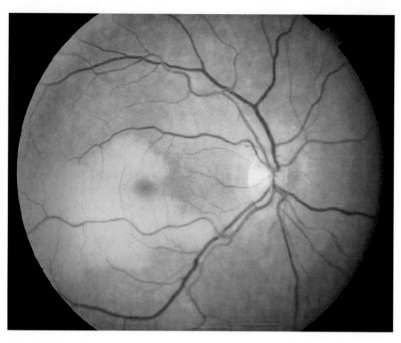

Fig 13 Retinal artery occlusion: the right eye is showing inferotemporal branch retinal artery occlusion with a cherry-red spot and surrounding retinal oedema and pallor. Visual loss is profound and may be total.

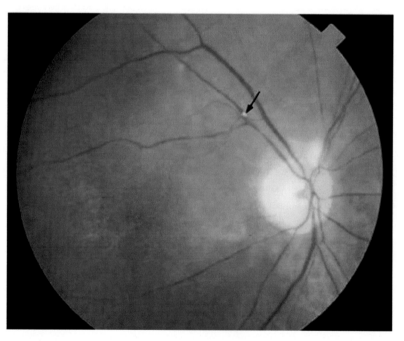

Fig 14 Branch retinal artery embolus (a Hollenhorst plaque): a well-defined refractile opacity is seen in the superotemporal branch artery at the first bifurcation (indicated by the arrow). There is also a cotton-wool spot at the edge of the optic disk at 1 o'clock.

Medical Masterclass Third edition

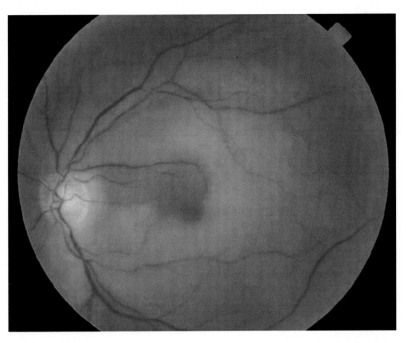

Fig 15 Retinal artery occlusion with macular sparing as a result of a patent cilioretinal artery. The central macula/fovea is perfused, but there is surrounding retinal pallor with oedema that causes a 'cherry-red patch' rather than a 'cherry-red spot'. The visual acuity in this eye recovered to 6/9, but with a permanently restricted peripheral field.

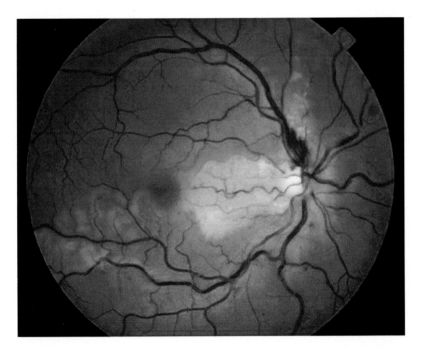

Fig 16 Cilioretinal artery occlusion. This right eye shows retinal oedema between the optic disc and macula, the opposite of Fig 15. Visual acuity is poor and there is a large central scotoma that will persist.

> other tests (eg haemoglobin electrophoresis and coagulation studies) – especially in younger patients with no other identifiable risk factors and as directed by clinical suspicion

> electrocardiogram (ECG) and chest radiograph – looking for arrhythmia or evidence of hypertension or valvular heart disease

> carotid Doppler studies and echocardiography – important in identifying a remediable source of emboli that may also threaten the brain

> fluorescein angiography – may be of value in atypical situations (Fig 17).

Differential diagnosis

The clinical features of a central retinal artery occlusion are difficult to confuse with other causes of acute unilateral visual loss such as a central retinal vein occlusion, retinal detachment or acute ischaemic optic neuropathy.

Treatment

 Hazard

Any treatment undertaken more than an hour after the onset of retinal artery occlusion is unlikely to improve visual recovery and it should be emphasised to patients that any visual improvement is a bonus.

No treatment has been shown to be effective in restoring vision and randomised controlled studies are lacking. Most treatments attempt to improve ocular perfusion either by lowering intraocular pressure or by vasodilatation.

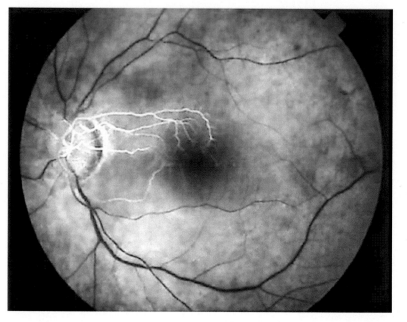

Fig 17 Fluorescein angiogram corresponding to Fig 15. Fluorescein dye, which appears white, fills the central cilioretinal circulation in contrast to the non-perfused retinal arteries and veins, which appear black.

Emergency interventions:

> Ocular massage – may dislodge an embolus if performed in the very early stages, and is easy to do.

> Paracentesis of the anterior chamber – the removal of aqueous humour with an insulin syringe (after instilling povidone–iodine solution) can dramatically reduce intraocular pressure.

Longer-term treatments:

> Address any identifiable risk factors – smoking, hypertension, coagulopathy or hyperlipidaemia.

> Anticoagulate – for embolic thrombus from the heart. If there is no embolic thrombus from the heart then consider clopidogrel or aspirin.

> Carotid stenosis – patients shown to have >70% carotid occlusion should be considered for carotid endarterectomy.

Complications

Long-term ocular complications after retinal artery occlusions are uncommon and much fewer than after retinal vein occlusion. Iris neovascularisation may occur, leading to neovascular glaucoma (see Section 2.4), but retinal neovascularisation is rare. The risk of a similar event in the second eye is very small, unless there is bilateral carotid disease or a cardiac source for emboli.

Prognosis

Of affected eyes, 30% recover visual acuity of 6/60 or better, although 5% have no light perception in the affected eye. Retinal artery occlusion is associated with serious life-threatening conditions that determine the overall mortality.

2.4 Retinal vein occlusion

Aetiology

Retinal vein occlusion occurs when the central retinal vein (central retinal vein occlusion (CRVO)) or one of its branches (branch retinal vein occlusion (BRVO)) become obstructed as a result of thrombosis within the lumen, often preceded by changes within the vessel wall. Hypertension, diabetes, hyperlipidaemia, hyperviscosity syndromes, hypercoagulability and raised intraocular pressure all predispose to this condition. Occlusion within the central vein usually occurs at the optic disc itself, and branch vein occlusion at an arteriovenous crossing.

Epidemiology

Retinal vein occlusion is the second most common retinal vascular disease after diabetic retinopathy.

Clinical presentation

Presenting symptoms result either from the onset of the occlusion or from the development of complications. Vein occlusions are usually unilateral and, if bilateral, rarely simultaneous.

The commonest presentation is with a sudden onset of painless loss of vision. BRVO causes visual loss when the macula is involved. If the macula is spared, the occlusion may be an incidental finding. Painless loss of vision may also arise (uncommonly) from vitreous haemorrhage as a complication of an ischaemic CRVO. A red, painful eye may (rarely) result from the late complication of neovascular (rubeotic) glaucoma.

Physical signs

In CRVO there are widespread flame and blot retinal haemorrhages (Fig 18), often with cotton-wool spots (microinfarcts) throughout the retina. This is in stark contrast to the sectoral distribution observed in BRVO (Fig 19). A relative afferent pupillary defect (RAPD) is indicative of significant retinal ischaemia, as are numerous cotton-wool spots. A BRVO will produce a corresponding visual field defect, but not a RAPD because much of the retina remains perfused and healthy.

Widespread ischaemia (irrespective of cause) leads to up-regulation of vascular endothelial growth factor (VEGF). VEGF acts as a stimulus for new blood growth at the optic disc, retina and iris. Development of new vessels in the former two locations may lead to bleeding and/or tractional retinal detachment, hence a vitreous haemorrhage may be suspected clinically as a result of obscuration of the red-light reflex during ophthalmoscopy (Fig 2).

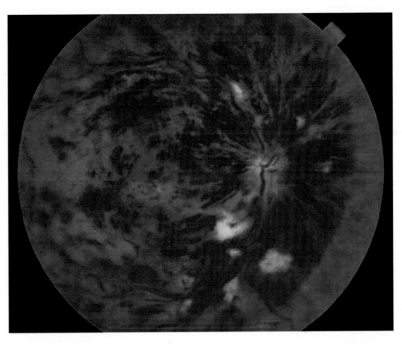

Fig 18 Central retinal vein occlusion with characteristic 'bloodstorm' appearance and cotton-wool spots.

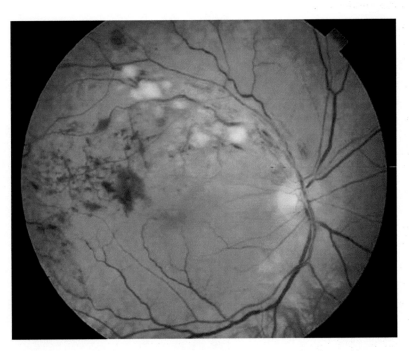

Fig 19 Branch retinal vein occlusion in a sector above the fovea. Vision may be affected, depending on changes at the fovea itself, such as haemorrhage or oedema.

Development of iris neovascularisation may lead to bleeding into the anterior chamber (hyphaema). Subsequent invasion into the anterior chamber angle may lead to obstruction of aqueous outflow resulting in a dramatic increase in intraocular pressure known as neovascular (rubeotic) glaucoma. Since raised intraocular pressure further impedes ocular perfusion, the anterior structures of the eye lose their function. As a consequence, the cornea becomes hazy, the conjunctiva red and the eye extremely hard to palpation.

Patients with retinal vein occlusion are generally those at high risk of atheromatous vascular disease, hence cardiovascular examination is appropriate, looking in particular for hypertension, vascular bruit(s) and at peripheral pulses.

Investigations

These should be directed at establishing the aetiology of the venous occlusion: the younger the patient, the greater the chance of finding a cause. The following tests are recommended as routine:

> full blood count (FBC)

> inflammatory markers – erythrocyte sedimentation rate and C-reactive protein

> blood glucose, electrolytes, renal/liver/ bone and lipid profiles.

The British Society of Haematology does not recommend routine thrombophilia screening in patients presenting with a vein occlusion in the absence of systemic symptoms/signs. Notwithstanding, if the patient has a family history of venous thromboembolic events, or has raised inflammatory markers, then further tests are warranted as follows:

> serum immunoglobulins / protein electrophoresis, urinary Bence–Jones proteins and (if indicated) plasma viscosity

> thrombophilia screen.

Specific ophthalmological investigations include:

> intraocular pressure estimation

> fluorescein angiography – this may be helpful in cases where there is diagnostic uncertainty. It is mainly used to demonstrate the site of occlusion, the degree of retinal ischaemia, and determine the risk of complications (Fig 20).

Differential diagnosis

Characteristic CRVO and BRVO are readily distinguished from most other causes of retinal haemorrhage. Bilateral CRVO is rare and may be mimicked by severe non-proliferative diabetic retinopathy. Myeloproliferative disorders such as Waldenström's macroglobulinaemia may produce retinal changes similar to bilateral CRVO. Hypertensive retinopathy may also need to be considered.

Key point

If you see retinal haemorrhages, always check the blood pressure (BP).

Treatment

Key point

Emergency treatments for retinal vein occlusion, such as haemodilution and anticoagulation, are of no reliable benefit.

Identifiable risk factors should be treated to reduce the risk of systemic complications and retinal vein occlusion in the other eye.

Central retinal vein occlusion

Patients presenting with a central vein occlusion complicated by macular oedema may receive injections of an anti-VEGF agent (which is first line) or corticosteroid into the vitreous of the eye. VEGF is one of the key cytokines that are raised in eyes that have developed a CRVO, and in addition to promoting neovascularisation it mediates vascular leakage leading to macular oedema. Corticosteroids inhibit VEGF to an extent, and they also reduce vascular permeability, but they are

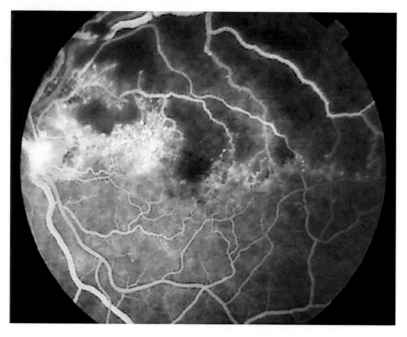

Fig 20 Fluorescein angiography in superior BRVO showing darker areas where there is loss of capillary circulation and profound retinal ischaemia.

associated with more ocular side effects (glaucoma and cataract) and hence are employed either in patients who cannot receive anti-VEGF agents immediately (stroke / myocardial infarction (MI) within the preceding 3 months, or pregnancy) or when anti-VEGF treatment has failed. These agents are usually administered on a monthly basis initially.

For those patients who have developed significant neovascularisation, the aim of treatment is to prevent further sequelae (especially neovascular glaucoma) rather than improve vision. Pan retinal photocoagulation is the treatment of choice in such cases.

Branch retinal vein occlusion

For patients harbouring a BRVO in the absence of macular oedema, observation will suffice. In the presence of macular oedema, patients are offered either intravitreal anti-VEGF agents or corticosteroids. Unlike its CRVO counterpart, macular oedema secondary to BRVO may be amenable to focal laser photocoagulation in selected cases.

Prevention

It is advised that oestrogen-containing hormone replacement therapy and oral contraceptives should not be commenced in women with a history of retinal vein occlusion.

Complications

Permanent visual impairment from macular damage from macular oedema is more common in CRVO than in BRVO, but the disparity has greatly reduced since the advent of local anti-VEGF and corticosteroid therapies. Uncommonly, retinal and iris neovascularisation may occur secondary to significant retinal ischaemia, leading to vitreous haemorrhage and/or neovascular (rubeotic) glaucoma.

Prognosis

The prognosis of BRVO is better than CRVO, with approximately 50% of untreated BRVO versus 20% of untreated CRVO cases retaining a visual acuity standard ≥6/12 after 1 year. The prognosis is much worse in eyes complicated by severe ischaemia, with over 90% having a final visual outcome of 6/60 or worse. Treatment success seems to be positively correlated with early treatment.

Key point
Since early treatment with local therapies may lead to a better long-term visual outcome in patients with CRVO and BRVO, these patients should be seen by an ophthalmologist within 2 weeks for further assessment.

2.5 Optic neuritis

Aetiology

Optic neuritis may present in isolation, but ultimately more than 50% of patients who have it will develop clinical evidence of multiple sclerosis (MS).

Clinical presentation

There is a rapid onset (over a couple of days) of moderate-to-severe loss of vision that is often associated with pain on eye movement. Visual loss may increase during the first week and then slowly recover, although improvement in acuity may be incomplete. Vision may be worse when the patient's body temperature is increased after a hot bath or exertion – Uhthoff's phenomenon.

Rarely, optic neuritis may be bilateral and associated with a transverse myelitis causing paraparesis or paraplegia (neuromyelitis optica). It may also occur 1–3 weeks following a systemic infection (parainfectious optic neuritis), or be secondary to a systemic inflammatory disease such as sarcoidosis.

Key point
The overall risk of developing MS following a single episode of optic neuritis is 50%.

Physical signs

Reduced visual acuity, reduced colour perception (red in particular) and reduced perceived brightness are commonly reported by patients suffering from optic neuritis. A relative afferent pupillary defect is typical in unilateral cases. Although the optic disc may appear swollen (Fig 4), it is important to note that the optic disc will appear normal in two-thirds of cases (a situation in which the examiner sees nothing and the patient nothing at all!). In some cases, the peripheral retinal veins appear to exhibit a whitish outline (sheathing), which indicates coexisting phlebitis (sometimes observed in patients with MS). Although patients with optic neuritis may possess any type of unilateral visual field defect, the central area is often affected.

Patients presenting with signs and symptoms suggestive of optic neuritis should receive a neurological examination looking in particular for evidence of cerebellar or spinal cord disease.

Investigations

Investigation is usually not necessary at first presentation in a previously healthy patient (unless corticosteroid treatment is planned) because the prognosis for visual recovery is good. An MRI may show features suggestive of demyelination and visual evoked potentials may show delay and/or reduction in amplitude. The risk of developing clinically definite MS increases if abnormal white matter abnormalities are detected radiologically.

Differential diagnosis

The main differential to consider is a non-arteritic, anterior ischaemic optic neuropathy, but here the visual loss is usually sudden, painless and often noticed on waking. Furthermore, patients with this condition tend to be older and possess vascular risk factors. Those who also complain of headaches, jaw claudication and/or constitutional symptoms should be considered to be suffering from the arteritic variant and treated and investigated as such. An altitudinal visual field defect affecting either the superior or inferior half of the patient's visual field is typical in anterior ischaemic optic neuropathy.

Nutritional or toxic optic neuropathies such as those caused by ethambutol, amiodarone, linezolid, quinine or vitamin B_{12} deficiency tend to be more insidious in onset and are often bilateral.

If a patient has recently suffered from an infection, a parainfectious optic neuritis may occur. This is more common in children and typically occurs 1–3 weeks after the infected episode.

Treatment

If the visual loss or pain is severe, intravenous methylprednisolone should be administered (1 g/day for 3 days) because it will ensure visual function recovers more rapidly and the pain is controlled. An alternative is oral methylprednisolone 500 mg/day for

5 days. Oral prednisolone (1 mg/kg) should not be used because the Optic Neuritis Study Group found this to be associated with an increased risk of new episodes of optic neuritis.

There is no proven visual benefit from the use of corticosteroids in the long term in patients harbouring a typical optic neuritis. By contrast, patients suffering from an autoimmune optic neuritis such as a neuromyelitis optica spectrum disorder require long-term immunosuppression.

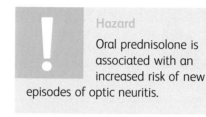

Hazard

Oral prednisolone is associated with an increased risk of new episodes of optic neuritis.

Prognosis

Visual recovery after a first episode is normally good or complete; recurrent episodes may be associated with progressive visual impairment that can be profound. Corticosteroid treatment only hastens recovery during acute episodes and does not improve the ultimate visual outcome. The risk of a similar event in the second eye is appreciable but low. The development of MS is associated with increased mortality.

2.6 Ischaemic optic neuropathy in giant cell arteritis

Aetiology

Giant cell arteritis is an inflammatory disorder of unknown aetiology affecting small to medium-sized arteries of the head and neck. It is characterised by disruption of the internal elastic lamina, with an inflammatory cell infiltrate of giant cells, lymphocytes and plasma

cells. Visual loss is most commonly caused by involvement of the posterior ciliary arteries, resulting in acute anterior ischaemic optic neuropathy (AION). In rare cases, a posterior ischaemic optic neuropathy may develop whereby the optic nerve appearance is normal but there is a dramatic loss of vision in the presence of a relative afferent pupillary defect (RAPD) (ie similar to a retrobulbar optic neuritis minus the pain and associated with more severe visual loss).

It is extremely rare in people younger than 60 years, and is twice as common in women. It was first described by Sir Jonathan Hutchinson in 1890, some 2 years after the description of polymyalgia rheumatica by William Bruce – the two syndromes constituting the opposite extremes of a single clinical disorder.

Clinical presentation

Systemic symptoms include scalp tenderness and headache, pain on chewing (jaw claudication), proximal muscle weakness or stiffness, and general malaise.

Visual loss, usually unilateral and severe, occurs in about 5–10% of cases. Altitudinal field loss may be seen (Fig 21). A central retinal artery occlusion may also occur and a patient may have symptoms of amaurosis fugax. Coexisting ischaemia of the other cranial nerves may give rise to ocular motility defects leading to binocular diplopia. Rarely, occipital blindness may occur as a result of involvement of the vertebrobasilar circulation.

Physical signs

Visual acuity is severely reduced, often to hand movements or light perception, and there is a relative afferent pupillary defect. The optic disc is pale and swollen, and there are often haemorrhages at the disc margin (Fig 22).

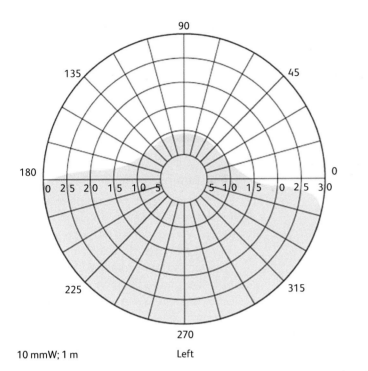

10 mmW; 1 m   Left

Fig 21 Inferior altitudinal field defect in giant cell arteritis with ischaemic optic neuropathy. The field of the right eye was normal. Uniocular altitudinal defects are secondary to an anterior lesion, in either the retina or the optic nerve.

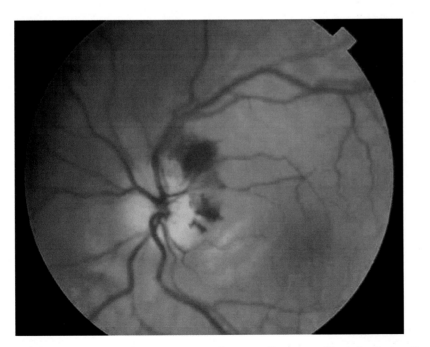

Fig 22 Optic disc in the acute stage of giant cell arteritis. The infarcted optic nerve head is pale and swollen with blurred and haemorrhagic margins. Visual loss is usually irreversible.

The temporal arteries may be tender and pulseless, although clinically normal arteries may be pathologically involved. Uncommonly, eye movements may be impaired as a result of involvement of cranial nerves III and VI.

Investigation

The important tests are:

> Inflammatory markers – erythrocyte sedimentation rate (ESR) and C-reactive protein (CRP): a normal ESR does not reliably exclude giant cell arteritis, although a normal CRP effectively does (there is only one documented case report with normal CRP pre-corticosteroid).

> Temporal artery biopsy, or a biopsy of another clinically involved artery such as facial or occipital – this should be performed within a week of starting steroids whenever possible to avoid compromising the histology. A positive biopsy is absolute confirmation of the diagnosis. This is important since patients often require corticosteroids for a period of at least 18 months.

A full blood count (FBC) may show a normochromic/normocytic anaemia.

Key point

> A normal CRP (before steroids) effectively excludes giant cell arteritis.

> A positive biopsy is absolute confirmation of the diagnosis.

> A patient presenting with amaurosis fugax with raised inflammatory markers and no symptoms or signs to account for these (eg infection or malignancy) should be considered to have giant cell arteritis until proven otherwise.

Differential diagnosis

The major differential diagnosis is between a non-arteritic AION and a retinal artery occlusion. It is important to establish the diagnosis because steroid therapy is necessary for giant cell arteritis. In cases of doubt, corticosteroids should be administered pending the outcome of investigations.

Treatment

Key point

The primary aim of treatment in cases of giant cell arteritis is to suppress the arteritis and minimise the risk of damage to the fellow eye or other organs.

Immediate

Urgent corticosteroid treatment should be initiated immediately after blood has been taken for ESR and CRP. Oral prednisolone in a dose of 1 mg/kg per day is appropriate. In patients with ophthalmic signs or symptoms, intravenous methylprednisolone may be considered and has been advocated by the British Society for Rheumatology and British Health Professionals in Rheumatology although the evidence for this modus operandi is by no means unequivocal.

Short term

The corticosteroid dose is tapered according to the response of clinical features, such as headache, and a fall in ESR and CRP. This can usually be achieved by 10 mg decrements every 2–4 weeks until receiving 30 mg, then by 5 mg decrements to 10 mg followed by a much more cautious reduction in 1 mg steps.

Longer term

The median duration of steroid therapy for giant cell arteritis is 2 years, so it is important to begin prophylaxis against osteoporosis. It is unusual for giant cell arteritis to recur after successful treatment, unless corticosteroids have been withdrawn too quickly. Since there is a significant risk of long-term complications with the treatment, it is more appropriate that the follow-up of patients with giant cell arteritis is undertaken by a physician or a medical ophthalmologist. Ocular side effects of corticosteroids include cataract and raised intraocular pressure (leading to glaucoma). The latter ocular side effect is more likely to be encountered with corticosteroids delivered locally to the eye rather than administered orally or parenterally.

Prognosis

Visual recovery is uncommon in the presenting eye. Unfortunately, some patients lose vision in the second eye within a week of initiating treatment.

2.7 Diabetic retinopathy

Aetiology

Retinopathy takes time to develop and is extremely rare before puberty or at presentation in those with type 1 diabetes, but after 10 years about 80% of patients have detectable retinopathy. By contrast, retinopathy is established in up to 25% of patients at the time of diagnosis in patients with type 2 diabetes, the onset of which is difficult to ascertain as patients may be asymptomatic for a considerable period of time before the diagnosis is established. Retinopathy is a consequence of chronic hyperglycaemia, and poor diabetic control is positively correlated with the severity of retinopathy.

Clinical presentation

Diabetic retinopathy is asymptomatic until sight-threatening complications occur, by which time the disease is in an advanced state. When symptoms do arise, gradual blurring of vision is more common than acute loss, unless there is a vitreous haemorrhage or the patient suddenly becomes aware of the problem and panics. Sight-threatening yet asymptomatic retinopathy must therefore be detected by screening. Diabetic maculopathy is the commonest cause of visual loss.

Key point

With regards to diabetic retinopathy it is important to remember:

> Patients with type 1 diabetes are more likely to develop proliferative disease than maculopathy – the reverse applies to those with type 2 diabetes.

> In type 2 diabetes, retinopathy may already be established at the time of diagnosis.

> Prevention of retinopathy is far better for the patient than laser treatment when retinopathy is established.

Examination

It is essential to examine the fundus through well-dilated pupils using at least 1% tropicamide combined with 2.5% phenylephrine drops to enable proper assessment of the macula – the central area between the major retinal vessels, temporal to the optic disc. Diabetic retinopathy is classified as follows.

Mild, non-proliferative (Background)

This is characterised by microaneurysms and haemorrhages, sometimes referred to as 'dots and blots' (Fig 23). Leakage from these can result in retinal oedema and hard exudates, but this is asymptomatic unless the fovea at the centre of the macula is involved (maculopathy). Cotton-wool spots may be observed in addition to venous loops.

Maculopathy (exudative or ischaemic)

Clinically significant oedema, hard exudates (Fig 24) or ischaemia may affect the macula, either alone or in combination. The critical area is within a disc diameter (1.5 mm) of the central fovea. Hard exudates are easily recognised, but retinal oedema and ischaemia are difficult to see by routine ophthalmoscopy and are more readily identified by optical coherence tomography (OCT) and fluorescein angiography. Maculopathy may coexist with non-proliferative and proliferative retinopathy.

Moderate, non-proliferative

With increasing ischaemia, retinal haemorrhages become more extensive in one quadrant and more cotton-wool spots become visible. Venous beading (Fig 25) may be present in one quadrant and early intraretinal microvascular abnormalities (IRMAs) may also be present. The latter represent arteriovenous shunts and resemble new blood vessels

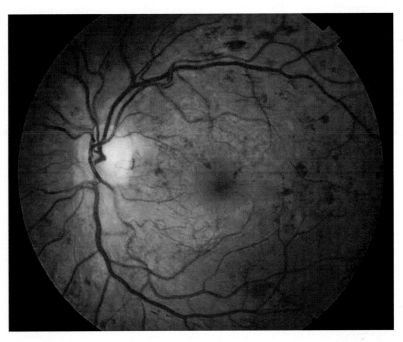

Fig 23 Mild, non-proliferative diabetic retinopathy with dot and blot haemorrhages, although there is no hard exudate.

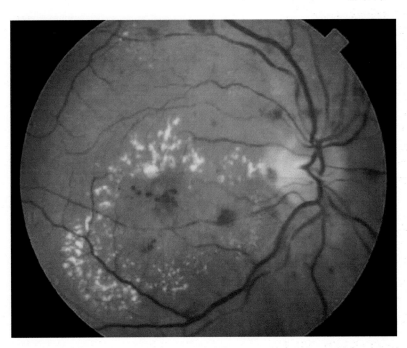

Fig 24 Diabetic maculopathy with hard exudates in a circular or circinate pattern at the fovea. In this instance, vision will already be reduced as the fovea is involved.

(neovascular vessels). Unlike their neovascular counterpart, IRMAs appear flat clinically and do not leak fluorescein during fluorescein angiography.

Severe, non-proliferative
This stage of severe retinopathy, although asymptomatic, indicates significant retinal ischaemia. The signs include multiple cotton-wool spots, large haemorrhages (more than half a disc in diameter) in all four quadrants of the retina, venous beading (Fig 25) in at least two quadrants, and extensive IRMAs in one quadrant.

Proliferative
The hallmark of this stage of retinopathy is the growth of new vessels (neovascularisation) from the surface of the retina at the disc (Fig 26) and/or elsewhere along the vascular arcades (Figs 27 and 28). Traction on new vessels may result in preretinal (Fig 29) and vitreous haemorrhages (Fig 2), and contraction may lead to retinal detachment.

Patients with diabetic retinopathy clearly require assessment by clinical examination (and investigation) for other evidence of microvascular or macrovascular disease.

Differential diagnosis
People with diabetes are at increased risk of retinal vein occlusion, which can usually be distinguished from diabetic retinopathy by the greater extent of haemorrhage and asymmetry of findings. Occasionally, in the presence of significant carotid stenosis, diabetic retinopathy may be very asymmetrical, with more severe retinopathy in the eye ipsilateral to the stenosis.

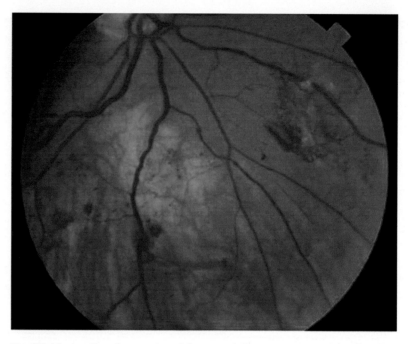

Fig 25 Venous beading and proliferative diabetic retinopathy with a fan of new vessels at 2 o'clock.

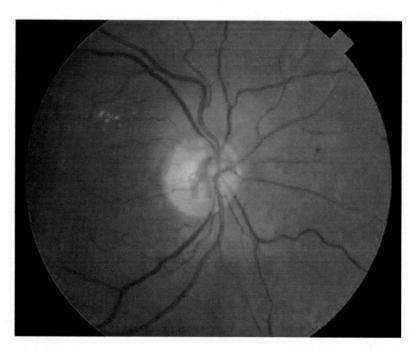

Fig 26 New vessels on the optic disc.

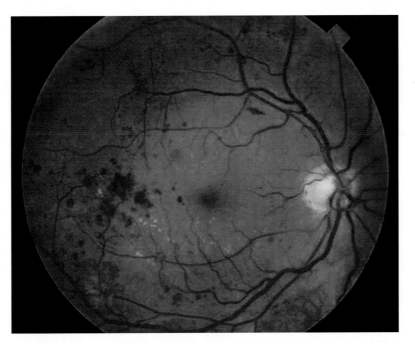

Fig 27 New vessels inferotemporal to the macula. Large blot haemorrhages temporal to the fovea are indicative of retinal ischaemia in the watershed area.

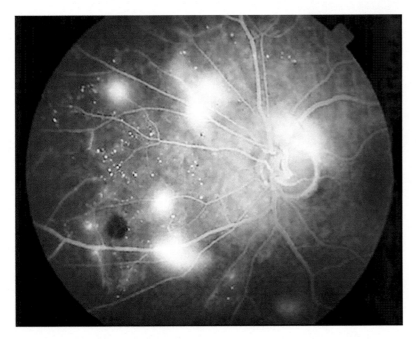

Fig 28 Fluorescein angiography of proliferative retinopathy showing profuse focal leakage of fluorescein (white patches) from retinal new vessels.

Investigation

Fluorescein angiography can be useful if clinical findings are unclear or if focal treatment is to be accurately targeted. Ocular ultrasonography can be helpful in detecting whether the retina is detached or if it cannot be visualised because of vitreous haemorrhage or a cataract.

Treatment

Maculopathy that does not involve the centre (fovea) may be treated by laser photocoagulation, either focally or as a 'grid', the primary goal being maintenance of vision by sealing leaking areas close to the fovea. However, when the maculopathy involves the fovea, intravitreal anti-vascular endothelial growth factor (VEGF) agents (the same as those employed in the management of central retinal vein occlusion (CRVO) and branch retinal vein occlusion (BRVO)) are injected on a monthly basis. If this treatment fails or the patient is unable to attend the eye clinic frequently, a corticosteroid implant can be injected into the vitreous cavity, which may last up to 3 years, but these implants are highly cataractogenic.

Proliferative retinopathy is treated by a more extensive scatter, or panretinal, laser (Fig 30). However, there are ongoing trials assessing the efficacy of anti-VEGF agents to address this form of retinopathy, which – if proven to be effective – will spare some patients some of the deleterious effects of laser photocoagulation such as reduced peripheral field of vision (with the attendant risk of not meeting the standards for driving) and poor night vision. Vitreous haemorrhage and advanced retinal fibrosis with detachment may require surgical treatment by vitrectomy and retinal microsurgery.

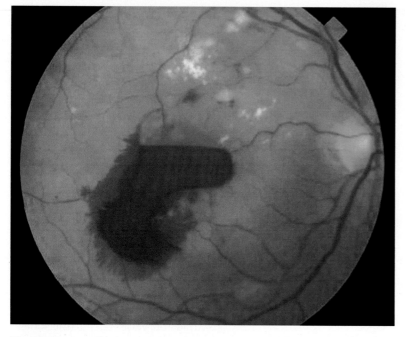

Fig 29 Preretinal haemorrhage showing a horizontal fluid level as a result of bleeding from new vessels.

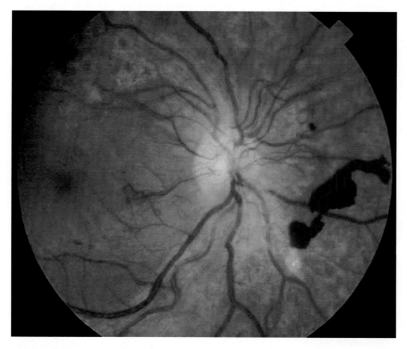

Fig 30 Proliferative diabetic retinopathy with focal scars produced by panretinal photocoagulation. Persisting obvious new vessels can be seen on the optic disc.

Patients must stop smoking, and assessment and optimisation of diabetic and blood pressure (BP) control are critically important.

Complications

Irreversible visual loss from untreatable or unresponsive maculopathy or proliferative disease is a common complication. Less frequent is neovascular (rubeotic) glaucoma caused by neovascularisation of the iris and obstruction to the drainage mechanism of the eye.

Prognosis

Key point

Risk of loss of vision depends on the stage of diabetic retinopathy. The approximate percentage of eyes that will lose useful vision irretrievably within 5 years if not treated rises from 3% for those with background retinopathy, through 20% for those with exudative and 30% for those with preproliferative, up to 50% for those with proliferative.

In the UK and USA, diabetic retinopathy is still the most common reason for patients to be certified as either sight impaired (formerly referred to as partially sighted) or severely sight impaired (formerly referred to as blind) in the working age group. In addition to the visual morbidity, diabetic retinopathy is also associated with an increased morbidity and mortality from other diabetic complications, including hypertension, ischaemic heart disease, peripheral vascular disease, cerebrovascular disease, peripheral neuropathy and nephropathy.

Prevention

Primary

The most important means of preventing blindness from diabetic retinopathy in both types 1 and 2 diabetes is good diabetic control, as proven by well-conducted clinical trials in the UK and USA. Other risk factors to be addressed include hypertension, hyperlipidaemia and smoking.

Secondary

The risk of visual loss from diabetic retinopathy can be reduced by undergoing regular eye examination by a trained observer such as an optometrist, physician or GP, or by retinal photography. If sight-threatening retinopathy is identified, treatment by laser photocoagulation will reduce the risk of blindness from maculopathy and proliferative disease by about 60%. Patients with background retinopathy or no retinopathy at all should be examined once a year, and preproliferative eyes more frequently than that – every 3–6 months.

3 Investigations and practical procedures

3.1 Optical coherence tomography

Principle

Optical coherence tomography (OCT) is a non-invasive technique of imaging either the anterior or posterior regions of the eye. It is analogous to ultrasonography but utilises light rather than sound waves. Its predominant use in ophthalmology is for imaging the posterior segment of the eye, when it is used in diagnosing retinal disorders and monitoring their treatment (Figs 31–36). It is also used in the field of neuro-ophthalmology: imaging of the optic nerve aids in the diagnosis of optic neuropathies and assessing response to treatment.

3.2 Fluorescein angiography

Principle

The retinal circulation is normally impervious to fluorescein because of the blood–retinal barrier, similar to the blood–brain barrier. Transit through the retina and choroid can be recorded either on film, digitally, by video or by direct observation. Indocyanine green angiography, a very similar technique, gives a better assessment of choroidal disease.

Indications

To enable assessment of the retinal circulation in a variety of diseases, in particular to determine the presence and degree of leakage (Fig 28) and ischaemia (Fig 20) within the retina.

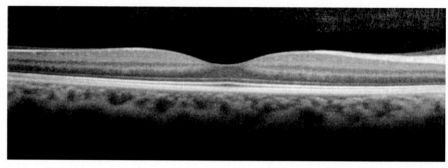

Fig 31 OCT image of normal macula.

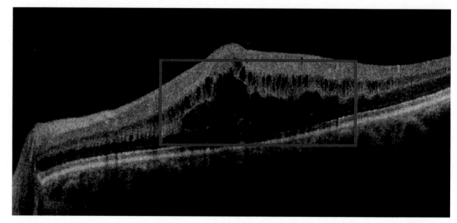

Fig 32 OCT image of macular oedema (note the intraretinal fluid within the red box).

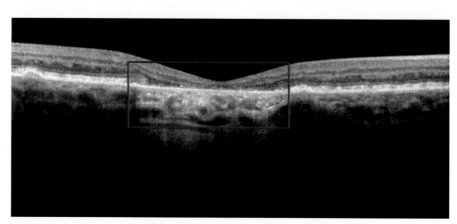

Fig 33 OCT image of dry age-related macular degeneration (note the absence of photoreceptors within the red box).

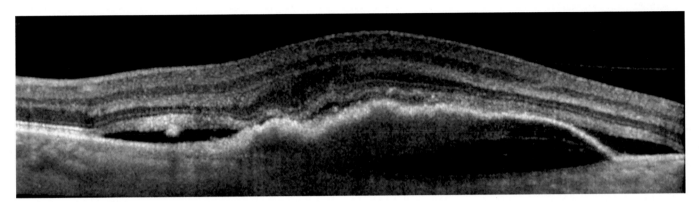

Fig 34 OCT image of wet age-related macular degeneration.

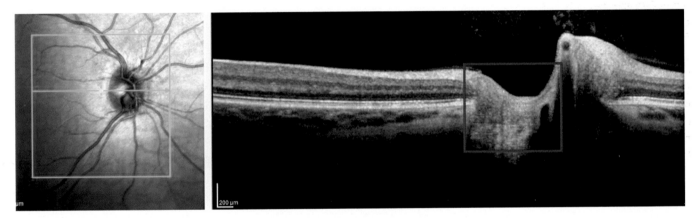

Fig 35 OCT of normal optic disc (note the optic cup within the red box).

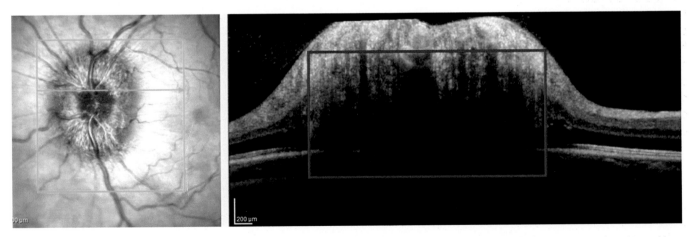

Fig 36 OCT image of papilloedema (note elevation compared with Fig 35). Note the large hyporeflective space within the red box.

Contraindications

Contraindications are previous allergy to fluorescein, recent myocardial infarction and pregnancy (relative).

Practical details

Before the procedure

Written informed consent should be obtained and the patient warned that their skin and urine will be discoloured for 24 hours. Resuscitation facilities must be available. The pupils should be fully dilated.

The procedure

The dye (3 mL of 20% or 5 mL of 10% sodium fluorescein) is rapidly injected into an antecubital vein with the patient seated at the camera. Venous access must be secure because extravasation is painful. A series of photographs or continuous video is recorded over the initial minute and then periodically over the next 5–10 minutes as the dye enters the eye and is distributed throughout the circulation.

Complications

Complications are transient nausea or vomiting (occurs in 5% of patients), local extravasation and thrombophlebitis, anaphylaxis and circulatory shock. Mortality is less than one in 200,000.

3.3 Temporal artery biopsy

Indications

This is used to establish the diagnosis of giant cell arteritis (cranial or temporal arteritis) in patients presenting with symptoms or signs suggestive of this condition.

Contraindications

There are no contraindications, except known extracranial–intracranial collateral circulation via the superficial temporal artery.

Practical details

A temporal artery biopsy should be performed as follows:

1 Written informed consent should be obtained.

2 The procedure should be performed under aseptic conditions in a designated clean area or operating room. The required equipment is: fine-toothed skin forceps, sharp and blunt scissors, skin retractors (cats' paws), scalpel (a D15 scalpel is ideal), suture forceps, absorbable and non-absorbable sutures, and local anaesthetic (a dental syringe is ideal for administration).

3 Identify the frontal branch of the temporal artery where it runs across the forehead, and mark its course with an indelible pen for about 3 cm.

4 Infiltrate the skin with the local anaesthetic in two parallel lines adjacent to, but not directly over, the artery.

5 Remove any overlying hair, cleanse the skin with 5% povidone–iodine solution (or equivalent) and then drape with sterile towels or plastic adhesive drape.

6 Incise the skin with the scalpel along the skin mark.

7 Dissect the subcutaneous tissues to expose the artery for the length of the skin incision. Avoid injury and pathological artefact to the artery by minimising any direct handling.

8 Ligate the ends of the artery and any branches with 5/0 chromic catgut (or similar suture), then excise the artery specimen.

9 Close the skin in two layers and dress the wound.

10 Place the arterial specimen in fixative and send for histopathology.

11 External, non-absorbable skin sutures can be removed at 5–6 days.

Complications

Haemorrhage can occur early or late in the procedure and is the result of either inadequate ligation or secondary infection. The chance of the latter occurring is increased by concomitant steroid therapy. It has been known for the facial nerve to be biopsied in error.

Medical ophthalmology: Section 4

4 Self-assessment

4.1 Self-assessment questions

MRCP(UK) Part 1 examination questions

Question 1

Clinical scenario

A 40-year-old Caucasian woman presented with a 5-day history of progressive pain (which woke her from her sleep) that radiated to her forehead and redness in her right eye. Her vision was unaffected and her pupil reactions were normal. The appearance of her right eye is shown (Fig 37).

Question

What is the most likely diagnosis?

Answer

A acute angle-closure glaucoma

B anterior scleritis

C anterior uveitis

D conjunctivitis

E episcleritis

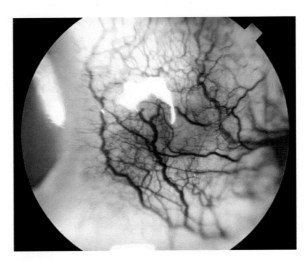

Fig 37

Question 2

Clinical scenario

A 35-year-old Caucasian woman presented with a 2-day history of visual loss (6/60) in her left eye associated with pain on eye movements. There was a left, relative afferent pupillary defect. She was systemically well. Her left ocular fundus is shown (Fig 38).

Question

What is the most likely diagnosis?

Answer

A amblyopia

B central retinal artery occlusion

C functional visual loss

D multiple sclerosis

E retrobulbar optic neuritis

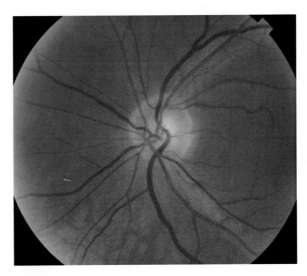

Fig 38

Question 3
Clinical scenario

A 30-year-old Caucasian woman was referred by her optometrist to the emergency department due to the appearance of her optic discs. The remainder of her ocular fundi appeared normal. She had been complaining of headaches for the past 2 months, which were precipitated with coughing and worse when she lay supine. Her previous medical history was unremarkable and she took no regular medications. On examination her body mass index (BMI) was 40 kg/m^2 (normal range 18–25) and her blood pressure (BP) was 170/100 mmHg (normal value 135/85). Neurological examination was normal except for the appearance of her optic discs (Fig 39 shows her left optic disc; the right was similar). Her visual acuities were 6/6 in each eye.

Question

What is the most likely diagnosis?

Answer

A cerebral space-occupying lesion

B cerebral venous thrombosis

C giant cell arteritis

D hypertensive emergency

E idiopathic intracranial hypertension

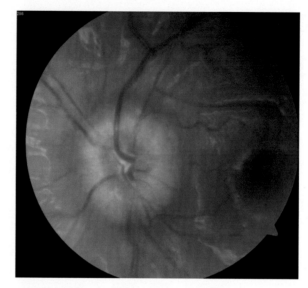

Fig 39

Question 4

Clinical scenario

A 40-year-old Greek man presented with recurrent chest infections and blurred vision in his right eye. The appearance of his right ocular fundus is shown (Fig 40); the left ocular fundus displayed similar but less severe changes.

Question

Which test would be diagnostic in this case?

Answer

A haemoglobin A$_{1c}$ (HbA$_{1c}$)

B haemoglobin (Hb) electrophoresis

C HIV serology

D lipid profile

E Mantoux test

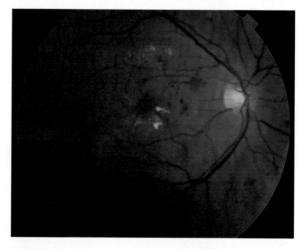

Fig 40

Question 5

Clinical scenario

A 25-year-old Caucasian man presented with a 6-week history of malaise, unintentional weight loss and fever. He appeared anxious and his BP was 160/100 mmHg. His left ocular fundoscopic findings are shown (Fig 41).

Question

What is the most likely cause for his ocular findings?

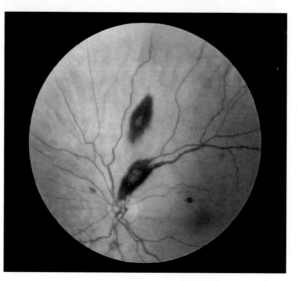

Fig 41

Answer

A cholesterol embolisation

B cytomegalovirus infection

C hypertensive retinopathy

D infective endocarditis

E toxoplasmosis

Question 6

Clinical scenario

A 70-year-old Caucasian woman developed an abrupt, severe, right-sided headache associated with blurred vision and vomiting following treatment for an acute exacerbation of chronic obstructive pulmonary disease (COPD). Her right eye was red and her pupil was unreactive. Her eye movements were full.

Question

What is the most likely diagnosis?

Answer

A acute, angle-closure glaucoma

B acute, anterior uveitis

C aneurysmal third nerve palsy

D cluster headache

E keratitis

Question 7

Clinical scenario

An 80-year-old Caucasian man who had been admitted to a care of older people ward as a result of recurrent falls complained of distorted vision in both of his eyes, which had been increasing gradually over the preceding 6 months. His medical history was noteworthy for type 2 diabetes mellitus and hypertension. The appearance of his left ocular fundus is shown (Fig 42).

Question

What is the most likely ocular diagnosis?

Answer

A atrophic, age-related macular degeneration

B diabetic maculopathy

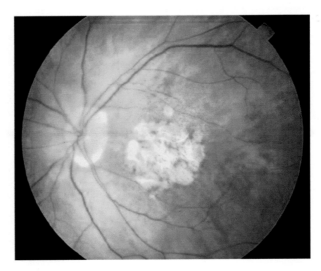

Fig 42

C exudative, age-related macular degeneration

D hypertensive retinopathy

E retinitis pigmentosa

Question 8

Clinical scenario

A 50-year-old Caucasian man was noted to have glycosuria. His haemoglobin A1c was 60 mmol/mol (normal range 20–42). His right ocular fundus findings are shown (Fig 43).

Question

What is the most likely cause of this appearance?

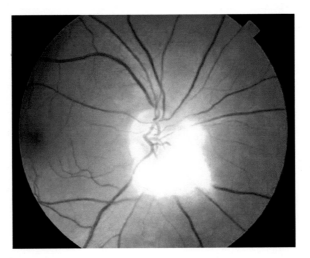

Fig 43

Answer

A anterior ischaemic optic neuropathy

B background diabetic retinopathy

C hypertensive retinopathy

D normal variant of no clinical significance

E ocular toxoplasmosis

Question 9

Clinical scenario

A 45-year-old Caucasian woman with type 1 diabetes mellitus attended for a routine outpatient clinic appointment. Her BP was 150/100 mmHg. She had no visual symptoms, but the appearance of her right ocular fundus was as shown in Fig 44. Her left ocular fundus was similar in appearance.

Question
What is the most likely diagnosis?

Answer
A background diabetic retinopathy

B hypertensive retinopathy

C lipaemia retinalis

D proliferative diabetic retinopathy

E severe, non-proliferative diabetic retinopathy

Question 10

Clinical scenario
A 72-year-old African-Caribbean man with end-stage renal failure of unknown cause attended the renal transplant clinic for routine review. He reported that his vision was 'not quite so good', but was unable to give further detail. His BP was 180/110 mmHg. Ophthalmoscopy of both eyes revealed the appearance shown in Fig 45.

Question
What is the ocular diagnosis?

Answer
A accelerated phase hypertension

B background diabetic retinopathy

C cataract

D cytomegalovirus retinopathy

E hypertensive retinopathy

MRCP(UK) Part 2 examination questions

Question 11

Clinical scenario
A 40-year-old Caucasian woman presented with a 5-day history of progressive pain (which awoke her from her sleep) that radiated to her forehead and redness in her right eye. Her vision was unaffected and her pupil reactions were normal. She also complained of swelling, pain and morning stiffness in the region of her metacarpophalangeal joints (MCP) joints. The appearance of her right eye is shown (Fig 37).

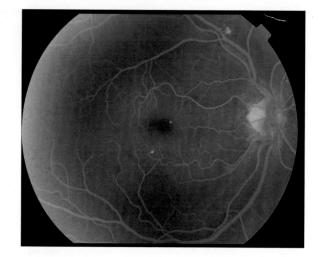

Fig 44

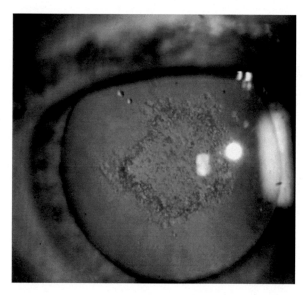

Fig 45

Question
What is the most likely underlying cause of her symptoms and signs?

Answer
A ankylosing spondylitis

B Behçet's disease

C granulomatosis with polyangiitis

D rheumatoid arthritis

E systemic lupus erythematosus

Question 12

Clinical scenario
A 25-year-old Caucasian man presented with a 3-day history of reduced vision in

his right eye associated with pain and photophobia. He gave a history of painful, recurrent mouth ulcers over the preceding 6 months, and had recently attended a genitourinary medical clinic for genital ulceration, where an infection screen had been negative. The appearance of his right eye is shown (Fig 46).

Question
What is the most likely underlying diagnosis?

Answer
A acute anterior uveitis

B Behçet's disease

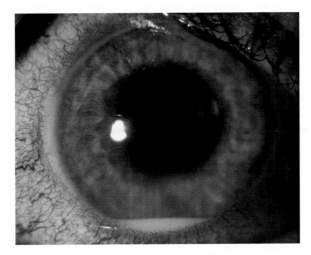

Fig 46

C Crohn's disease

D hypopyon

E *Treponema pallidum*

Question 13

Clinical scenario

A 75-year-old Caucasian man presented with acute loss of vision in his left eye. His medical history was noteworthy for diabetes and hypertension. Over the past month he had felt generally unwell and had lost 6 kg in weight because he had been unable to chew his food, although he remained able to drink. The appearance of his left optic disc is shown (Fig 47).

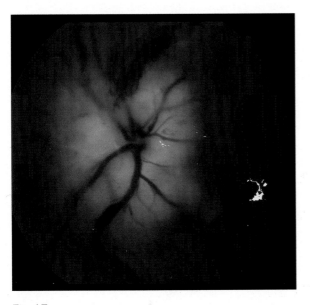

Fig 47

Question

What is the most appropriate immediate management?

Answer

A intravenous methylprednisolone

B lumbar puncture

C magnetic resonance imaging (MRI) of the head

D oral prednisolone

E temporal artery biopsy

Question 14

Clinical scenario

A 65-year-old Caucasian man presented with painless visual loss in his right eye.

He suffered from hypertension and glaucoma and was receiving treatment for both. He had been reviewed by his ophthalmologist 1 month previously, at which time his intraocular pressures had been well controlled. The appearance of his right ocular fundus is shown (Fig 48).

Question

What is the most appropriate management for his ocular condition?

Answer

A intravitreal anti-vascular endothelial growth factor (VEGF) inhibitor

B intravitreal corticosteroid

C lower his intraocular pressure

D observation

E optimise cardiovascular risk factors

Question 15

Clinical scenario

A 45-year-old Caucasian woman with a history of type 1 diabetes mellitus complained of reduced vision in her left eye when she attended for her annual check-up. Her medical history was also noteworthy for breast carcinoma and she was taking tamoxifen. Her left ocular fundus is shown (Fig 49).

Question

What is the most likely cause for her visual disturbance?

Answer

A background diabetic retinopathy

B choroidal metastases

C diabetic maculopathy

D proliferative diabetic retinopathy

E tamoxifen retinopathy

Question 16

Clinical scenario

A 40-year-old Asian man presented with acute kidney injury. Dipstick urinalysis revealed haematuria 2+ and proteinuria 2+. The appearance of his right ocular fundus is shown (Fig 50). His left ocular fundus was similar in appearance. Over the next 2 months his renal function,

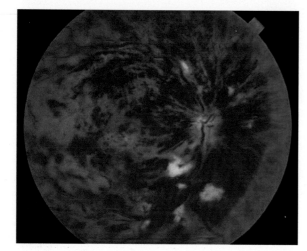

Fig 48

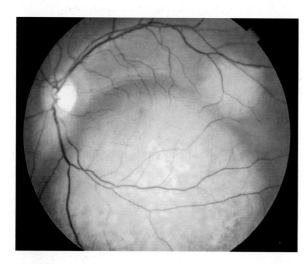

Fig 49

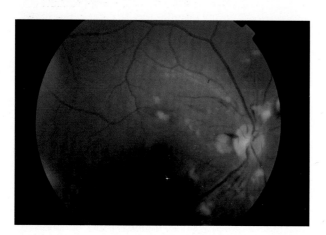

Fig 50

urinalysis and ocular appearance normalised.

Question
What treatment did he receive?

Answer
A antibiotics
B antihypertensive treatment
C anti-vascular endothelial growth factor (VEGF)
D insulin
E intraocular corticosteroids

Question 17

Clinical scenario
A 25-year-old Caucasian woman presented with a 2-day history of increasing discomfort in her right eye, which was particularly noticeable when it was exposed to bright lights. In addition, she had noticed a mild reduction in her vision. Her medical history was unremarkable, and she had no systemic symptoms of note. Her right pupil appeared to be smaller than her left pupil.

Question
What is the ocular diagnosis?

Answer
A acute anterior uveitis
B acute glaucoma
C episcleritis
D left Horner's syndrome
E right Horner's syndrome

Question 18

Clinical scenario
A 75-year-old Caucasian woman who had been admitted to a general medical ward with falls was noted to have nasal visual field loss on confrontation in each eye. The appearance of the right optic disc is shown (Fig 51). Her left optic disc was similar in appearance.

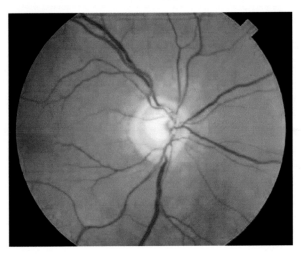

Fig 51

Question

What is the most appropriate diagnostic test?

Answer

A BP measurement

B computerised tomography (CT) scan of orbits and brain

C intraocular pressure measurement

D lumbar puncture

E MRI of the brain and orbits

Question 19

Clinical scenario

A 75-year-old Caucasian man was admitted to a general medical ward with an acute exacerbation of his COPD. On waking one morning he noticed a painless loss of vision in the inferior field of his right eye. His medical history was otherwise noteworthy for type 2 diabetes mellitus and hypertension.

Question

What is the most likely diagnosis?

Answer

A central retinal artery occlusion

B central retinal vein occlusion

C inferior branch retinal artery occlusion

D non-arteritic anterior ischaemic optic neuropathy

E occipital stroke

Question 20

Clinical scenario

A 58-year-old man with a history of hypertension and diabetes presented with sudden painless loss of peripheral vision in his left eye. The appearance of the left ocular fundus is shown (Fig 52).

Question

What is the ocular diagnosis?

Answer

A central retinal artery occlusion

B central retinal vein occlusion

C cilioretinal artery occlusion

D retinitis pigmentosa

E vitreous haemorrhage

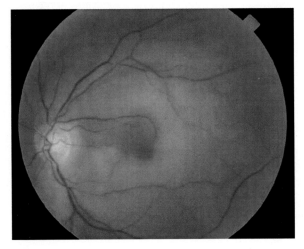

Fig 52

4.2 Self-assessment answers

Answer to Question 1

B: anterior scleritis

The pain associated with scleritis is typically progressive, often awakens the affected person from his/her sleep and radiates to the forehead on the same side as the affected eye. The pupil is spared differentiating it from other painful red eye causes such as acute glaucoma (dilated pupil) and anterior uveitis (small pupil). Episcleritis and conjunctivitis are usually associated with mild discomfort. In addition, a discharge is often associated with the latter.

Answer to Question 2

E: retrobulbar optic neuritis

The image demonstrates a normal ocular fundus. In the presence of a relative afferent pupil defect and pain on eye movements, this is very typical of retrobulbar optic neuritis. Functional visual loss may be suspected in patients with no demonstrable pupillary defect. Amblyopia (colloquially referred to as a 'lazy eye') develops in infancy and is secondary to an uncorrected refractive error, a strabismus or an anatomical defect (for example, a ptosis). Although multiple sclerosis is associated with retrobulbar optic neuritis, there are no other features in the scenario to suggest this disorder.

Answer to Question 3

E: idiopathic intracranial hypertension

The image reveals a swollen optic disc. In the context of normal visual acuities and symptoms of raised intracranial pressure, this most likely represents papilloedema which is defined as optic disc swelling secondary to raised intracranial pressure. In view of her raised body mass index (BMI), the most likely underlying diagnosis is idiopathic intracranial hypertension (formerly known as benign intracranial hypertension).

Answer to Question 4

A: haemoglobin A_{1c} (HbA_{1c})

The image displays features typical of diabetic retinopathy (hard exudates, microaneurysms, dot and blot haemorrhages). The test leading to the diagnosis is therefore HbA_{1c}.

Answer to Question 5

D: infective endocarditis

The image demonstrates a couple of haemorrhages exhibiting a pale centre. These are sometimes referred to Roth's spots and are classically associated with infective endocarditis, although they are also associated with anaemia (and secondary causes for this) and myeloproliferative disorders.

Answer to Question 6

A: acute, angle-closure glaucoma

Acute angle-closure glaucoma is associated with a rapid onset of redness, pain and a fixed, semi-dilated pupil that are secondary to the ischaemia induced by raised intraocular pressure. This condition can be induced following dilation of a patient's pupil in an eye

that is anatomically predisposed to reducing the outflow of aqueous fluid into the drainage structures (trabecular meshwork and canal of Schlemm in the anterior chamber angle). Ipratropium is an anticholinergic agent that may dilate a patient's pupils and place those susceptible of angle-closure glaucoma at risk of developing this ocular condition.

Answer to Question 7

A: atrophic, age-related macular degeneration

The pale yellow, well-demarcated area within the macula that is shown in the image is typical of retinal atrophy associated with the dry or atrophic form of macular degeneration. This, in combination with the wet or exudative form of the disease, remains the commonest cause of blindness in the Western world. Retinitis pigmentosa is often associated with pigmentary changes in the mid-peripheral aspect of the retina in addition to arteriolar attenuation and a pale optic disc. There are no microaneurysms or other abnormal vascular changes to support a vascular retinopathy such as diabetes or hypertension.

Answer to Question 8

D: normal variant of no clinical significance

The dense white opacity overlying the optic disc margin from 2 and 8 o'clock and obscuring the underlying retinal vasculature is due to myelinated nerve fibres. This is a congenital condition that is of no pathological consequence. Normally, myelination of nerves in the eyes cease behind the optic disc.

Answer to Question 9

C: lipaemia retinalis

The image reveals a fundus with very pale blood vessels in the absence of haemorrhages or any other vascular abnormalities. This is the typical appearance of lipaemia retinalis, which is associated with hypertriglyceridaemia.

The vision is often normal. High levels of chylomicrons account for the fundal appearance, which normalises on reducing the triglyceride levels.

Answer to Question 10

C: cataract

The image shows an early cataract against the red reflex. The granular appearance in the centre of the pupil is typical of a posterior subcapsular cataract due to the use of systemic corticosteroids.

Answer to Question 11

D: rheumatoid arthritis

The most likely underlying diagnosis is rheumatoid arthritis. Unlike episcleritis, scleritis is often associated with systemic disease, most commonly rheumatoid arthritis. Although granulomatosis with polyangiitis can cause scleritis, there are no features in the scenario suggestive of this. Ankylosing spondylitis is associated with anterior uveitis.

Answer to Question 12

B: Behçet's disease

The image demonstrates a hypopyon (pus in the anterior chamber). The most likely cause in this case is uveitis secondary to Behçet's disease in view of the history of recurrent painful mouth ulceration and non-infectious genital ulceration.

Answer to Question 13

A: intravenous methylprednisolone

The image demonstrates a chalky white, swollen disc, which, in the context of a patient suffering from constitutional symptoms and jaw claudication (leading to inability to chew solid foods) is indicative of arteritic, anterior ischaemic optic neuropathy secondary to giant cell arteritis. It would be appropriate to check inflammatory markers, anticipating that these would be raised, but intravenous corticosteroids should be commenced immediately in an attempt to prevent visual loss in the contralateral eye and the diagnosis should be confirmed via a temporal artery biopsy, which should be performed within 2 weeks of commencing corticosteroids to reduce the risk of obtaining a false negative result.

Answer to Question 14
A: intravitreal anti-vascular endothelial growth factor (VEGF) inhibitor

The image reveals multiple haemorrhages scattered throughout the entire ocular fundus associated with optic disc swelling. This is the classic appearance of a central retinal vein occlusion. The main cause of visual loss is macular oedema and this can now be treated with intravitreal injections of inhibitors that target VEGF. Anti-VEGF inhibitors are also employed in the management of branch retinal vein occlusions, diabetic maculopathy, and wet, age-related and myopic macular degenerations.

Answer to Question 15
B: choroidal metastases

The image demonstrates a well-defined, rounded and raised, mottled lesion that is typical of choroidal metastases secondary to breast carcinoma. These may be present in the absence of visual symptoms. Tamoxifen can affect the macular region and is typified by fine crystalline deposits, which are not demonstrated in this case.

Answer to Question 16
B: antihypertensive treatment

The presence of cotton-wool spots and flame – shaped haemorrhages but a paucity of microaneurysms is highly suggestive of a vascular retinopathy other than diabetes. Although the blood pressure (BP) was not given in the scenario, the presence of non-visible haematuria and proteinuria with acute kidney injury (AKI) and these ocular findings suggest that the patient had accelerated phase hypertension.

Answer to Question 17
A: acute anterior uveitis

A painful, red eye associated with a small (miosed) pupil and photophobia (discomfort with bright lights brought on by the involuntary, autonomic movements of an inflamed iris) are the hallmarks of acute anterior uveitis. Patients harbouring a Horner's syndrome (oculosympathetic paresis) may also harbour a red eye (to a lesser degree than its uveitis counterpart) with a small pupil, but they seldom exhibit photophobia.

Answer to Question 18
C: intraocular pressure measurement

The optic disc appearance demonstrated in the image reveals a large pale area within the optic disc known as cupping. This represents an area of the optic nerve that is devoid of retinal nerve fibres and is typical of chronic, open-angle glaucoma. The commonest visual field defects associated with this condition are nasal. The most appropriate test to ascertain the diagnosis is to measure the pressure.

Answer to Question 19
D: non-arteritic anterior ischaemic optic neuropathy

A central retinal vein or artery occlusion would cause a generalised reduction in the whole visual field. An inferior branch retinal artery occlusion would cause a superior visual field defect. An occipital stroke could cause an inferior visual field defect if it affected the superior calcarine fissure, but this would affect both eyes rather than one. The only ocular disease compatible with this presentation is a non-arteritic, anterior ischaemic optic neuropathy.

Answer to Question 20
A: central retinal artery occlusion

The appearance is of retinal artery occlusion with macular sparing as a result of a patent cilioretinal artery. The central macula/fovea is perfused, but there is surrounding retinal pallor with oedema that causes a 'cherry-red patch' rather than a 'cherry-red spot'.

Psychiatry

Authors

Dr A Ashby, Dr H Costello, Dr D Horton and Dr N Sarkar

Editor

Dr D Horton

Editor-in-Chief

Dr JD Firth

The psychiatry section of the second edition of Medical Masterclass was written by Dr MS Lipsedge and Dr V Kirchner (editor). This third edition of Medical Masterclass contains entirely new material, but many sections from the second edition have been retained and updated, and we gratefully acknowledge the contribution of these authors.

Psychiatry: Section 1

1 PACES stations and acute scenarios

1.1 History taking

1.1.1 Eating disorders

Letter of referral to medical outpatient clinic

Dear Doctor,
Re: Ms Alison Jones

I would be grateful for your opinion on this 17-year-old schoolgirl whose parents are concerned because she eats very little and is underweight. She denies that there is any problem at all, but her parents have told me that she refuses to join them for meals, weighs herself several times a day and exercises compulsively. As you can see she is painfully thin. I cannot find any obvious physical cause and would be grateful for your opinion, in particular to exclude a serious underlying medical problem.

Yours sincerely,

Introduction

Control and self-esteem are the issues that patients with eating disorders are usually struggling with. Eating and weight are things they sometimes feel in control of, although a lot of the time even that feels out of control. If they have suffered abuse then these feelings may be even stronger. Anyone telling them to eat and gain weight might be met with considerable hostility and putting undue pressure on them may arouse feelings of abuse. They often lack insight into the severity of their illness and will have strong, rigid thoughts about their appearance or weight. Approach the situation with empathy and understanding, and concentrate on winning her trust. It may initially be appropriate to address urgent medical complications, not the eating disorder itself. Eating disorders have the highest mortality of any psychiatric conditions, and the medical risk should not be underestimated. It is important to differentiate between anorexia nervosa and bulimia nervosa, as management is different for each.

Key point

***International statistical classification of diseases and health-related problems*, 10th edition (ICD-10) criteria for anorexia nervosa**

> body mass index (BMI) <17.5 or body weight >15% below expected, where BMI = weight $(kg)/(height\ in\ metres)^2$

> self-induced weight loss

> body image distortion with dread of gaining weight

> abnormalities of the hypothalamic–pituitary–gonadal axis are present (amenorrhoea in women; loss of sexual interest and potency in men)

> if its onset is prepubertal, then delayed puberty.

Key point

***Diagnostic and statistical manual of mental disorders (DSM)-V* criteria for anorexia nervosa**

> significantly low body weight

> intense fear of gaining weight or becoming fat

> disturbance in the way in which one's body weight or shape is experienced, undue influence of body weight or shape on self-evaluation, or persistent lack of recognition of the seriousness of the current low body weight.

Key point

ICD-10 criteria for bulimia nervosa

> recurrent episodes of overeating with large quantity of food eaten in short time

> persistent preoccupation with eating and craving to eat

> patient attempts to counteract the 'fattening' effects of food by one of more of the following: self-induced vomiting, purgative abuse, alternating periods of starvation, use of drugs (eg appetite suppressants, thyroid preparations, diuretics)

> morbid dread of fatness.

History of the presenting problem

Anorexia nervosa is a clinical diagnosis (see above) and other general medical conditions that may account for the weight loss must be excluded.

Focusing on the possible diagnoses of anorexia nervosa and bulimia nervosa, try to establish how much, what and how often she is eating by asking the patient to talk you through a day of usual eating and drinking – describe a typical day. Explore if she relates to these common behaviours/symptoms:

> intense fear of putting on weight

> strong belief of being overweight despite low body weight

> restriction of 'fattening' foods (eg butter, dairy products) from diet

> constantly thinking about food

> does not eat with family or in public places (already suggested in this scenario)

> binge eating and/or self-induced vomiting

> laxative and diuretic abuse

> ritualistic, excessive and possibly abnormal exercise

> amenorrhoea or irregular menstrual cycle

> self-image: ideal weight, 'What do you see when looking in the mirror?'

In most cases the diagnosis is clear and never in substantial doubt, but take care not to rush to conclusions immediately and enquire about bowel habit, abdominal bloating and other symptoms that might indicate malabsorption. Also check for symptoms that might indicate one of the diseases listed in the 'Key point' above.

Other relevant history

Ask the patient how old was she when the eating disorder started and how it has progressed. What does she believe set it off? How does it affect her life? Has she had previous medical complications? Has she received treatment in the past? Briefly clarify her family and social situation (especially in clinical practice where this is highly relevant).

Has she been abused physically, sexually or emotionally? Asking about abuse should only be done when you perceive that your relationship with her is such that she will not find such a question overwhelmingly intrusive, and in routine clinical practice this issue should clearly not be broached in the presence of anyone who might be or have been an abuser.

It is important to explore family dynamics and relationships and attitudes to the patient's eating habits: these may direct family interventions to address the eating disorder.

Collateral history

This will not be available in a PACES scenario, unless given in the letter of referral. However, the patient may feel ashamed of her eating pattern and therefore be unwilling to divulge information. In routine clinical practice her parents may be able to provide further details, but you should beware of making the patient feel colluded against.

Plan for investigation and management

In routine clinical practice, but not in PACES Station 1, investigations would follow physical examination, with the following elements of particular relevance: body weight / BMI; features to suggest anorexia nervosa (discoloured hands and feet, brittle nails, dry skin, hair loss from scalp, lanugo hair on the body, pallor, easy bruising (hepatic impairment), slow capillary refill, heart rate (bradycardia or tachycardia), low blood pressure, oedema, squat test (proximal myopathy), and (if vomiting) calluses on the knuckles, salivary gland enlargement and eroded dentition).

Investigations are necessary to identify medical complications and exclude other causes for weight loss, rather than to aid in making the diagnosis of anorexia or bulimia nervosa. Explain the need to exclude general medical causes for her symptoms, and since she may not herself be worried about her weight loss (in fact she might value it) it might be worth emphasising the amenorrhoea or poor temperature control as these are symptoms she might agree to having investigated.

Initial investigations would be blood tests, an electrocardiogram (ECG) and a chest X-ray. Those required for a patient with probable anorexia nervosa are shown in Table 1. Specific tests to exclude medical differential diagnoses (see the 'Key point' above) – eg anti-tissue transglutaminase antibodies for coeliac disease, HIV test – would be employed as clinically indicated.

General management goals for a patient with anorexia nervosa would include:

> treating medical complications

> restoring a more normal eating pattern

> providing information

> referral to psychiatric services or general practitioner (GP) so psychotherapy and family therapy can be initiated.

Although psychotherapy is the treatment of choice, there is no agreed 'best' psychological treatment for anorexia nervosa and the outcome is variable. Cognitive analytic or behavioural therapies, interpersonal psychotherapy and focal dynamic therapy are all psychological therapies that should be considered. Family interventions that directly address eating disorders are particularly useful in adolescents with anorexia nervosa.

Arrange a follow-up outpatient appointment to review test results, confirm with the patient that the diagnosis is a primary eating disorder and that specialist follow-up is in place.

Further discussion

Key point

Self-starvation is a serious life-threatening problem. The signs of starvation are:

> hypothermia

> lanugo hair

> loss of muscle mass

> dependent oedema

> bradycardia

> hypotension

> neuropathy.

Key point

If she is inducing vomiting, tell-tale signs are:

> salivary gland enlargement

> dental erosion

> calluses on the fingers/knuckles.

Anorexia nervosa – refusal of treatment

If the patient's situation is life-threatening and she adamantly refuses treatment, she must be assessed by a psychiatrist for consideration of treatment under the Mental Health Act 1983 (see Section 2.14).

Table 1	Routine investigations required in patients presenting with probable anorexia nervosa	

Investigation	Possible abnormalities
Electrolytes	Hypokalaemia
	Hypochloraemic alkalosis
	Renal failure
Calcium	Low
Phosphate	Low
Magnesium	Low
Liver function test	Low proteins
	Raised liver enzymes
Glucose	Low
FBC	Low white cell count
	Normochromic or iron-deficient anaemia
Erythrocyte sedimentation rate	Should be normal
Thyroid function test	Low triiodothyronine
ECG	Dysrhythmias
	T-wave changes, ST depression and lengthened QT interval
Chest X-ray	Small heart
	Osteoporosis

ECG, electrocardiogram; FBC, full blood count.

1.1.2 Medically unexplained symptoms

Dear Doctor,

Re: Ms Catherine Davies

Thank you for seeing this 45-year-old solicitor who presented with an 8-month history of feeling exhausted and unable to engage in any activity that required physical exertion. She has recently been spending up to 15 hours a day in bed and feels miserable because of not being able to do what she could previously. She has been off sick from work for the past 2 months. There is no history of mental illness. I cannot find any abnormality on examination. Her blood pressure is 120/80 mmHg. A range of blood tests including full blood count (FBC), erythrocyte sedimentation rate, urea and electrolytes, liver and bone function tests and thyroid function tests have all been normal.

Yours sincerely,

Introduction

Medically unexplained physical symptoms are common, with some falling into the category of somatic symptom disorders (previously known as somatoform disorders) (Table 2). In these conditions patients present with physical symptoms that are not explained by any medical condition and are assumed to have an underlying psychosocial cause.

Medically unexplained physical symptoms are often dismissed and patients feel they are not being taken seriously despite feeling very ill indeed.

It is important to note that to the patient these symptoms are real and often highly impairing. They are difficult to treat and often make doctors feel impotent and frustrated. Although psychological factors are assumed to be important, patients rarely accept a purely psychological explanation. It is also common to have 'functional overlay' of symptoms on a background of physical illness. A sensible approach is for physician and psychiatrist to work collaboratively. One physician should investigate possible medical causes and coordinate all investigations and care. An empathic but firm and sensible approach is essential. The involvement of a large number of doctors is likely to do more harm than good.

Functional symptoms, and somatic symptoms disorder, involve an unconscious converting of difficult feelings such as sadness, anger or frustration into physical symptoms. Think of it like a fuse blowing – a sort of 'off switch' for the mind that can be quite protective against, for example, low mood with suicide ideation. Patients often feel that medical professionals think they are making it up, or putting symptoms on. It is important to note that factitious disorder and malingering, in both of which physical symptoms are knowingly and deliberately feigned (for different reasons), are extremely rare in comparison, and these diagnoses should not be confused.

History of the presenting problem

A full medical and functional history is required, with any leads followed appropriately, but it is very likely that nothing convincing will emerge in the medical enquiry. Giving the patient enough time to talk about all their different physical symptoms is extremely important as the person is likely to have recurrently had the experience that they have not shared all their concerns, leading to a worry something important may have been missed.

Look for predisposing, precipitating and perpetuating factors. These may be biological, psychological or social. For example, a high-achieving person who is not reaching their self-imposed targets at work.

Ask the patient:

> When did the symptoms start?

> When did her mood change?

> What was the first symptom?

> Why does she think the symptoms are happening?

> In what sequence did symptoms develop?

> What was going on in her personal, family and work life just prior to the onset?

> Is she taking any medication that might have troublesome side effects?

> Does she have a history of mental illness, eg mood or eating disorders?

> Does she have alcohol or other substance misuse problems?

> How do the symptoms impair her quality of life?

Do look for symptoms of comorbid mental disorder such as low mood or anxiety, but it is not uncommon for people with functional symptoms to not have these, or even have a rather unexpected sense of not being worried about their severe physical impairment (often called 'la belle indifférence').

When asking about past history, factors such as similar symptoms within the family may have provided a model of illness behaviour. Periods of extended absence from school or work may indicate a predisposition to using physical symptoms to deal with psychological distress or social pressures. Enquire about the coexistence of other medically unexplained syndromes or idiosyncratic beliefs about her health, eg irritable bowel syndrome, fibromyalgia or beliefs about food allergies.

Table 2	DSM-V Psychiatric diagnoses for medically unexplained symptoms
Disorder	**Characteristic features**
Depression	Fatigue, weight loss and pain are common
Somatic symptom disorder[1]	Distressing somatic symptoms along with abnormal thoughts, feelings and behaviours in response to these symptoms
Functional neurological symptom disorder	One symptom simulating a disease, eg motor or sensory symptoms and seizures. Previously called conversion disorder
Illness anxiety disorder	Preoccupation with having a particular disease
Psychotic disorder	With somatic delusions and hallucinations
Factitious disorder	Previously called 'Munchausen's syndrome'. Person deliberately produces, feigns or exaggerates symptoms, with the motive being to attain the sick patient's role and the care associated with this
Malingering	Person deliberately fabricates symptoms for secondary gain such as the avoidance of criminal charges or for financial gain

1 The term 'somatic symptom disorder' is used in the *Diagnostic and statistical manual of mental disorders* (DSM)-V to encompass conditions previously known as somatisation / somatoform / pain disorders. The question of how patients with 'myalgic encephalomyelitis / chronic fatigue syndrome' should be classified remains a subject of much debate, with some arguing that it should be classified as a neurological condition and some as a psychiatric condition. Patients do not seem to be well served by arguments about terminology.

Plan for investigation and management

In routine clinical practice, but not in PACES Station 2, you would perform a full and thorough physical examination, reassuring the patient that any abnormal physical signs would be followed up, but in repeated encounters you should also explain that repeated examinations are not helpful unless new circumstances warrant it. Do make sure that the results of any tests done, regardless of the findings, are explained to the patient.

Tell the patient that a well-thought-out battery of investigations will be carried out as the next step (see below). This will reassure her – and also other doctors involved in her care – that possible physical causes are being taken seriously. However, if physical examination and investigations are negative, then in this patient a likely diagnosis is chronic fatigue syndrome; the criteria of which are listed in the following 'Key point'.

 Key point

Diagnostic criteria for chronic fatigue syndrome

Clinically evaluated, medically unexplained fatigue of at least 6 months' duration that is:

> of new onset

> not a result of ongoing exertion

> not substantially alleviated by rest

> a substantial reduction in previous levels of activity.

Along with the occurrence of four or more of the following symptoms:

> subjective memory impairment

> tender lymph nodes

> muscle pain

> joint pain

> headache

> unrefreshing sleep

> post-exertional malaise.

To successfully manage chronic fatigue symptoms it is essential to establish a collaborative relationship with the patient and use a comprehensive treatment approach, addressing physical disabilities and using psychological strategies. Establishing whether the illness-related behaviour has some secondary gain is helpful in understanding and resolving the situation (eg is there an intolerable situation at work?).

The following are management strategies that have been investigated:

> Graded exercise programmes and cognitive behavioural therapy are the only two treatments shown to be of definite benefit.

> No medications have been shown to be effective, but low-dose amitriptyline is sometimes used for chronic pain.

> Dietary supplements and nicotinamide adenine dinucleotide (NADH) have limited or unknown effectiveness.

> Immunotherapy is unlikely to be beneficial.

> Prolonged rest is ineffective and tends to be harmful.

Review the patient in outpatients on a regular basis, eg at 6-weekly intervals. It is important to ensure reliable communication with the other clinicians involved (GP and cognitive behavioural therapist). The reason for regular review is to pre-empt her making numerous urgent appointments and to provide reassuring, consistent clinical care.

Further discussion

What routine tests would be reasonable to request in this case?

Routine tests should include:

> urine dipstick for protein and sugar

> FBC and white cell differential

> C-reactive protein

> creatinine and electrolytes

> bone function tests (including calcium)

> liver function tests

> glucose

> creatine phosphokinase

> thyroid function tests

> autoantibodies profile, eg antinuclear factor and antiendomysial antibody

> chest X-ray

> electrocardiogram (ECG).

Other investigations will be guided by findings from history and examination, or by abnormalities detected on the routine tests listed above. It is important, but sometimes extremely difficult, to avoid a situation where every interaction with the patient leads to them producing a new symptom, which then triggers a new battery of tests. The mature physician, having taken details of the new history and repeated the physical examination if relevant, will say: 'I have followed what you have been saying, but I don't think that there's anything new to worry us here (assuming that there isn't). I don't think any more tests are needed.'

1.2 Communication skills and ethics

1.2.1 Panic attack and hyperventilation

Scenario

Role: you are a core medical trainee working in the emergency department.

Scenario: a 21-year-old university student is brought to the emergency department by her tutor with difficulty in breathing. She is very worried about her final examinations that start the next day because she has not completed her revision programme. In addition to the breathing difficulty she complains of palpitations, shakiness, sweating and pins and needles in her hands and around her mouth. She is distressed and tearful. Other than hyperventilation, a physical examination and investigations including chest radiography and electrocardiogram (ECG) are normal. You conclude that her symptoms are due to an anxiety state with hyperventilation.

Your task: to explain the psychological nature of her problems and suggest how matters might be helped.

Key issues to explore

> What are her fears and her own explanation of what is happening to her at present?

> Can she see the link between psychological distress and her physiological response?

Key points to establish

> Introduce yourself appropriately.

> Demonstrate good listening skills and an empathic approach.

> Explain the reassuring results of both the physical examination and the investigations.

> Elicit the patient's view of her anxiety symptoms – does she realise it's anxiety?

> Emphasise the link between anxiety and her physical symptoms, and explain the physiology of hyperventilation in terms she would understand: 'When you get anxious and worried your heart rate and breathing naturally speed up, and this has effects on the body. It can make you feel light-headed and dizzy, and this can make you feel more anxious which makes things worse – a sort of vicious cycle.'

> Reassure her that this is anxiety and not a more severe mental illness, and that it is understandable in her current stressful situation.

> Reassure her that her condition is not serious or life-threatening.

> Suggest simple strategies to manage the anxiety: 'We need to find a way of getting out of the vicious cycle. Sitting down and concentrating on taking slow breaths may help, sometimes breathing into a paper bag can help to slow the breathing down. Deliberately trying to think of something calm and pleasant is also useful.'

Appropriate responses to likely questions

Patient: am I going to die?

Doctor: no, I don't think that's at all likely – what are you worried you may die from?

Patient: I think I am going to have a heart attack or stop breathing altogether.

Doctor: I have done a physical examination and carried out tests including an ECG, which is an electrical tracing of your heart, and a chest X-ray. All of the results are normal and show that your heart and lungs are fine.

Patient: so what do you think is going on?

Doctor: I think you're having a panic attack, which is a common reaction to a very stressful situation.

Patient: will it come back?

Doctor: you might have more attacks like this one, but now that you know what is going on and understand the link between frightening thoughts and physical symptoms, you will feel less out of control if it does come back.

Patient: will these attacks get longer?

Doctor: no, I don't think that's likely: as you have seen today, the distressing feelings settled down quite quickly. The more you use the strategies we discussed to deal with them, the more likely you are to control them and prevent them.

Patient: what if these attacks do not go away?

Doctor: I think that they will – they almost always do. But if they didn't, we would then arrange for you to see a specialist. There are highly effective talking treatments, for example a treatment called cognitive behavioural therapy (CBT) can be very helpful.

Patient: are there any medicines that might help me?

Doctor: we do sometimes give medicines in the short term to help people with anxiety and panic attacks that are out of control, but this isn't usually necessary, and it's best to avoid using drugs if we can.

Patient: should I sit my exam tomorrow?

Doctor: that's something that you will have to discuss with your tutor.

In some ways it would be good if you could do so, because we know that one of the things that reinforces anxiety is avoiding the problem – whatever it is. Many people doing an exam feel that they haven't done as much revision as they should have done.

1.2.2 Self-harm

Scenario

Role: you are a core medical trainee working in the emergency department.

Scenario: Mrs Freda Smith, a 64-year-old widow, was brought to hospital after taking an overdose of her antihypertensives. She has a history of depression. Over the years she has become estranged from her children and increasingly isolated. She is not in contact with psychiatric services. You have assessed her mental state and found all the features of a depressive illness. She told you she had been planning this overdose for a long time and had been collecting the tablets to carry this out. She still wishes she was dead and is disappointed that she was found by her neighbour who called the ambulance. You have assessed her physical health and no further medical treatment is required for the overdose. She is anxious to go home and is reluctant to see a psychiatrist.

Your task: explain to Mrs Smith that she needs to speak to a psychiatrist and she would benefit from help from the mental health service.

Key issues to explore

> Address her concerns about seeing a psychiatrist.
> Explain that depression is a treatable illness.

Key points to establish

> Approach her empathically and above all avoid giving the impression that you are criticising or condemning her for the suicide attempt.
> Reassure her that you expect her to recover physically from the overdose.
> Establish why she does not want to see a psychiatrist.
> Explain that she is depressed and that this is a treatable condition.
> Prepare her for admission to a psychiatric ward.

Appropriate responses to likely questions

Patient: I am not mad so why do I need to see a psychiatrist?

Doctor: I haven't said that you are mad, but I do think that you need help. This has clearly been a difficult time for you.

Patient: you think I don't know what I am doing.

Doctor: no, that's not right: I don't think that. I think that you were feeling very miserable and you took the overdose to end those feelings of hopelessness.

Patient: I don't see how a psychiatrist could help me with that.

Doctor: you told me that you have been feeling miserable and lonely. The overdose shows how desperate you have been feeling. What you have is depression, which is an illness that can be treated. Psychiatrists specialise in this.

Patient: *what sort of treatments are there?*

Doctor: the commonly used treatments are a combination of talking therapies and antidepressant medication. Have you come across these treatments before?

Patient: *I have heard about antidepressants: I have heard they are addictive.*

Doctor: antidepressants have been used for many years and doctors have a lot of experience with them. They are effective in treating depression and they are not addictive in the sense that they don't make people feel as though they want to take more and more of them, and they don't cause euphoria – a feeling of being overly excited or happy.

Patient: *will I be locked up if I see a psychiatrist?*

Doctor: I think that you need treatment, and right now hospital might be the best place for you to get that treatment – even if that is not what you want. Once you feel better you may feel differently about being in hospital.

Patient: *how long would they keep me in hospital?*

Doctor: I'm not an expert in this – the psychiatrist will advise us – but treatments for depression take a few weeks to start working, so it is likely that you would be in hospital for a few weeks.

Patient: *if I try to leave, will you stop me?*

Doctor: I very much hope that you won't just walk out. I think that you are depressed and that we can help this. I very much hope that you will agree to talk to someone from the psychiatry team so that we can find out what they think would be best. But if you do try to go, I will insist that you see a psychiatrist even if that means stopping you from leaving.

1.2.3 Medically unexplained symptoms

Scenario

Role: you are a core medical trainee in a medical outpatient clinic.

Scenario: a 34-year-old woman has been followed up in the medical outpatient clinic. She presented with a 12-month history of fatigue. On examination there were no abnormal physical findings. A battery of laboratory investigations has been done and all have been normal or negative. There is no evidence of an underlying depressive illness.

She had suffered a brief flu-like illness about a week before the onset of her fatigue. She returned to work before she had fully recovered because she did not want to let her colleagues down. As things turned out, she was not able to cope with her job as a trader in an international bank and was sent on sick leave. She is an articulate woman who is a perfectionist and sets herself high standards. She is convinced that the virus has damaged her immune system and is still making her ill. She spends most of the day either in bed or resting on a couch. Any attempt to do tasks that are physically demanding, for example climbing up the stairs, causes her breathlessness, rapid heartbeat and weakness of her legs. She attributes this to an ongoing disturbance of her immune system. She has spent a lot of time and money pursuing complementary therapies, including high doses of vitamins and trace elements. A diagnosis of chronic fatigue syndrome has been made by the consultant in charge of her care.

Your task: to explain her illness to her and introduce a treatment approach of graded exercise and cognitive behavioural therapy.

Key issues to explore

> Explore her explanatory model for her illness and offer an alternative.

> Introduce the idea of graded exercise and explain its rationale.

> Introduce the idea of cognitive behavioural therapy.

> Encourage problem solving that will enable her to get back to work.

Key points to establish

> Summarise the position both in terms of her history and investigations.

> Acknowledge the distressing and real nature of her symptoms and disabilities.

> Acknowledge her own explanatory model, ie her conviction that all her symptoms are caused by a damaged immune system.

> Reassure her that there is no laboratory evidence of any ongoing disturbance to her immune system.

> Offer her an alternative explanatory model, gently suggesting a link between physical symptoms and distress, and a continued lack of exercise. It can be helpful to explain this as a spectrum: all human emotions are associated with physical symptoms, so much so that it has become part of everyday language, such as 'butterflies in the stomach' in anxiety, or feeling 'gutted' when we mean we feel sad but actually do have that very physical sinking feeling.

> Explain how graded exercise and talking therapies could help, regardless of the underlying cause.

Appropriate responses to likely questions

Patient: *I'm sure that the problem is with immune system, isn't it?*

Doctor: it may be that your immune system was affected when you had the viral infection a year or so ago, but there's no evidence that this is the main problem now. The tests we've done, including looking for markers of immune system activation in the blood, are all normal, which is very reassuring.

Patient: if my immune system is back to normal, why do I feel so exhausted?

Doctor: for the past year you have been spending most of your time in bed or on the sofa. This means that your body has got out of condition, so any exertion – even very minor exertion – makes you feel fatigued for a long time afterwards.

Patient: why does any physical effort make me feel much worse?

Doctor: when you don't exercise your muscles they become very weak, the opposite to what happens when you train in the gym. Your heart also becomes unfit, so any exertion will cause it to beat rapidly. The same goes for your breathing. So over the past year the combination of your muscles, heart and lungs becoming weaker is now causing you to feel exhausted all the time.

Patient: can I have a second opinion?

Doctor: yes, you could, but I honestly don't think that it would help you. I think the best thing would be to develop a plan for how we can help you to build up your exercise capacity and get back to doing the things that you want to do. But if you do want a second opinion, your GP could make a referral, and – if it would be helpful – we could offer them some suggestions as to who might be appropriate. I could talk with my consultant about this.

Patient: so what would you recommend?

Doctor: I think that the most helpful treatments would be graded exercise therapy and cognitive behavioural therapy. If you were willing to consider these, I would find out how you could best access them and let you know.

Patient: in the self-help group that I subscribe to, they say that there are bound to be underlying problems with my immune system and it may take me another year or 2 to recover.

Doctor: we know from experience that the longer you remain inactive the harder it is to recover. People who make an early start to a graded exercise programme combined with cognitive behavioural therapy begin to recover more quickly.

Patient: I am receiving income protection benefit and the insurers and my employers are pressurising me to return to work, but I cannot possibly do that at the moment. What should I do?

Doctor: at what point do you see yourself returning to work?

Patient: I would need to be completely recovered to cope with my job.

Doctor: that is looking at things in an 'all or nothing' way, and it would be very difficult to do after having had such a long time off. Have you been in touch with the bank's occupational health department? If not, I think you should. Their business would be trying to find a way by which you could get back to work, probably working reduced hours in the first instance.

1.3 Acute scenarios

1.3.1 Acute confusional state

Scenario

A middle-aged man develops an acute confusional state after coronary artery bypass graft surgery. His mental state had appeared normal on admission, but 48 hours after the operation he has pulled out his intravenous line, refuses to allow the nurses anywhere near him, and is cowering in a corner of the ward. He is clearly terrified and suspicious, and accuses the staff of trying to kill him.

Introduction

The most likely diagnosis is an acute confusional state (delirium), but occasionally patients might develop a brief psychosis or a severe affective (mood) disorder after major surgery. It is important to consider alcohol withdrawal and delirium tremens.

> **Key point**
>
> **Key features of an acute confusional state**
>
> > clouding of consciousness, which may fluctuate
>
> > disorientation in time, place and person
>
> > impaired grasp of their situation and diminished attention
>
> > reversal of the sleep–wakefulness cycle
>
> > the confusion worsens at night, but with a lucid interval in the morning.

Common causes of an acute confusional state

After coronary artery surgery, delirium following a lucid interval is probably due to metabolic disturbance, medication, sleep deprivation or alcohol withdrawal. Common causes of delirium are shown in Table 3.

History of the presenting problem

Review of clinical records

You know the patient was mentally well prior to the surgery. Think of what may have happened during the surgery and look at the perioperative records: were there, for instance, problems with the anaesthetic or with the surgery that might have affected cerebral perfusion or caused a cerebrovascular event?

People are commonly confused and disorientated as they recover from

Table 3   Common causes of an acute confusional state

Common causes	Conditions
Systemic	Infection (eg pneumonia, septicaemia and urinary tract infection) Respiratory or cardiac failure Electrolyte imbalance Metabolic disorder (eg hypoglycaemia, renal or hepatic failure) Severe hypotension due to reduced cardiac output secondary to myocardial infarction, pulmonary embolus or arrhythmia Severe anaemia
Intracranial	Cerebrovascular accident Postictal state
Drug-induced	Steroids, theophylline or beta-blockers Drug intoxication (eg with analgesics) Withdrawal of alcohol or benzodiazepines
Other	Pain Urinary retention

anaesthetic. What has happened to this man? Look at the following:

> Nursing and medical notes: did he gain lucidity within the expected time frame? Have there been any postoperative medical problems, eg bleeding?

> Drug charts: what medication has he been given in the last 48 hours? Analgesics are a common cause of confusion.

> Observation and fluid charts: has he been hypotensive, and what fluids has he been given?

Discussion with nursing colleagues
The nursing staff are likely to be the main source of information in a case such as this, although any relatives that are present may give a useful history and for a variety of reasons may be keen to do so. Ask the nurses if the patient has had vomiting and/or diarrhoea. In addition, inquire about early warning signs of impending delirium, for example:

> daytime drowsiness

> if there was a lucid interval in the morning, which might have given a misleading impression of normality during the morning ward round.

Other relevant history
Try to establish the underlying cause of the delirium by looking for information in the notes and/or asking relatives. The most important issues are:

> to estimate the patient's usual daily alcohol intake

> whether there has been increasing absent-mindedness and progressive impairment of memory over the preceding 6–12 months or so, indicating dementia with superimposed delirium

> has this happened before in other contexts?

Consider the risks, both to the patient (pulling out drips, refusing treatment, reduced oral intake, etc) and to others on the ward (aggression to staff or other patients). In clinical practice, ensure you discuss this with ward staff and consider contacting hospital security.

Other less likely possibilities should also be considered. Has there been a recent head injury (unlikely in this context, but you need to consider the possibility of subdural haematoma)? Is there a history of a previous psychiatric disorder that might point towards a relapse of schizophrenia or mood disorder

precipitated by the psychological stress of the operation? Is there a history of seizures? (Rarely a presentation such as this can be due to a prolonged complex partial seizure or prolonged ictal state.)

Examination
Physical examination
You would clearly want to perform a physical examination of the patient to look for evidence of conditions listed in Table 3, but in the immediate circumstances this will not be possible in the normal manner. Note any evidence of focal neurology (eg dysphasia, impairment of movement of one or more limbs). As and when the situation changes and he becomes less resistant to nursing or medical attention, perhaps after the administration of sedation, complete a full examination, as described in relevant scenarios in the *Acute medicine* book.

Examination of mental state
Look for features to establish the diagnosis of delirium:

> General appearance – the patient generally appears more frightened than hostile, although he may act aggressively in self-defence against an

imaginary enemy. In some cases the patient will appear apathetic and withdrawn rather than agitated: this is hypoactive delirium, which can be mistaken for depression.

> Behaviour – the patient is commonly restless and may pluck at the bedclothes, and they may attempt to escape from the ward. In contrast to this picture of 'noisy' delirium, a patient may be withdrawn and underactive, and it might only be on close questioning that the clinician learns that they are disorientated and unable to grasp what is going on around them.

> Changes in speech and thinking – the patient's speech may be incoherent. There may be fleeting and sketchy ideas of persecution or ideas of reference (eg the ward television is showing a police drama which the patient interprets to mean that he is about to be arrested). Delusional themes might include the patient being convinced that he is being held in prison, or that staff are trying to poison him.

> Mood – this is often changeable and can fluctuate from intense fear and agitation to milder forms of anxiety, depression and irritability.

Key point

In delirium there is clouding of consciousness. This helps to distinguish delirium from the agitation of severe depression or the excitement of mania, in which consciousness is unimpaired.

> Perceptual disturbances – there may be illusions and hallucinations. The latter are mainly visual but can also be auditory and tactile. A telephone wire may be perceived as a snake, while the ringing of a telephone might sound like a fire alarm.

> Cognitive function – there is disorientation in both time and place, and misidentification of members of staff or members of his own family. The patient is likely to appear dazed and unclear about his surroundings: he has difficulty in grasping what is happening around him, his attention to what is going on around him is greatly reduced and he tends to drift off. His attention span is also decreased (unable to correctly repeat seven digits listed to him).

> Tests of cognitive function – in this particular patient testing is very likely to be impossible, but in a less disturbed and somewhat more cooperative patient you could ask them to recite the days of the week and then the months of the year in reverse order. Another test of attention and concentration is to serially subtract seven from 100 or three from 20. Other general tests of cognitive function that are commonly used are the Abbreviated Mental Test and the Mini Mental State Examination. When interpreting the patient's performance on these tests, you need to take into account their educational attainment and fluency in the language of the examination.

> Insight – this fluctuates with the patient's level of consciousness. After the episode the patient will have little recollection of what he thought, how he behaved and how he was treated.

Key point

In assessing a patient with an acute confusional state you should always try to perform a full physical examination (after sedation if necessary), looking for evidence of any of the conditions listed in Table 3. This may be very difficult to do: your notes in the clinical record must detail your findings or explain the circumstances that prevented thorough examination.

Investigations

These should be performed (after sedation if necessary) to establish the presence of any of the conditions listed in Table 3. In the absence of obvious clinical clues, which would direct investigations, the tests shown in Table 4 would be appropriate when possible.

Management

The patient with delirium is often unable to cooperate with nursing and medical care. He might refuse medication and investigations. He may become dehydrated or sustain an injury when falling or fighting.

The priorities are:

> Keep the patient from harming himself and others: one-to-one nursing care is indicated, preferably with a single nurse on each shift rather than a succession of nurses 'dropping in'. Keep the patient in touch with his surroundings: a window increases awareness of the contrast between day and night, and a clock may help orientation to time. Consider relaxing visiting time rules to allow familiar people, family members, to be around to help reassure.

> Establish and treat the cause of the delirium if possible, eg electrolyte imbalance, dehydration, infection or anaemia.

> Review all current medication and withdraw any that can be stopped.

Remember to consider the legal framework under which the patient is being detained in the hospital and treated. Usually this will be the Mental Capacity Act 2005, but this legal area is under review, hence ask for up-to-date advice from the hospital safeguarding adults team, or liaison psychiatry service.

Table 4	Investigations to determine the cause of an acute confusional state		
Investigation		**Comment**	
ECG		Has he had an infarct or developed an arrhythmia?	
Glucose (finger-prick test plus laboratory)		Hypoglycaemia is common after surgery	
Electrolytes and calcium		Hyponatraemia is common postoperatively	
Renal and liver function		Acute kidney injury is common postoperatively	
FBC and erythrocyte sedimentation rate		Looking for anaemia or evidence of infection	
Culture of urine, blood and sputum			
Pulse oximetry and arterial blood gases			
Chest X-ray			
CT head scan		If focal neurological signs are present and/or no other obvious explanation for confusion	

Other tests as determined by clinical findings or results from initial investigations

CT, computerised tomography; ECG, electrocardiogram; FBC, full blood count.

Sedatives and tranquilisers

For severe agitation associated with delirium, consider using haloperidol (2.5–5 mg *per os* (PO) or intramuscular (IM)) or olanzapine (5 mg PO or IM). Try to avoid benzodiazepines which can make disorientation worse. Use lower doses in older people.

In cases of delirium tremens, administer chlordiazepoxide 30 mg four times a day (reducing dose regime) to prevent withdrawal seizures, and parenteral vitamin B to prevent development of Wernicke's encephalopathy.

Key point

Delirium is an urgent situation and the staff have a clear duty of care. If the patient clearly lacks the capacity to give meaningful consent or refuses potentially life-saving investigation and treatment, then treatment can be given in their best interests. If more than emergency interventions are required because the problems persist, then it would be advisable to call in the duty psychiatrist to discuss the use of the Mental Health Act.

1.3.2 Self-harm

Scenario

A 30-year-old, unemployed woman is brought into the emergency department after taking an unknown quantity of paracetamol and vodka 90 minutes earlier. She is alert and tearful. She is able to tell the triage nurse that she was feeing desperate because her partner had left her and she had just been evicted for rent arrears. Some years ago she took an overdose and cut her wrists after one of her children was taken into care.

Introduction

Intentional self-harm leads to about 100,000 hospital admissions in England and Wales every year and its incidence is increasing. During the 10-year period following any episode of self-harm, the risk of suicide is increased to 30-fold higher than that expected in the general population, with the first 6 months being the period of greatest risk.

Key point

Self-harm and risk of suicide

> After an episode of self-harm, 1% of patients kill themselves in the year that follows. Try to remember this at the most difficult times, for example at 3am in the acute admission ward, when a face familiar to you presents again – don't fall into the trap of minimalising such cases.

> One-fifth to one-quarter of patients who die by suicide have presented to a general hospital following episodes of self-harm in the year before their death.

The highest suicide rate occurs in people aged over 75, but the rate among young men has increased greatly over the past 20 years. Men tend to use violent means such as hanging; women are more likely to kill themselves by self-poisoning with drugs. Most people who commit suicide have a psychiatric disorder such as depression (15% lifetime risk of suicide), schizophrenia (10% lifetime risk) and alcohol addiction (3.4% lifetime risk). Risk factors for suicide can be split into static (fixed) and dynamic (amenable to change) factors.

History of the presenting problem
Preparation for the overdose

> Had she planned the overdose for some time or did she take it on impulse?
> Where did she get the pills from?
> Had she taken precautions to make sure that she was alone and undisturbed?
> Did she leave a suicide note?
> Had she given away her most treasured possessions or made other preparations for her death, eg funeral plans, sending children/pets to stay elsewhere?
> Did she research suicide methods online?
> What triggered her to take the overdose at that time?

During and after the overdose

> What was her intent?
> What did she think would happen?
> Who called for help? Did she resist this?
> How does she feel about it now?
> Does she still have suicidal thoughts, plans or intent?

Hazard

Patients are not experts in pharmacology

When evaluating risk do not assume that a small overdose of a relatively safe drug necessarily implies minimal lethal intent: the patient might think that a few temazepam tablets are as dangerous as a handful of digoxin pills.

Psychiatric symptoms

Screen for symptoms of major mental illness such as depression or psychosis. Ask about mood, loss of interest or enjoyment, sleep, appetite, thoughts of guilt or worthlessness, hopelessness and ongoing suicidal thoughts or ideas. Ask about hallucinations or delusions, particularly depressive delusions such as guilt or nihilism. Ask about substance use.

Other relevant history
Assessment of the short-term risk of a further suicide attempt

Increased risk of suicide – does she have a psychiatric disorder that puts her at risk of suicide? Chronic, painful, disabling or life-threatening illnesses also increase the risk. This patient has a history of self-harm, which makes her more vulnerable to future suicide attempts, as would a family history of suicide. She has also recently separated from her partner, is in debt and has lost her home – recent events of this type are risk factors.

Reduced risk of suicide – explore protective factors such as the quality of her social support network. Other protective factors include a sense of responsibility, having children or pets in the home, employment and problem-solving skills or alternative coping strategies. Strong religious belief is a protective factor, but beware the stigma that is often associated with suicide when it is regarded as something forbidden – people may have left it far later in their illness to seek help.

Collateral history

Because suicidal people are often reluctant to reveal information, speaking to someone else who

knows her well may tell you more about the suicide attempt and her personal circumstances. This would also help you to assess whether she has an impulsive or aggressive personality, which is important because these traits are known to be additional risk factors.

Hazard

Difficulties in the assessment of suicide risk

> The degree of suicide intent can fluctuate. After self-harm events there can be a sort of elation about being alive, probably a very human survival trait, that does not always last.

> Gravely suicidal patients can deliberately conceal their intentions – they may appear misleadingly calm after they have made a firm but undisclosed plan to kill themselves.

Management

The immediate priority in any patient presenting with self-harm is dealing with the physical consequences of the self-harm. In this case this would include managing paracetamol poisoning by establishing blood levels, monitoring liver function and administering acetylcysteine.

The second priority is to prevent further episodes of self-harm. All patients who have harmed themselves should have an assessment by the duty liaison psychiatry team to determine whether admission or discharge with follow-up are appropriate.

Hazard

Recognition of the patient at high risk

> Patients who discharge themselves from the emergency department before psychosocial assessment have three times the rate of repetition of self-harm.

> Failure to resolve precipitating circumstances and failure to establish a rapport with the medical staff are two things that should alert you that a patient is still at high risk.

> Patients with untreated psychiatric illness or substance misuse are at especially high risk.

Refusal of life-saving treatment or psychiatric assessment

First, evaluate her capacity to make an informed decision. Explain the risks to the patient of not receiving treatment and then see if she understands what you have explained. Is she able to retain the information and does she believe it? Is she able to weigh it up in the balance when making her decision? Is she able to communicate her decision to you? Remember capacity is decision and time specific.

After this, record your assessment of her capacity, including the reasons why you have come to your decision (rather than just a yes/no). If she lacks capacity to decide to stay in hospital, she can be detained in hospital and receive life-saving treatment in her best interests under the Mental Capacity Act 2005. It is good practice to enlist the support of family or friends. If she presents as a risk to herself or others and presents with a mental disorder, and if she is admitted to a medical ward, she could be held in hospital under Section 5(4) or Section 5(2) of the Mental Health Act 1983.

1.3.3 Complications of alcohol use in hospital

Scenario

A 54-year-old man is admitted to hospital in a neglected state. He appears anxious, agitated, shaky and sweaty. He reports that he stopped drinking alcohol 2 days previously.

Introduction

Alcohol abuse and dependence

The *Diagnostic and statistical manual of mental disorders* (DSM)-V criteria for alcohol abuse and dependence (alcohol use disorder) are based on the patient's answers to a series of questions (see the following 'Key point').

Key point

Diagnosis of alcohol use disorder

A score of 1 is assigned to each question for which 'yes' is the answer.

In the past year, have you:

1 had times when you ended up drinking more, or longer, than you intended?

2 more than once wanted to cut down or stop drinking, or tried to, but couldn't?

3 spent a lot of time drinking, or being sick or getting over other after effects?

4 wanted a drink so badly you couldn't think of anything else?

5 found that drinking, or being sick from drinking, often interfered taking care of home / family, or caused problems with your education or job?

6 continued to drink even though it was causing trouble with your family and friends?

7 given up or cut back on activities that were important or interesting to you, or gave you pleasure, in order to drink?

8 more than once got into situations while or after drinking that increased your chances of getting hurt?

9 continued to drink even though it was making you depressed/anxious, or adding to another health problem? Or after having had a memory blackout?

10 had to drink much more than you once did to get the effect you want? Or found that your usual number of drinks had much less effect than before?

11 found that when the effects of alcohol were wearing off you had withdrawal symptoms (eg trouble sleeping, shakiness, restlessness, nausea, sweating, palpitations, seizure) or sensed things that were not there?

Score	Alcohol use disorder
2–3	Mild
4–5	Moderate
6 or more	Severe

Withdrawal symptoms

The DSM-V criteria for alcohol withdrawal symptoms are shown in the following 'Key point'.

Key point

Diagnosis of alcohol withdrawal

Requires *two or more of the following*, developing within several hours to a few days after an individual stops drinking:

> insomnia

> autonomic symptoms – eg sweating, palpitations

> increased hand tremors – 'the shakes'

> psychomotor agitation – physically restless, cannot stop moving

> anxiety

> seizures – typically generalised tonic–clonic

> hallucinations – auditory, tactile or visual.

Safe alcohol consumption

The UK Chief Medical Officers (2016) published guidelines for both men and women are as follows:

> To keep health risks from alcohol to a low level it is safest not to drink more than 14 units a week on a regular basis.

> It is best to spread drinking evenly over 3 or more days (if you do drink as much as 14 units a week).

If people drink 14 or more units of alcohol a week, then their lifetime risk of dying from an alcohol-related condition is at least 1%.

History of the presenting problem

Key point

Developing a helpful therapeutic relationship

> A grasp of his current social circumstances and supports will help this man feel understood as a person and may give insight into why he continues to drink.

> A blaming, moralistic attitude focusing exclusively on alcohol abuse will result in a frustrating, ineffective therapeutic relationship.

The important aspects to try to establish are:

> When was his last drink?

> What is he drinking?

> What is the strength?

> How much? How many units per week (see Table 5)?

> How often?

> When in the day?

> Does he relate drinking to any particular pattern or situation?

> Does he drink alone or with people?

Other relevant history

Related to alcohol abuse

The age he started drinking and why may reveal continuing psychological reasons for drinking: problem drinking would have started later.

Impact of drinking – explore with the patient the negative social effects of heavy drinking such as drinking and driving offences, accidents or injuries, and losing jobs or partners (in addition to the medical consequences).

Relapses – discuss precipitants of previous relapses.

Withdrawal symptoms – has he had these before, and what was their outcome? This may help to predict what happens now.

Family history – a family history of alcohol abuse may indicate a genetic propensity and/or exposure to a heavy drinking micro-culture where alcohol is routinely used as an inappropriate coping device.

Previous treatment for alcohol abuse – examining the outcome of previous treatment programmes and why they failed may help him to overcome obstacles to abstinence.

Table 5 Units of alcohol in common beverages, where 1 unit of alcohol contains 8 g of ethanol	
Type of drink	**Units of alcohol**
Pint of lager	2
Pint of extra-strong lager	5
150 mL glass of wine	1
One shot of spirits (25 mL)	1

Associated psychiatric conditions

One-third of people with alcohol dependence also have another mental illness, most commonly a mood disorder, an anxiety disorder or an antisocial personality disorder. Suicide is also commonly associated with alcohol.

Associated medical conditions

Conditions that are associated with alcohol abuse and dependence are:

> oesophagitis

> gastritis

> gastric ulcer

> alcoholic hepatitis and cirrhosis

> oesophageal varices

> pancreatitis

> cardiomyopathy

> thiamine deficiency – Wernicke–Korsakoff syndrome

> neuropathy

> head injuries (subdural haematoma)

> cerebellar atrophy.

Examination

Look for signs of:

> withdrawal (see above)

> infection (especially pneumonia)

> malnutrition

> possible medical complications of alcohol abuse (see above)

> confusion, ie being disorientated, having impaired attention and registration, etc.

If he is confused, conditions to consider include:

> hypoglycaemia

> delirium tremens, which can occur within 72 hours of his last drink

> Wernicke's encephalopathy

> postictal state – but before attributing seizures to alcohol withdrawal, exclude other causes such as hypoglycaemia, hyponatraemia, hypomagnesaemia and other central nervous system pathology, eg subdural haematoma. In cases of delirium exclude other medical conditions including infection and hepatic failure

> head injury.

Key point
Wernicke's encephalopathy

Classical presentation is with:

> ophthalmoplegia (horizontal and vertical nystagmus, weakness/paralysis of lateral rectus muscles and weakness/paralysis of conjugate gaze)

> ataxia

> confusion.

Hazard
Wernicke's encephalopathy

> caused by thiamine deficiency

> if missed and not treated with parenteral thiamine, it will result in death or permanent neurological and cognitive damage.

Management

Aside from treatment of intercurrent medical issues, the important aspects are as follows:

> General – nurse the patient in a well-lit, quiet environment, with one-to-one nursing if required.

> Treatment of withdrawal symptoms – give a 7–10-day course of diazepam or chlordiazepoxide, usually orally. Occasionally intravenous treatment is required for seizures. Never use intramuscular injection because of erratic absorption. Initially titrate the oral dose until symptoms are controlled, then taper the dose until stopping.

> Thiamine supplementation – give parenterally if there is a risk of Wernicke's encephalopathy.

> Consider hypoglycaemia – monitor for and prevent.

> Fluids and diet – treat dehydration; give a high-calorie, high-carbohydrate diet.

> Antipsychotics – avoid because they lower the seizure threshold.

Key point
Refer the patient to alcohol services for follow-up, support, advice and cognitive behavioural therapy; and also to a psychiatrist if comorbid mental illness is present.

1.3.4 Complications of intravenous drug use in hospital

Scenario
A 29-year-old woman has been admitted to a surgical ward for drainage of an abscess on her forearm. She uses heroin intravenously and says that she is about to go into opioid withdrawal.

History of the presenting problem

History of substance misuse

Important points to elucidate are:

> What substances is she using? (This list may be extensive.)

> Since when?

> By what method?

> How much?

Heroin can be smoked, injected or snorted, and may be used in conjunction with other opioids. Ask her to describe any withdrawal symptoms she may be experiencing or has experienced in the past. Has she developed tolerance? Does she have any plans to kick her habit?

Opioid use disorder

The *Diagnostic and statistical manual of mental disorders* (DSM)-V criteria for opioid use disorder are shown in the following 'Key point'.

Key point

Diagnosis of opioid use disorder

Requires a problematic pattern of opioid use leading to clinically significant impairment or distress, as manifested by *two or more of the following* occurring within a 12-month period:

1 Opioids are often taken in larger amounts or over a longer period than was intended.

2 There is a persistent desire or unsuccessful efforts to cut down or control opioid use.

3 A great deal of time is spent in activities necessary to obtain the opioid, use the opioid, or recover from its effects.

4 Craving, or a strong desire / urge to use opioids.

5 Recurrent opioid use resulting in failure to fulfil major role obligations at home, work or in education.

6 Continued opioid use despite persistent or recurrent social or interpersonal problems caused or exacerbated by the effects of opioids.

7 Important social, occupational or recreational activities are given up or reduced because of opioid use.

8 Recurrent opioid use in situations in which it is physically hazardous.

9 Continued opioid use despite knowledge of having a persistent or recurrent physical or psychological problem that is likely to have been caused or exacerbated by the substance.

10 Tolerance, as defined by a need for markedly increasing amounts of opioids to achieve intoxication / desired effect, or a markedly diminished effect with continued use of the same amount of an opioid.

11 Withdrawal, as manifest by a characteristic withdrawal syndrome (see the 'Key point' below), or that opioids (or a closely related substance) are taken to relieve or avoid withdrawal symptoms.

Score	Opioid use disorder
2–3	Mild
4–5	Moderate
6 or more	Severe

Withdrawal symptoms

The DSM-V criteria for opioid withdrawal symptoms are shown in the following 'Key point'.

Key point

Diagnosis of opioid withdrawal

A – Either of the following:

> cessation of (or reduction in) opioid use that has been heavy and prolonged (several weeks or longer)

> administration of an opioid antagonist after a period of opioid use.

Together with:

B – three or more of the following, developing within minutes to several days after criterion A:

> dysphoric mood

> nausea or vomiting

> muscle aches

> lacrimation or rhinorrhoea

> pupillary dilation, piloerection or sweating

> diarrhoea

> yawning

> fever

> insomnia.

Other relevant history

Social issues

Ask the patient about her current social circumstances and social supports. What was happening in her life at the time her drug abuse started? Does she have children or might she be pregnant? Does she have a safe place to live? How does she fund her drug habit? Understanding these issues will help establish a therapeutic alliance as well as giving you a more holistic view of her problems.

Medical complications of drug abuse

Chronic liver disease and its complications, endocarditis and HIV are the most common serious conditions seen with intravenous drug use.

Examination

People with drug-dependence problems may present in a demanding and overwhelming manner, but do not let this put you off from establishing objective evidence of drug use if this can be obtained safely (if it cannot, the notes you make in the clinical records should explain why you could not do this).

Aside from checking vital signs (hypertension, tachycardia and temperature dysregulation are typical in opioid withdrawal), weight (body mass index – people who use drugs are frequently malnourished) and performing a general physical examination, look for:

> evidence of drug abuse – needle track marks, discoid scars from subcutaneous injection, burn marks on fingers and neglected self-care

> signs of opioid withdrawal – as listed above.

Investigation

Urine test kits are now available in most emergency departments that will tell you within 10 minutes whether any drug or its metabolites are present in any urine sample. They usually just indicate the presence or absence of a drug, not the amount.

In this woman with an obvious septic focus it will be appropriate to check full blood count (FBC), glucose, electrolytes, renal / bone / liver function tests, C-reactive protein, clotting screen, blood cultures and (with appropriate consent) for hepatitis B and C, HIV and syphilis; also to swab the abscess.

Further tests may be required if there are specific indications, eg echocardiography if there is a suspicion of endocarditis.

Management

Key point
Always get advice from a substance misuse specialist.

In addition to drainage of the abscess, appropriate antimicrobial therapy and treatment of any other medical problems, the question to be tackled is 'how should opioid withdrawal be prevented or treated?'.

Hazard
Poly-substance abuse
This is common among heroin users, but does not necessarily mean dependence on all the substances. Withdrawal symptoms from one substance may be altered by the presence of others.

Methadone

If you have determined that the patient is dependent on opioids and is in withdrawal, then she will need methadone substitution to relieve her symptoms. If she is pregnant this is mandatory as opioid withdrawal is associated with spontaneous abortion and fetal death.

If you can, establish her methadone dose from her prescribing drug team or dispensing pharmacy, and when she last collected a script. If you have no other collateral information, initially prescribe 10 mg methadone bd and monitor 4-hourly for withdrawal symptoms. Increase by 5–10 mg increments if withdrawal symptoms occur, up to a maximum of 20 mg bd in the first 24 hours. Determine how much methadone is required over a 24-hour

period, and then that dose can be given as a single or divided dose.

Beware of overdosing her as this could result in respiratory arrest. Remember that she may be getting opioids from an alternative source while she is in hospital, so look for signs of intoxication and ensure that naloxone is available in case this occurs.

Hazard
Methadone can cause fatal respiratory depression at a dose of 30 mg, or even lower if combined with other opioids, alcohol or benzodiazepines. Remember:

> never give a methadone dose equivalent to what the patient reports they are using (Table 6)

> never prescribe methadone to occasional opioid users

> seek advice from a specialist in substance misuse.

Other treatments for withdrawal symptoms

Clonidine and lofexidine are centrally acting agents used to dampen down sympathetic tone, thereby reducing the severity of withdrawal symptoms. Try to avoid the use of benzodiazepines as these are frequently also abused.

Opioid withdrawal

An acute admission unit is not a suitable setting to embark on an opioid withdrawal programme. Aim to stabilise the dose of methadone the patient is receiving and then refer them to a drug rehabilitation unit if withdrawal is deemed appropriate. Withdrawal should take 10–14 days. If discharging the patient to the community, ensure their methadone will be prescribed for supervised administration in an appropriate setting, and share information about treatment in hospital with the treating drug team.

Drug	Dose	Methadone equivalent
Street heroin	1	1
Pharmaceutical heroin	10 mg tablet or ampoule	20 mg
Morphine	10 mg ampoule	10 mg
Dihydrocodeine (DF 118)	30 mg tablet	3 mg
Buprenorphine hydrochloride	200 μg tablet	5 mg
	300 μg ampoule	8 mg
Codeine phosphate	15 mg tablet	1 mg
J Collis Browne 100 mL	10 mg extract of opium	10 mg

Table 6 Equivalent opioid doses

1 Purity varies, hence it is impossible to make an accurate estimate.

Other matters

This may be the only contact she has with medical services, so try to provide her with some information about safer drugs use (harm minimisation), the availability of services and the dangers of HIV and hepatitis.

Refer her to a psychiatrist if comorbidity is suspected. Encourage attendance at a drug rehabilitation unit or community substance misuse service (methadone cannot be used without this). Strategies used here include motivational interviewing, cognitive behavioural therapy, methadone maintenance or withdrawal programmes, inpatient treatment programmes, drug substitution and assistance with social problems. Naltrexone may be used to prevent relapse.

1.3.5 The frightening patient

Scenario

A tall and physically intimidating man is brought to the emergency department by the police. He appears dishevelled, is shouting abuse and lashing out at anyone who approaches him.

Introduction

Key point

If you are concerned that a patient might be violent:

> Do not take any risks.

> Never see them alone.

> Call back-up, eg hospital security and/or police.

> Remove your tie, scarf or necklace.

> Make sure that you and other staff always have easy access to an exit door.

> Remove other patients from the area.

> Remove potential weapons from the area.

> Do not let back-up, eg hospital security and/or police, leave until you feel the situation is safe.

> Check for concealed weapons.

Violent behaviour is most often exhibited by men, individuals under 30 years, and associated with access to weapons, and drug and alcohol abuse. Remember, however, that pain or nausea, anxiety about physical symptoms (or a relative or friend), and the long waits associated with attending an emergency department, may also have triggered angry feelings in anyone!

The approach and management will be different in each case and the more information you can gather about the person the better you will be equipped to make good decisions in a calm and rational manner. Look at past notes, including asking for information from the liaison psychiatry team. Some people react in an angry and blaming way to the feelings of uncertainty and loss of control that may accompany an illness. People with mental illness might be aggressive because they are very frightened by their symptoms, although violence is far more commonly associated with alcohol or drug use, and far less common in mental illness than the media would suggest.

Understanding and reassurance go a long way to resolve these situations. While being rigidly authoritarian may just escalate matters, clear boundaries about acceptable behaviour, given in a calm and reasonable voice, can be containing for an agitated or frightened person.

Key point

Violence with intent to harm others should always be reported to police. If a person is in custody after committing a crime, and presents to the emergency department, the police should stay with the person until they are medically fit to return to custody – illness should not circumvent criminal process.

History of the presenting problem

Recognising that information you are able to gain from the patient may be sparse and that you may have to rely on collateral information from family, friends, the police and medical notes, etc, what questions are you going to ask?

If possible, find out:

> What is he normally like?

> When did this behaviour start?

> Did anything precipitate it?

> What was he doing when he was found by the police?

> Has he threatened or injured anyone?

> Has he destroyed property?

> Has he used drugs or alcohol?

> What has he been saying?

> Has he been making sense?

Having established information about the incident that led to the patient's arrest, what further information about him do you need to determine the underlying cause of his violent behaviour? Enquire:

> Has he got any medical conditions, eg epilepsy or diabetes?

> Is he normally on medication and is he compliant?

> Has he received treatment for a mental illness?

> Does he have a history of aggressive behaviour?

> Does he have a history of drug and alcohol abuse?

> Has he been arrested or convicted in the past?

> If the violence is thought to be as a result of mental illness then consider the following:

>> delirium / acute confusional state (see Section 1.3.1)

>> mood disorders (see Section 2.13)

>> psychotic disorders (see Section 2.4).

Examination

The patient's general appearance may give clues to an underlying condition. What he is saying may indicate that he is confused or deluded. If he is behaving bizarrely or appearing to respond to hallucinations, then this may suggest the presence of delirium or psychosis.

It is imperative to try to get his cooperation to do a physical examination, or as much of one as he can tolerate, to look for an underlying physical condition. But if this is not possible you should record precisely why in the medical notes. Write down exactly what is said by the patient, including expletives!

Investigations

It may not be possible to perform any investigations before sedation is administered. If you are able to get the patient to cooperate, then only do what is absolutely necessary as excessive demands may irritate him. The following should certainly be considered:

> check for drug abuse – urine drug screen (see Section 1.3.4)

> check for alcohol abuse – breathalyser test or saliva alcohol test

> check for delirium – always check finger-prick blood glucose, and

perform those tests listed in Section 1.3.1 that are indicated and possible. If the tests cannot be done, then your notes should explain precisely why, eg 'patient would not allow venepuncture (told me to "xxxx off")'.

Management

Key point

Remember first and foremost not to risk your safety or that of other patients and hospital staff, and:

> keep a calm, reassuring appearance

> be pleasant, clear and firm: do not make promises you cannot keep, and do what you say you are going to do

> do not bargain with, argue with or threaten him, but do listen to his concerns and expectations – among the shouting there may be some things you can help with or change

> minimise confrontational, direct eye contact, and be aware of your posture (do not cross your arms, for example, as this appears defensive)

> maintain a safe distance – do not invade his body space; stay a leg's length away

> offer food and drink (cooled tea, not hot!)

> reassure the patient and let him know that you appreciate how frightened or angry he must be and say that you would like to help. It can sometimes be helpful to reflect how you feel, to say you are frightened, as often this comes as a surprise to the person and will defuse the situation

> praise any attempts at self-control, no matter how minor

> try to establish a rapport.

Physical restraints

These should not be used and may be construed as assault. The police or staff trained in control and restraint may restrain him if necessary, but beware of positional asphyxia if a patient's movement or breathing is in any way restricted. Particularly hazardous is restraining the patient lying face down and applying pressure downwards on his back as this impairs breathing. If physical restraint is unavoidable, his vital signs must be continuously monitored.

Sedation

Always offer oral sedation first, then intramuscular (IM) only if necessary. Start with lorazepam 1–2 mg *per os* (PO) or IM, maximum 4 mg in 24 hours (0.5–1 mg, maximum 2 mg in 24 hours in older people). If this is not effective, then add haloperidol in an initial dose of 1–5 mg PO or IM (0.5–2.5 mg in older people); maximum 20 mg PO or 12 mg IM in 24 hours.

Hazard

Giving sedation
Heart disease – caution must be taken if antipsychotics are required in patients with heart disease.

Electrocardiogram (ECG) – always attempt to obtain an ECG before administration in all patients who are antipsychotic naïve, and if this is not possible, document why.

Total dose – beware the total dosage of all antipsychotics given – eg if 50% of the maximum dose of olanzapine is given regularly, only 50% of the maximum dose of haloperidol should be given prn. If you give more than this to treat extreme agitation, document why this was needed on the balance of risks and benefits.

In extreme situations, sedation can be administered compulsorily as an emergency treatment under common law to contain the situation. The patient should immediately be assessed for treatment and admission under the Mental Health Act 1983 (see Section 2.14) if there is suspicion of an underlying mental disorder.

Reduction of aggression in emergency departments

Do not keep agitated patients waiting. Encourage patients to air their grievances. Keep patients and their relatives or friends informed about what you are doing. Staff in high-risk areas should receive training in control and restraint. There should be better security measures (eg video surveillance and security staff) in these areas. The design and layout of clinics should be relaxing and pleasant, but with security in mind.

2 Diseases and treatments

2.1 Dissociative disorders

Psychopathology

There is a temporary but drastic modification of a person's character or sense of personal identity, usually to avoid emotional distress although also occurring at times of extreme emotion, eg religious experiences or drug intoxication.

Epidemiology

The exact prevalence is unknown. Dissociative disorders are more common in women and adolescents / young adults. They may occur in epidemics, especially in children. Dissociative amnesia is the most common, whereas fugue is rare. Dissociative identity disorder is less frequently diagnosed in the UK than in the USA. In the UK the symptoms are often felt to fit in better with the concept of personality disorder. As an isolated symptom depersonalisation is very common, but as a recurrent persistent problem it is rare.

Clinical presentation

Dissociative disorders present in different ways and the features of recognisable syndromes are described in Table 7.

Differential diagnosis

Conditions that may present with dissociative symptoms include:

> schizophrenia

> temporal lobe epilepsy

> depression

Table 7 Types of dissociative disorders

Type	Characteristics
Amnesia	Sudden inability to recall periods of an individual's past or their own identity
Fugue	Travel away from usual surroundings, amnesia for past identity and sometimes even the assumption of a new identity
Identity disorder	Presence of two or more distinct identities / personality states
Depersonalisation	Mental processes or body are perceived as unreal, remote or automatised – the individual is in a 'dream-like state'

> head injury

> delirium

> dementia

> drugs

> acute stress disorder.

Treatment

Treatment needs to be tailored to the individual and the following are guiding principles: treat any underlying medical and psychiatric illnesses that may be the primary problem; identify and address stressors; use psychological interventions to help the person process and integrate stressful feelings.

Prognosis

Dissociative amnesia and fugue usually recover as abruptly as they started and recovery is usually complete with few relapses. Dissociative identity disorder is often associated with borderline personality disorder and usually has a chronic course, which is seldom with a complete resolution of symptoms.

2.2 Somatic symptom and related disorders

Psychopathology

It is thought that somatic symptom disorders occur due to a psychological mechanism, in which an unacceptable or unbearable emotional/psychological state is converted into physical symptoms as a defence mechanism. It occurs more commonly in cultures and individuals who do not recognise or communicate emotion, and in children (such as tummy aches before going to school).

Epidemiology

The prevalence of somatic symptom disorder is thought to be around 5–7% in the general population. It is more common in females and children. In outpatient medical populations, the 6 month–1 year prevalence of illness anxiety disorder is between 3% and 8%, and it affects males and females equally. The precise prevalence of functional neurological symptom disorder is not known, but studies suggest that it is found in about 5% of referrals to neurology clinics.

Clinical presentation

The diagnostic categories for these disorders are outlined above (see Section 1.1.2). Somatic symptom disorder involves a persistent, distressing preoccupation with one of more somatic symptoms (such as pain, burning sensations, fatigue or palpitations). This may coexist with other medical conditions. The patient has high levels of anxiety about their health and may attribute minor or normal bodily sensations to a serious illness.

Illness anxiety disorder includes a preoccupation with having a particular serious disease, such as cancer, with associated disproportionate anxiety or distress. It can be differentiated from somatic symptom disorder partly by an absence, or only minimal, somatic symptoms, ie the patient is largely asymptomatic. They may seek repeated investigations, not accepting medical reassurance that they do not have the illness.

Functional neurological symptom disorder, previously called conversion disorder, presents with one of more symptoms of altered motor or sensory function in the absence of a recognised neurological condition. This might include limb paralysis, abnormal movements such as tremor, speech or swallowing difficulties, and non-epileptic attack disorder (NEAD). A common feature of conversion disorders is 'la belle indifference' – a surprising lack of concern about their presenting symptoms.

Key point

> Somatic symptom disorder involves one or more somatic symptoms.

> Functional neurological symptom disorder involves one or more motor or sensory disturbance.

> Illness anxiety disorder involves a preoccupation with having a specific illness.

Treatment

Psychological treatments are the mainstay of treatment, with cognitive behavioural therapy (CBT) and interpersonal therapy most often used. Initially patients are unlikely to accept a purely psychological explanation and may refuse to engage with psychological therapy. It is helpful to link physical symptoms with the patient's subsequent distress or anxiety so that they feel psychological therapy may help with these, in spite of their continued belief in a physical explanation of their symptoms.

Medication should not be routinely used, but low-dose tricyclic antidepressants are sometimes used for chronic pain disorders.

Patients with somatic symptom disorders may end up accumulating a large number of medication treatments, such as analgesics. It is important to bear this in mind and rationalise medications as far as possible. Liaison psychiatry services may offer a neuropsychiatry or persistent physical symptoms clinic which might assist with this.

Prognosis

Persistent somatic symptoms are associated with demographic features (female sex, older age, fewer years of education, lower socio-economic status, unemployment), a reported history of sexual abuse or other childhood adversity, concurrent chronic physical illness or psychiatric disorder. Patients who can accept the diagnosis and engage in psychological treatment at an earlier stage do better.

2.3 Dementia

Psychopathophysiology

Dementia is characterised by the features shown in the 'Key point' below.

Key point

Features of dementia
> memory impairment
> impairment in several other cognitive domains (such as language, perception or executive function)
> a decline from previous levels of functioning
> mood and behaviour changes
> no impairment of consciousness.

Epidemiology

In community residents, 5% of those aged over 65 years and 20% of those aged over 80 years have dementia, comprising 50% due to Alzheimer's disease, 10–20% due to dementia with Lewy bodies and 10–20% due to vascular dementia.

Huntington's disease affects women and men equally, and is usually diagnosed in the late 30s and 40s. Prion diseases, eg Creutzfeldt–Jakob disease (including new variant type), are rare, and the age of onset depend on the age at exposure to the prions and the incubation period. HIV and head injury affect a younger population. Minor cognitive problems due to HIV are common and acquired immune deficiency syndrome (AIDS) dementia complex is the AIDS-defining illness in about 4.5% of cases.

Clinical presentation

The typical clinical presentations of the different types of dementia are shown in Table 8.

Key point

Executive dysfunction
Problems with planning, organisation, sequencing and abstraction; all of which are functions of the frontal lobe. This can also lead to disinhibited behaviours.

Table 8 Clinical presentation of dementia

Types of dementia	Clinical presentation
Alzheimer's disease	Gradual onset and decline. Features include: forgetfulness, lack of spontaneity, disorientation, depressed mood, deterioration in self-care, dysphasia, apraxia, agnosia and executive dysfunction
Vascular dementia	Presence of vascular disease elsewhere and/or vascular risk factors. Course is typically with stepwise progression. More pronounced mood lability or personality change is common, otherwise the features are largely similar to Alzheimer's disease
Lewy body dementia	Fluctuating cognition, visual hallucinations, Parkinsonism, sensitivity to antipsychotic drugs, falls / transient loss of consciousness / syncope and delusions
Frontotemporal dementia	Personality changes, executive dysfunction, deterioration in social skills, emotional blunting / apathy, disinhibition and expressive dysphasia. Typically earlier age of onset (<70)
HIV	Forgetfulness, slowness, poor concentration, problem-solving difficulty, apathy and neurological abnormalities
Huntington's disease	Depression, irritability, anxiety, paranoia, choreoathetosis, memory impairment and problems with executive functioning (single autosomal dominant gene on chromosome 4)
Prion diseases	Myoclonic jerks, seizures, ataxia, with periodic electroencephalogram activity and progressive cognitive impairment. Pulvinar sign on MRI head

MRI, magnetic resonance imaging.

Differential diagnosis

Exclude reversible cause of cognitive dysfunction:

> 'pseudodementia' due to depression
> delirium
> alcohol
> hypothyroidism
> syphilis
> vitamin B_{12} deficiency
> normal pressure hydrocephalus
> subdural haematoma.

Treatment

Consider the following:

> social support
> occupational therapy (OT) and physiotherapy assessment and interventions
> behavioural problems managed through behavioural and environmental modifications. Rarely a short course of low-dose

antipsychotic drugs may be used as an adjunct if behavioural disturbance is severe. Also antidepressants can be used to treat low mood and regulate sleep

> cholinesterase inhibitors in mild–moderate Alzheimer's disease, eg donepezil, rivastigmine and galantamine
> memantine (reversible N-methyl-D-aspartate antagonist) may be used in severe Alzheimer's disease, or where cholinesterase inhibitors are no longer helpful.

Complications

Be aware that the complications of dementia are not only medical, but are also social and behavioural problems that include:

> distress of caregivers
> social isolation
> self-neglect
> risk of personal injury, eg accidents, falls and wandering

> vulnerability to exploitation
> aggression and other behavioural problems.

Prognosis

Alzheimer's disease has a variable course, but death usually occurs within 5–8 years of onset. Except for dementia due to head injury, all dementias are progressive – but in some their progression can be halted temporarily (eg HIV and Alzheimer's disease) or permanently (eg hypothyroidism and syphilis).

Key point

Normal-pressure hydrocephalus

Head injury predisposes to this condition, which is characterised by:

> progressive dementia
> urinary incontinence
> gait disturbance
> enlarged ventricles.

Prevention

Consider the following:

> genetic counselling (Huntington's)

> cardiovascular disease prevention and treatment

> intellectual stimulation.

Factors found to reduce risk in research (although not used clinically):

> antioxidants, eg vitamin E and selegiline

> hormone replacement therapy in Alzheimer's disease

> non-steroidal anti-inflammatory drugs (NSAIDs) in Alzheimer's disease.

Important information for patients

People with dementia should be encouraged to plan early for the eventual cessation of driving. Also financial planning needs to be done. At earlier stages, while they retain capacity, they may wish to consider a lasting power of attorney for financial and/or health decisions to be made in future, or an advance directive.

2.4 Schizophrenia, delusional disorder and antipsychotic drugs

2.4.1 Schizophrenia

Aetiology/psychopathology

Schizophrenia is currently believed to be a neurodevelopmental disorder. There is strong evidence of genetic risk, eg identical twins have a 48% chance of concordance. An individual with a first-degree relative who has schizophrenia has a roughly 5–10% lifetime risk of developing schizophrenia. A number of genetic loci have been implicated; importantly 22q11 deletion (velocardiofacial syndrome) is associated with psychosis in up to 30% of cases.

Structural changes seen in MRI studies include decreased volume of areas such as the parahippocampus, thalamus, superior temporal gyri and frontal lobes. Neurohistology shows reduced synaptic markers. Functional MRI (fMRI) shows reduced activity in the frontal cortex, with one theory being that schizophrenia arises due to aberrant connectivity.

Older neurotransmitter theories focused on defects in the dopamine system, specifically increased dopamine function in the striatum and mesolimbic pathway, but newer theories include defects in glutamate neurotransmission involving the hippocampal N-methyl-D-aspartate receptors.

There is evidence of an approximately twofold increased relative risk of psychosis, including schizophrenia, among people who smoke cannabis regularly, but no direct causal link has been established. It is well known that cannabis use may precipitate a relapse of psychotic symptoms in individuals with such a susceptibility.

Epidemiology

Statistics are:

> prevalence – 0.5–1.5% of the general population

> incidence – 0.5–5 per 10,000 individuals per year

> median age at onset – early- to mid-20s for men, and late 20s for women

> three to five times more common in migrants

> twofold increased risk if urban born.

Clinical presentation

All psychotic disorders share the presence of delusions and/or hallucinations. A delusion is a false, fixed belief which is held with conviction despite a lack of evidence, and which is out of keeping with the patient's cultural, social or religious background. A hallucination is a perception in the absence of an external stimulus, which

may occur in any sensory modality. Often prodromal negative symptoms are apparent in the history.

According to *Diagnostic and statistical manual of mental disorders* (DSM) criteria for a diagnosis of schizophrenia, at least two characteristic symptoms must be present for at least 1 month. Typical features of schizophrenia are shown in Table 9. *International statistical classification of diseases and health-related problems*, 10th edition (ICD-10) divides symptoms into Schneiderian first-rank (delusions; auditory hallucinations; thought echo, insertion, withdrawal or broadcast) and second-rank symptoms (hallucinations in other modalities, neologisms, catatonia, negative symptoms). Diagnostic criteria according to ICD-10 refer to one first-rank symptom being present or two or more second-rank symptoms.

Differential diagnosis

Other disorders presenting with schizophrenia-like symptoms include the following:

> schizoaffective disorder – concurrent mania or severe depression or prominent mood symptoms during the illness course

> delusional disorder – encapsulated delusions with minimal hallucinations

> acute and transient psychotic disorder – less than 1 month's duration

> shared psychotic disorder (*folie à deux*) – a person without psychosis taking on the psychotic symptoms of someone else

> due to general medical condition, eg high-dose steroids

> drug-induced psychosis, eg amphetamine intoxication

> affective disorder – delusions and hallucinations may occur in severe depression or mania; affective symptoms become severe at onset and precede mood-congruent psychotic symptoms.

Table 9 Core symptoms of schizophrenia

Symptoms	Characteristics
Delusions	Persecutory delusions are most common. Delusions of reference involve things having a special significance for the individual, eg a news story is a hidden message to them
Hallucinations	Most commonly auditory. May take the form of a running commentary or third-person discussion about the patient – usually derogatory
Delusions of thought control	Belief that their thoughts are being inserted, withdrawn or broadcast to others
Delusions of passivity	Belief that their actions, movements, thoughts or sensations are being controlled by someone or something other than themselves
Thought disorder	Loss of normal structure of thinking leading to disorganised or incoherent speech
Negative symptoms	Blunted affect, apathy, poverty of speech, attentional impairment and poor motivation
Disorganised behaviour	Excitement, stupor and mutism

Treatment

This is a complex illness that needs a comprehensive treatment approach. Always obtain collateral information. Physical examination and special investigations are needed to exclude concurrent medical problems. A useful approach to treatment is to use the 'biological, psychological and social' guidelines in Table 10.

Key point

The impacts of parents or caregivers

High expressed emotion (ie criticism), hostility and over-involvement of parents or caregivers towards people with schizophrenia is a significant risk factor for relapse.

Complications

Hazard

Suicide

Of patients with schizophrenia, 10% die by suicide and up to 50% attempt suicide.

Table 10 Biological, psychological and social approach for the treatment of schizophrenia

Approach	Treatment
Biological	Antipsychotic medication
Psychological	Cognitive therapy Crisis management Social skills training Coping with voices groups
Social	Family therapy Vocational rehabilitation Psycho-education, eg recognising early signs of relapse

Prognosis

Prognosis is variable and difficult to predict for any individual. Estimates are as follows: 10–15% have a good prognosis; 10–15% have a chronic, unremitting course; the remainder vary from occasional to frequent relapses.

Predictors of poor outcome:

> male sex

> obstetric complications

> abnormal premorbid personality

> low IQ (premorbid cognition)

> single (social isolation)

> early age at onset

> insidious onset

> substance abuse

> family history of schizophrenia

> absence of obvious precipitant

> urban setting

> poor insight and compliance

> predominantly negative symptoms.

2.4.2 Delusional disorder

Epidemiology

Delusional disorder is less common than schizophrenia. It can occur at any age, but onset is most frequent between 34 and 45 years. Prevalence is 0.03% in the general population.

Clinical presentation

Patients usually do not perceive themselves as having a mental illness and they generally do not present themselves for treatment. Their delusions frequently have internal logic and are systematised. They may have olfactory and tactile hallucinations that provide confirmatory evidence to their beliefs, but hallucinations are generally not prominent. Apart from the delusions and their ramifications, the patient's functioning is not markedly impaired. However, the condition should be taken seriously as patients may be at risk of impulsivity, suicide and homicide. The different subtypes of delusional disorder are shown in Table 11.

Key point

Risk factors for delusional disorder include:

> social isolation

> stress of immigration/exile

> family history

> personality disorder.

Differential diagnosis

The following conditions present with either delusional thinking or preoccupations that can be confused with delusional thinking.

> schizophrenia and other psychotic disorders (see Section 2.4)

> mood disorders

> dementia (see Section 2.3)

> somatoform disorders (see Section 1.1.2)

> obsessive–compulsive disorder (see Section 2.9)

> neurological disorders, eg after head injury

> substance abuse (see Section 1.3.4).

Table 11   Different subtypes of delusional disorder

Subtype	Typical preoccupation
Somatic type	Undiagnosed disease
Persecutory type	Conspiracy
Grandiose type	Missionary zeal
Jealous type	Morbid jealously (Othello syndrome)
Erotomanic type	Impossible love relationship (de Clérambault's syndrome)

Treatment

Reassurance, compassion and support. Cognitive behavioural therapy may ameliorate delusional thinking. Antipsychotic medication and selective serotonin reuptake inhibitors (SSRIs) have been shown to be of some value. Hospitalise the patient if there are concerns about aggression, suicide, homicide or extreme impulsivity.

Hazard

Morbid jealously carries a significant risk of violence, and concurrent alcohol abuse increases this risk.

Prognosis

Often a chronic lifelong problem; 30–50% of cases go into remission.

2.4.3 Antipsychotics

General principles

Antipsychotic medications are primarily effective for positive symptoms, such as delusions and hallucinations, with little effect on negative symptoms. As well as treating an acute psychotic episode, antipsychotics also significantly reduce relapse rates.

The main mechanism of action of antipsychotics is through blocking dopamine receptors. The atypicals also act by blocking serotonin receptors in the striatal system and the frontal cortex, hence there are fewer extrapyramidal side effects and greater efficacy for negative symptoms.

Antipsychotics can be divided into low-potency, high-potency and atypical drugs (Table 12).

Key point

Clozapine – more effective than other antipsychotics and used in treatment-resistant cases.

Hazard

Clozapine – significant risk (0.8%) of agranulocytosis; regular monitoring of full blood count is mandatory.

Indications

The main indication is for psychosis, and use in any other condition (Table 13) must be carefully considered because these drugs have severe side effects that can be permanent, most notably tardive dyskinesia.

Table 12 Subgroups of antipsychotics

Subgroup	Examples	Discussion
Low-potency drugs	Chlorpromazine	Generally associated with more anticholinergic, antihistaminergic and α-adrenergic blocking side effects. Therefore more epileptogenic and cardiotoxic (prolonged QT interval)
High-potency drugs	Haloperidol and trifluoperazine	Associated with greater extrapyramidal side effects
Atypical drugs	Risperidone, olanzapine, quetiapine, amisulpiride and aripiprazole	Far fewer side effects Weight gain and sedation can be problematic Can lead to a metabolic syndrome, ie hypertension, diabetes and hyperlipidaemia
Long-acting antipsychotic injection	Atypical: paliperidone, risperdal, aripiprazole, olanzapine Typical: clopixol, haloperidol, depixol	IM injections given every 1–4 weeks, or depot injections such as paliperidone which can even be given once every 3 months May increase compliance and evidence of fewer relapses than with oral medication
Clozapine		Clozapine is more effective than other antipsychotics and is used in patients who have failed treatment with two other antipsychotics: 30% of treatment-resistant patients will respond to clozapine by 6 weeks, a further 20% by 3 months, and an additional 10–20% by 6 months On clozapine, 2.7% of patients develop neutropenia and 0.8% agranulocytosis: monitoring involves weekly FBC for the first 18 weeks, then fortnightly for 1 year and monthly thereafter (according to NICE guidelines)

FBC, full blood count; IM, intramuscular; NICE, National Institute for Health and Care Excellence.

Table 13 Other conditions in which antipsychotics are used

Condition	Example of antipsychotic
Anxiety	Low doses used
Impulsivity	Low doses used
Tourette's syndrome	Aripiprazole or risperidone
Nausea	Prochlorperazine
Chronic hiccoughs	Chlorpromazine
Infant opioid withdrawal	Chlorpromazine
Emergency sedation	Haloperidol

Key point

Antipsychotics
When using these drugs, remember:

> Always use the lowest dose possible.

> Start with a low dose and slowly titrate up until therapeutic effect is achieved.

> Always be aware of side effects.

> Do not use more than one antipsychotic at a time.

Hazard
Use antipsychotics judiciously because of the risk of tardive dyskinesia.

In general, atypical antipsychotics are used as first-line treatment as they have a better side-effect profile and similar efficacy to typical antipsychotics. Clozapine is the only antipsychotic with superior efficacy, but its use is limited to patients who have not responded to two previous antipsychotics due to the risk of agranulocytosis and need for blood test monitoring.

Contraindications

> drowsiness, confusion, coma due to central nervous system depressants

> bone-marrow suppression

> phaeochromocytoma

> if at all possible avoid use in patients who are pregnant or breastfeeding.

Complications

Side effects

Side effects of antipsychotics are common. Many can be understood by dopamine blockade effects on other dopaminergic pathways:

> tuberoinfundibular pathway – increased prolactin release

> nigrostriatal pathway – extrapyramidal side effects

> mesocortical pathway – cognitive impairment and reduced motivation.

Side effects are listed and briefly described in Table 14: some can be severe and even life-threatening.

Hazard
The most important adverse effects of antipsychotics include:

> agranulocytosis

> neuroleptic malignant syndrome

> acute dystonia

> tardive dyskinesia

> akathisia.

2.5 Personality disorder

Psychopathology

The essential feature of a personality disorder (PD) are impairments in personality (self and interpersonal) functioning and the presence of pathological personality traits. The *Diagnostic and statistical manual of mental disorders* (DSM)-V criteria for diagnosis are shown in the following 'Key point'.

Key point

Diagnosis of PD (DSM-V)

The following criteria must be met:

> An enduring pattern of inner experience and behaviour which deviates markedly from the expectations of the individual's culture. This is manifested in two (or more) of the following areas:

> > cognition (eg ways of perceiving/interpreting self or others)

> > affectivity (eg range, intensity, lability or appropriateness of emotional response)

> > interpersonal functioning

> > impulse control.

> This pattern is inflexible and pervasive across a broad range of situations.

> This pattern leads to significant distress of impairment.

> The pattern is stable and of long duration, and its onset in adolescence or early adulthood.

> The impairments are not solely due to the direct physiological effects of a substance (eg a drug of abuse), or a medical condition (eg severe head trauma) or another mental disorder.

PD is often accompanied by a history of being abused or having behavioural disturbances during childhood. There are different types of PD (Table 15).

Epidemiology

The prevalence ranges between 2% and 13% in the general population. There are gender differences: antisocial PD is diagnosed more frequently in men; histrionic, borderline and dependent PDs are diagnosed more frequently in women.

Clinical presentation

A diagnosis needs a longitudinal view of a person's lifelong behaviour patterns. Difficult and odd behaviour in reaction to a stressful situation can easily be confused with a PD.

Key point
A thorough risk assessment, including the following factors, must always be assessed in a person who has a PD:

> deliberate self-harm

> aggression

> violence

> impulsivity

> suicide.

Comorbid mental illness is frequently present, eg depression, drug dependence, alcohol dependence and anxiety disorders.

Before subclassification of PD can be made it is essential to ensure that symptoms meet the criteria for a PD in the first place, including an early onset, enduring symptoms which cause functional impairment, and distress to self and/or others in different situations.

The most commonly encountered PD in medical settings is borderline PD. These individuals frequently present with impulsive acts of self-harm, emotional instability, impatience, and explosive outbursts of anger. Other features include chronic feelings of emptiness, a disturbance in the patient's own self-identity, intense or unstable pattern of relationships, impaired interpersonal functioning, fear of abandonment, and impulsivity. One should be aware of the intense frustration and splitting

Table 14 Side effects of antipsychotics

Side effect	Characteristic
Extrapyramidal symptoms	Stiffness, tremor, hypersalivation, acute dystonia, akathisia, tardive dyskinesia
Anticholinergic symptoms	Blurred vision, constipation, urinary retention, dry mouth, confusion, agitation and seizures
Antihistaminic symptoms	Sedation
α-Adrenergic blocking	Orthostatic hypotension
Leukopenia	Agranulocytosis can occur with all antipsychotics, but has a higher incidence with clozapine
Increased prolactin secretion	Amenorrhoea, galactorrhoea and sexual dysfunction Osteoporosis if long term
Metabolic syndrome	Weight gain, hypertension, diabetes and hyperlipidaemia
Obstructive jaundice	Thought to be due to additives in old phenothiazine preparations Associated with thioridazine at doses above 600 mg/day
Allergic dermatitis and photosensitivity	
Neuroleptic malignant syndrome	Muscle rigidity, hyperthermia, fluctuating level of consciousness and autonomic dysfunction, leucocytosis and elevated creatine phosphokinase

Table 15 Classification of personality disorders in DSM-V

Cluster	Types	Characteristics
A	Paranoid,[1] schizoid[1] and schizotypal[2]	Often appear odd or eccentric
B	Antisocial[2] (dissocial[3]), borderline[1] (emotionally unstable personality disorder[3] – impulsive and borderline types), histrionic[1] and narcissistic[1]	Often appear dramatic, emotional and erratic
C	Avoidant,[1] dependent[1] and obsessive–compulsive[2] (anankastic[3])	Often appear anxious or fearful

1 Recognised in DSM and *International statistical classification of diseases and health-related problems*, 10th edition (ICD-10).
2 Recognised only in DSM.
3 Recognised only in ICD-10.

within the care team (eg saying one thing to one doctor and something else to another) that often arises and see this as part of the patient's disorder.

In ICD-10 borderline PD is referred to as emotionally unstable personality disorder (EUPD) and subclassified into impulsive and borderline types. Patients with EUPD can sometimes be misdiagnosed as having bipolar disorder due to mood fluctuation, but a key difference is that in bipolar disorder mood episodes are sustained, while in EUPD mood can fluctuate within minutes or hour.

Treatment

Psychotherapy remains the mainstay of treatment. The success rate of patients recovering sufficiently to no longer meet the diagnostic criteria for PD can be as high as 52%. Types of psychotherapy used include psychodynamic therapy, cognitive behavioural therapy, interpersonal therapy, dialectical behavioural therapy and group therapy. Certain PDs tend to be resistant to treatment, eg antisocial PD.

Aside from treatment of comorbidities, drug treatments are only occasionally effective in reducing problematic behaviours and should be prescribed in a specialist setting only. The following have been found to have some limited efficacy:

> antipsychotics and selective serotonin reuptake inhibitors (SSRIs) at low doses for impulsive, deliberate self-harm behaviour

> mood stabilisers

> carbamazepine for aggressive behaviour.

Treatment approach can be based on DSM cluster:

> cluster A – consider antipsychotic treatment

> cluster B – consider mood stabiliser, typically lamotrigine or quetiapine; consider lithium or carbamazepine for extreme risk

> cluster C – consider antidepressant.

Key point
Drug treatments can be effective when they are used to treat a comorbid illness, eg depression, and problem behaviours may abate.

Prognosis

The course of PD is variable, but as a general rule it ameliorates with age and may even remit. Completed suicide occurs in 8–10% of patients with borderline PD.

2.6 Psychiatric presentation of physical disease

Epidemiology

Psychiatric symptoms are common in general medical conditions, eg on general medical wards 15–25% of patients experience delirium; 30–50% of patients with epilepsy have a psychiatric difficulty at some time.

Clinical presentation

When medical conditions have psychiatric symptoms as part of their presentation, it is necessary to decide whether the psychiatric symptoms are a result of the medical illness, part of a separate mental disorder and/or a psychological reaction to having an illness (see Section 2.7).

Key point
Symptoms should be elicited that identify serious mental illness or distress, which would need to be addressed urgently. These symptoms include:

> hopelessness

> thoughts of suicide

> guilt

> loss of interest

> severe insomnia

> psychosis.

Common mental disorders that may be the result of an underlying medical condition or medication are as follows:

> delirium

> dementia

> amnesia

> mood disorders

> anxiety disorders

> sleep disorder

> sexual disorders.

Medical conditions that commonly present with symptoms and signs of mental disorder:

> epilepsy

> degenerative disorders, eg Parkinson's, Huntington's and Wilson's diseases

> brain tumours

> head trauma

> demyelinating disorders

> infectious disease, eg syphilis, encephalitis, meningitis, Creutzfeldt–Jakob disease and HIV (acquired immune deficiency syndrome (AIDS))

> autoimmune disorders, eg systemic lupus erythematosus

> endocrine disorders, eg thyroid, pituitary and adrenal disease

> metabolic disorders, eg hepatic, uraemic, hypoglycaemic encephalopathies and porphyria

> nutritional disorders, eg thiamine and niacin deficiencies

> toxins, eg organophosphates and heavy metals.

Key point
Other comorbid problems that may complicate the picture:

> alcohol and drug abuse

> personality disorders

> factitious disorders and malingering

> medication, eg steroids may induce psychosis.

Treatment

A general principle is to address medical problems as far as possible before attempting to treat any psychiatric symptoms or suspected mental disorders, because these may resolve. However, circumstances may be such that recovery from the medical condition is dependent on the person's mental health and their ability to cooperate, in which case the psychiatric symptoms should be treated early. For example, a person with diabetes may find their motivation to remain compliant with treatment is poor because they are depressed.

Key point

Psychiatric treatments in physical illness

Treatments are the same as would be used in patients who did not have concurrent physical illness, but be aware of drug interactions and adverse effects, eg anticholinergic effects of tricyclic antidepressants.

Treatment strategies to help alleviate psychiatric symptoms are as follows:

> Use an empathic, reassuring approach.

> Ensure the patient's physical needs are met, eg hydration and nutrition.

> Provide information about illness, investigations, treatments and their likely effects to help allay any fears and anxieties.

> The nursing environment should be well lit, quiet and tranquil.

> Invite the patient's family or other people who are familiar to visit.

> Hypnotics and anxiolytics should only be used if the patient is not responding to the above treatment strategies.

If there is concern that the patient is severely depressed or psychotic, a psychiatric opinion should be sought immediately. Otherwise a psychiatric assessment may be helpful in identifying the psychological processes that are affecting recovery and compliance.

2.7 Psychological reactions to physical illness (adjustment disorders)

Aetiology/psychopathology

When considering the possibility of a psychiatric disorder in a physically ill person, think of the possible interactions between mind, body and behaviour (Table 16).

The commonest reactions to physical illness and disability are adjustment disorders. These are generally seen in primary care, but 5–20% of psychiatric outpatients may present with this clinical picture. The stressor is usually much less intense and severe than in cases of post-traumatic stress disorder. The onset should be within 1 month or so of the stressful event. Predisposing factors include personality disorder or immature personality.

Epidemiology

Males and females are equally affected.

Clinical presentation

Presentation is usually with severe subjective distress and emotional disturbance (this is based on the clinician's own subjective judgement), with impairment of social functioning and performance.

The onset is within 1 month of a significant life change, leading to continued unpleasant circumstances.

Symptoms, which are not sufficiently severe to justify a more specific diagnosis such as major depression, include:

> depressed mood

> tearfulness and/or hopelessness

> nervousness

> anxiety

> worry

> inability to cope or plan ahead

> disability in performance of daily routine.

The usual duration is a maximum of 6 months, but symptoms can last longer in a chronic disabling medical condition.

Table 16 Possible interactions between the mind and physical illness

Relationship with physical illness	Clinical example
Coincidental	A person with schizophrenia contracts pneumonia
Causal	Physical illness causing psychiatric disorder, eg hypothyroidism causing depression
Reactive	Anxiety and depression are the commonest reactions to threatening or progressive illness
Iatrogenic	Treatment of physical illness causes a psychiatric disorder, eg L-dopa causing delirium
Reciprocal	Failure to mobilise after a stroke causing or caused by depression
Compliance	Poor compliance, eg in the depressed diabetic or in the patient with memory impairment
Somatisation	Psychiatric illness presents as a physical one
Denial	A psychological defence mechanism by which frightening news, eg a diagnosis of cancer, is excluded from conscious awareness and the patient behaves as if they are unaware of the distressing facts

Diagnosing depression in physical illness

Approximately 30% of cancer patients develop depression, a generalised anxiety disorder or an adjustment disorder within the first 2 years of diagnosis, but only a small proportion of this morbidity is recognised and treated.

Key point

Depression in physical illness

Be aware of:

> dismissing depression as an understandable reaction to severe illness

> biological symptoms being unreliable, hence use the Hospital Anxiety and Depression (HAD) Scale (Fig 1)

> depressive cognitions, eg 'I deserve to be ill' or 'I am not worth treating'; also a loss of interest in other people

> suicidal ideas

> when asking about anhedonia, there is not much to enjoy in hospital, but ask about, for example, when family visit

> tearfulness (especially in men)

> indecisiveness

> any past history of depression.

The diagnosis of depression in patients with physical illness can be complicated by the presence of fatigue, loss of appetite and sex drive, and insomnia.

These symptoms can also be the typical biological symptoms of depression. Therefore, it is helpful to use the HAD Scale that excludes somatic symptoms and concentrates on the psychological symptoms of depression and anxiety (Fig 1). This self-rating scale has only 14 items and is easy to complete and to score. It was designed specifically for use in non-psychiatric hospital departments. A score of 11 or more on either the anxiety or the depression subscale indicates 'caseness' (the range on each subscale is 0–21).

Treatment

Encourage discussion and ventilation of feelings to help overcome denial and avoidance. Teach a problem-solving technique (see the following 'Key point'), which is applied collaboratively with the patient, who takes responsibility for the process, thereby enhancing their sense of autonomy and control.

Key point

Problem-solving technique

Problem solving is a straightforward counselling technique with the following components:

> listing the problems

> selecting one specific problem to focus on

> listing alternative courses of action

> evaluating each action plan

> selecting and implementing the most promising course of action

> evaluating results of the trial

> repeating the process until positive results are obtained.

Complications

Complications of adjustment disorders include:

> decreased compliance with medical treatment

> increased length of hospital stay

> impaired performance at work

> disruption of social relationships

> increased risk of suicide attempts and suicide.

2.8 Anxiety disorders

Anxiety is familiar to everyone as an adaptive response to external threat. Normal fear and apprehension are accompanied by an increased activity of the sympathetic nervous system in preparation for 'fight or flight'. Anxiety becomes pathological when it is excessive, prolonged or recurrent, and/or focused on bodily sensations (Table 17).

Morbid anxiety can be either:

> generalised (generalised anxiety disorder (GAD) – see below)

> episodic (panic disorder – see Section 2.8.2)

> situational (phobias – see Section 2.8.3).

The distinction between these is shown in Table 18. See also Section 1.2.1.

2.8.1 Generalised anxiety disorder

Aetiology/psychopathology

Release of noradrenaline, eg by yohimbine, increases anxiety. γ-Amino butyric acid inhibits anxiety.

There may be an underlying anxious personality disorder (see Section 2.5) with long-standing persistent and pervasive feelings of tension, apprehension and inferiority, along with an intense fear of disapproval and rejection.

The precipitating event is generally a threat to the person's security in a relationship or at work, or being given the diagnosis of a serious physical illness. Thus, 'danger events' (ie the expectation of loss or deprivation) precede anxiety, whereas depression tends to be preceded by actual loss.

This questionnaire will help you to let us know how you are. Read each item and underline the response which comes closest to how you have felt in the last few days. Don't take too long over your replies, your immediate reaction will probably be more accurate than a long thought-out response.

I feel tense or 'wound up'

Most of the time ☐
A lot of the time ☐
From time to time, occasionally ☐
Not at all ☐

I still enjoy the things I used to enjoy

Definitely as much ☐
Not quite as much ☐
Only a little ☐
Hardly at all ☐

I get a sort of frightened feeling as if something awful is about to happen

Very definitely and quite badly ☐
Yes, but not badly ☐
A little, but it doesn't worry me ☐
Not at all ☐

I can laugh and see the funny side of things

As much as I always could ☐
Not quite so much now ☐
Definitely not as much now ☐
Not at all ☐

Worrying thoughts go through my mind

A great deal of the time ☐
A lot of the time ☐
From time to time but not often ☐
Only occasionally ☐

I feel cheerful

Not at all ☐
Not often ☐
Sometimes ☐
Most of the time ☐

I can sit at ease and feel relaxed

Definitely ☐
Usually ☐
Not often ☐
Not at all ☐

I feel as if I am slowed down

Nearly all the time ☐
Very often ☐
Sometimes ☐
Not at all ☐

I get a sort of frightened feeling like 'butterflies' in my stomach

Not at all ☐
Occasionally ☐
Quite often ☐
Very often ☐

I have lost interest in my appearance

Definitely ☐
I don't take as much care as I should ☐
I may not take quite as much care ☐
I take just as much care as ever ☐

I feel restless as if I have to be on the move

Very much indeed ☐
Quite a lot ☐
Not very much ☐
Not at all ☐

I look forward with enjoyment to things

As much as ever I did ☐
Rather less than I used to ☐
Definitely less than I used to ☐
Hardly at all ☐

I get sudden feelings of panic

Very often indeed ☐
Quite often ☐
Not very often ☐
Not at all ☐

I can enjoy a good book or radio or TV programme

Often ☐
Sometimes ☐
Not often ☐
Very seldom ☐

Fig 1 Hospital Anxiety and Depression Scale. Four options follow each statement: the best response (least anxious or depressed) scores 0; the worst response (most anxious or depressed) scores 3.

Table 17 Comparison of normal and morbid (pathological) anxiety

Feature	Normal anxiety	Morbid (pathological) anxiety
Reaction to a threat	Proportionate	Excessive
Duration	Brief	Prolonged
Focus of attention	Towards the external world	Morbid preoccupation with a physiological response, eg rapid heartbeat means imminent heart attack

Table 18 Distinction between GAD, panic disorder and phobias

Diagnosis	Characteristics of morbid anxiety
GAD	Continuous, pervasive and persistent ('free floating' and situation specific)
Panic disorder	Episodic with intense unpredictable panic attacks lasting about 30 minutes. Can occur in any situation
Phobias	Situation specific

GAD, generalised anxiety disorder.

Anxiety reactions are more likely to occur where there is lack of social support due to separation, divorce or bereavement. Some physical disorders and drugs may mimic generalised anxiety disorder (GAD) (Table 19).

Epidemiology

The 6-month prevalence is 2.5–6.5%. The Office for Population Censuses and Surveys National Survey of Psychiatric Morbidity found that in the week before they were interviewed nearly 3% of the population had a GAD and over 7% had a mixed anxiety–depression.

GAD is twice as common in females. Rates of neurotic disorders such as anxiety are much commoner in those with lower socio-economic status. Onset is commonest in late adolescence and early adulthood.

Table 19 Medical disorders and drugs that may cause anxiety

Medical disorders	Hyperthyroidism
	Hypoglycaemia
	Cardiac dysrhythmia
	Phaeochromocytoma
	Respiratory dysfunction
Prescribed drugs	Selective serotonin reuptake inhibitors
	Sympatheticomimetics
Recreational drugs	Caffeine
	Amphetamine
	Cocaine
	LSD
Drug withdrawal	Alcohol
	Benzodiazepines
	Opiates

Clinical presentation

Anxiety states are characterised by a combination of psychological and somatic symptoms. Psychological symptoms are shown in the following 'Key point'.

Key point
Psychological symptoms of GAD

> an inappropriate and excessive sense of apprehensiveness and dread that impairs everyday functioning

> excessive fear of loss, illness, death, accidents, losing control and going insane

> irritability, restlessness, worrying, poor concentration and insomnia

> thoughts of impending personal catastrophe.

Somatic symptoms arise from autonomic arousal, muscle tension and hyperventilation (Table 20). Hyperventilation causes a low PCO_2 and alkalosis.

GAD can affect various systems of the body:

> cardiac – palpitations

> pulmonary – hyperventilation, tightness in chest and breathlessness

> gastrointestinal – dry mouth, difficulty in swallowing, 'butterflies in the stomach', nausea and frequent bowel motions

> urinary – frequency

> neurological – headache, light-headedness, paraesthesia around mouth and in hands, tremor and muscle aches

> autonomic – sweating, shakiness, feeling too hot or cold and erectile impotence.

Table 20 Somatic symptoms of anxiety

Somatic symptom	Signs
Autonomic arousal	Palpitations
	Muscle tremor
	Sweating
	Epigastric discomfort
Muscle tension	Constricting headaches
	Backache
Hyperventilation	Paraesthesia
	Headache
	Dizziness
	Faintness

Treatment

Cognitive behavioural therapy is the safest and most effective treatment. Be circumspect with benzodiazepines – these should only be used in periods of crisis and for no longer than 2–4 weeks. Selective serotonin reuptake inhibitors (SSRIs) are the first-line medication. Beta-blockers might help to reduce tremor or palpitations. As second line, pregabalin (alone or in combination) can be used for patients who have not responded to first-line treatments, and augmentation with low-dose atypical antipsychotic (specifically quetiapine) has hypnotic, anxiolytic and antidepressant effects.

Complications

> Anxiety disorders are associated with increased mortality due to suicide as well as alcohol and smoking-related disorders.

> Dependence on benzodiazepines, hypnotics and alcohol.

Prognosis

Good prognostic indicators:

> a stable premorbid personality

> development of acute symptoms in response to transitory stress

> good social/family support.

There is a poor prognosis with:

> chronic or severe symptoms

> agitation, depersonalisation or conversion symptoms

> suicidal preoccupations

> persistent social/occupational factors

> inadequate social support.

Hazard
Do not forget ...
Patients with an anxiety disorder might:

> have an underlying medical disorder (see Table 19)

> have a concurrent depressive illness

> present with somatic rather than psychological symptoms

> later develop a depressive illness

> self-medicate with alcohol or other substances.

2.8.2 Panic disorder

Aetiology/psychopathology

Panic disorder consists of recurrent bouts of intense and rapidly escalating anxiety associated with the unrealistic anticipation of imminent personal catastrophe. The condition is probably caused by an interaction between biochemical and psychological events, perhaps from a biochemical abnormality associated with poorly regulated autonomic responses.

Panic disorder is five times commoner in first-degree relatives than in the general population.

Psychological factors

Patients with panic disorder are more likely than those with generalised anxiety disorder (GAD) to make alarming deductions from the physical symptoms of anxiety. According to this cognitive hypothesis, there is a vicious circle of fear (Fig 2) that intensifies the autonomic response so that the patient interprets an increase in their heart rate as a sign of an imminent heart attack, which in turn heightens their anxiety and further accelerates their heart rate.

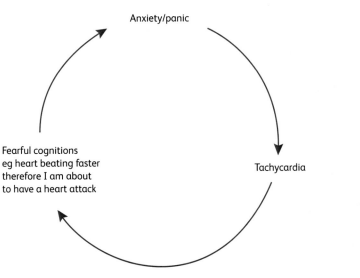

Anxiety/panic

Fearful cognitions
eg heart beating faster
therefore I am about
to have a heart attack

Tachycardia

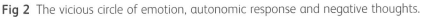

Fig 2 The vicious circle of emotion, autonomic response and negative thoughts.

Epidemiology

There is a lifetime prevalence of 1.5%, with the onset usually before the age of 40. There is a female to male ratio of 2:1.

Clinical presentation

The patient experiences repeated unexpected bouts of severe anxiety that can occur in any situation and are not restricted to certain places. The physical and psychological symptoms of panic disorder are similar to those of GAD, but are episodic and more intense. Common symptoms of a panic attack are shown in the following 'Key point'. There is an overwhelming fear of loss of control and of imminent death, generally from a heart attack. As the disorder progresses, individuals often worry excessively about having panic attacks or their possible consequences (eg losing control or having a heart attack), and often begin to avoid situations in an attempt to prevent attacks (such as avoiding supermarkets or unfamiliar places).

Key point

Symptoms of panic attacks

1 palpitations, pounding heart, or accelerated heart rate

2 sweating

3 trembling or shaking

4 sensations of shortness of breath or smothering

5 feelings of choking

6 chest pain or discomfort

7 nausea or abdominal distress

8 feeling dizzy, unsteady, light-headed, or faint

9 chills or heat sensations

10 paresthesias (numbness or tingling sensations)

11 derealisation (feelings of unreality) or depersonalisation (being detached from oneself)

12 fear of losing control or 'going crazy'

13 fear of dying.

Differential diagnosis

Panic attacks can occur in the course of GAD, agoraphobia, social anxiety disorder, depression and alcohol withdrawal. In these cases panic attacks would be expected, and so would not be diagnosed as panic disorder. The diagnosis of panic disorder depends on the attacks being recurrent and unexpected (out of he blue).

Treatment

Provide reassurance and explanation by describing the interaction between fear and overactivity of the sympathetic nervous system. Give the patient a simple diagram of the vicious circle that develops when fear caused by the physical symptoms of anxiety intensifies their thoughts of imminent catastrophe (Fig 2).

Antidepressants have anti-panic effects, but cognitive behavioural therapy is as effective as antidepressants and has a lower relapse rate. Benzodiazepines are to be avoided in the longer-term treatment of a panic disorder because of the risk of dependence.

Selective serotonin reuptake inhibitors (SSRIs) are first-line treatment, but be aware of rebound anxiety when the antidepressant is withdrawn as well as common gastrointestinal and sexual side effects. They may also cause increased anxiety at the initiation of treatment, and using low doses with slow titration is recommended. Propranolol can be a useful adjunct to treat physical symptoms of panic. Other classes of antidepressant can be used if SSRIs are not tolerated, including mirtazapine and venlafaxine.

Complications

Major depressive disorder occurs in at least half of those who have panic disorder. Agoraphobia is a common complication. Some patients become dependent on alcohol as a form of self-medication, and benzodiazepine dependence is not uncommon.

Prognosis

The course tends to fluctuate. Even with treatment 20–30% of patients with panic disorder are symptomatic at 6-year follow-up.

2.8.3 Phobic anxiety disorders

Aetiology

The cardinal features of phobias are fear and avoidance. The fear is disproportionate to the circumstances and the patient recognises this. Despite this insight, the phobic patient feels intensely anxious at the very thought of a particular situation (anticipatory anxiety). Phobias are classified as specific (simple), blood/injection/injury, agoraphobia and social phobia.

Specific (simple) phobias

Simple phobias can sometimes be traced to a single traumatic incident such as being stuck in a lift or underground train, being attacked by a vicious dog, or having been involved in a road traffic accident. Specific phobias might sound trivial but they can severely impair performance at work and in social life (eg due to inability to travel by plane). Specific phobias include familiar fears of spiders, snakes, heights, flying and thunder.

Blood/injection/injury phobia

Blood/injection/injury phobia can occur after a traumatic medical incident, and is the most important phobia in the hospital setting. Triggers include the sight of blood, injury or medical apparatus – especially syringes and needles. There might also be excessive fear of contamination. These phobias can lead to a delay in seeking medical help, refusal to have blood tests, or reluctance to submit to any invasive medical procedure.

Blood/injection/injury phobia is associated with an unusual physiological response. Whereas other specific phobias are associated with an acceleration of the heart rate on exposure to the focus of fear and avoidance, those suffering from blood/injection/injury phobia have a strong vasovagal response with deceleration of their heart rate and a fall in blood pressure (BP), which could lead to syncope.

Agoraphobia

Agoraphobia sometimes follows one or two isolated panic attacks occurring in a public, crowded or confined space. The patient's fear of further episodes subsequently discourages them from leaving home. This avoidance behaviour prevents habituation and perpetuates the condition. The phobia is reinforced by the conviction that further potentially harmful panic attacks will occur if they venture out again.

Social phobias

Social phobias tend to occur in shy and unconfident people, and might be precipitated by an embarrassing incident. Thus, a sensitive person whose credit card is rejected due to a computer error might subsequently be afraid to sign cheques in public because they fear that their anxious tremor will be noticed.

Epidemiology

The epidemiology of various phobias is shown in Table 21.

Clinical presentation

The phobic patient experiences both the psychological and the somatic symptoms of morbid anxiety in specific circumstances. Even the anticipation of those situations provokes anxiety and this leads to avoidance. Patients may postpone seeking treatment until there is a change in their domestic or occupational circumstances which forces them to seek help. For example, the social phobic may be given the responsibility of making a public presentation; an agoraphobic may lose

Table 21 Epidemiology of phobias

	Age of onset, general	Male:female ratio	Other features	Prevalence in population (%)
Specific phobias	From childhood	Female > male	Might follow traumatic event, eg being trapped in a lift	10
Blood/injury/injection phobia	From childhood	Female > male	Vasovagal reaction and a positive family history	Not known
Agoraphobia	Age 20–40	Female > male	Often associated with panic attacks	3
Social phobia	Mid-teens	Female = male		2.5

a relative who used to do his or her shopping; while a blood/injection/injury phobic might develop severe anaemia and need to have laboratory tests.

Agoraphobia

Agoraphobics fear and avoid any situation from which escape might be difficult or embarrassing (see the following 'Key point').

Key point

Features of agoraphobia

Agoraphobic people are afraid of:

> leaving home

> going into crowded places (eg supermarkets)

> using public transport

> collapsing, having a convulsion or fainting

> going mad

> being incontinent in a public place

> having a heart attack without access to immediate help.

Social phobia

Social phobia is the fear and avoidance of social situations (eg restaurants, parties, public speaking and committee meetings). In social phobia the fear is that others will regard the person as socially clumsy or will notice his or her anxiety-induced tremulousness or sweating. The core fear is of negative evaluation by others.

Differential diagnosis

A delusional disorder (see Section 2.4.2) has to be excluded in both social phobias and agoraphobia:

> Does the patient have insight? In social phobia, the person retains insight and recognises that the fear that other people will observe them and judge them critically is excessive and disproportionate. The person is aware that their discomfort derives from his or her own self-consciousness. By contrast, the paranoid person suspects that other people regard them with unjustified hatred and malevolence.

> Why won't the patient go out? Both agoraphobic and paranoid people will be afraid to venture out of their homes, but the agoraphobic is housebound because he or she fears his or her own anxiety and panic, while the paranoid person locates danger in other people's actions and intentions.

Patients with dysmorphophobia (body dysmorphic disorder) might also eschew social events and public places.

Patients with a depressive episode may have negative beliefs about themselves, leading to low self-esteem and avoidance of social situations. It may also lead to reduced motivation and energy levels causing the patient to remain at home, mimicking agoraphobia.

Treatment

Cognitive behavioural therapy is the treatment of choice for all phobic anxiety. Techniques including flooding and graded exposure are important, and there is emerging experience of the use of virtual reality for specific phobias. Selective serotonin reuptake inhibitors (SSRIs) are first-line treatment in social anxiety disorder, similar to other anxiety disorders.

Complications

> dependence on alcohol and benzodiazepines

> social withdrawal and isolation

> impairment of family, occupational and social functioning.

Prognosis

Without treatment phobias tend to follow a chronic course.

2.9 Obsessive–compulsive disorder

Aetiology/psychopathology

There is a possible genetic contribution to obsessive–compulsive disorder (OCD). A significant proportion of sufferers have a previous personality that is characterised by extreme punctuality, orderliness and cleanliness. OCD can be accompanied by soft neurological signs. The obsessive symptoms can also occur in a number of organic disorders including Huntington's chorea and Tourette's syndrome. OCD can follow head injury and encephalitis. Studies of cerebral metabolic function show an association between obsessive–compulsive symptoms and striatal and orbitofrontal activity.

Acute onset OCD in young people has been linked with PANDAS (paediatric autoimmune neuropsychiatric disorder associated with streptococcal infections), and some adults with OCD have been found to have autoantibodies to targets in the basal ganglia.

Epidemiology

The prevalence is 1.3% of the general population. Men and women are equally affected.

Clinical presentation

Obsessions

These are unwanted, distressing and intrusive thoughts, images or impulses which the patient recognises as coming from their own mind. They are involuntary and the sufferer tries to suppress them, but this resistance only heightens their frequency and intensity. Both the obsessions themselves and the attempts to resist them cause severe anxiety. Clinical features are shown in the following 'Key point'. The content of obsessions (thoughts or images) is often obscene, sadistic or blasphemous. The patient might have recurrent ruminations about danger, disaster, disease or contamination, and may demonstrate 'magical undoing' such as believing not turning a switch off could cause a loved one to die in a car crash.

> **Key point**
>
> **Clinical features of obsessions**
>
> - recurrent
> - unbidden
> - unwelcome
> - distressing
> - resisted
> - cannot be got rid of
> - accompanied by anxiety
> - lead to 'cancelling out' rituals.

Compulsions

These are stereotyped actions which are carried out to neutralise either the anxiety caused by obsessional urges and images or their imaginary disastrous consequences. They are not inherently pleasurable and the patient only does the act to reduce anxiety.

Compulsive rituals include repetitive washing of one's hands, cleaning and checking, which provides temporary relief from the anxiety caused by the obsession itself or its feared consequences, eg that a blasphemous thought might cause a beloved relative to develop a malignant disease. Compulsive rituals are often performed a specific number of times. Many patients have obsessional doubts (*folie du doute*) which make them feel uncertain about whether they have actually carried out their rituals, so they then feel compelled to repeat this activity.

Obsessions and compulsions can occur in the course of a depressive illness and might remit on recovery from the depression.

Differential diagnosis

The main differential diagnoses to be considered are phobias and paranoid delusions: consider the characteristics shown in Table 22. Psychosis is also a major differential of OCD where the origins of obsessions and rituals are externally perceived by patients, eg rituals may be deemed secondary to passivity phenomenon or as a result of command auditory hallucinations and obsessions due to thought insertion.

Table 22	The differential diagnosis of OCD		
	OCD	**Phobia**	**Paranoid delusions**
Focus of fear	Fear of consequences of obsessions or of failure to carry out compulsive rituals	Fear and avoidance of specific situations which induce marked anxiety	Fear of danger to self from imaginary enemies
Insight	Retained (the patient partly recognises that their fears are irrational and absurd)	Retained (the patient is aware that their fear is disproportionate to objective danger)	Absent (the patient is absolutely convinced that the danger is real and they do not try to suppress their unusual thoughts)

OCD, obsessive–compulsive disorder.

Key point

Of patients with major depression, 30% have obsessional symptoms while 30% of patients with OCD also suffer from major depression.

Treatment

This consists of either behaviour therapy and/or pharmacotherapy.

Behaviour therapy

This treatment consists of exposure to the environmental triggers that provoke compulsive rituals (eg contact with dirt), combined with prevention from carrying out the ritual activity such as compulsive handwashing (prolonged exposure and response prevention). This treatment produces long-lasting improvement in up to two-thirds of patients. Behaviour therapy can be supplemented by cognitive therapy which teaches the patient to challenge the content of the obsessions.

Medication

Serotonergic antidepressants such as clomipramine and selective serotonin reuptake inhibitors (SSRIs) (higher doses may be needed than in other conditions) reduce obsessive–compulsive symptoms, especially where there is concurrent clinical depression. The prognosis is more favourable if OCD is secondary to depression. Second-line treatment can include augmentation of antidepressant treatment with antipsychotics.

Complications

Severe depression.

Prognosis

The course tends to be chronic.

2.10 Acute stress reactions and post-traumatic stress disorder

These conditions are produced by exceptionally stressful and life-threatening events.

> Acute stress reactions tend to develop rapidly and are short-lived.

> Post-traumatic stress disorder (PTSD) runs a more protracted course.

Adjustment disorders (Section 2.7) are provoked by major adverse life events which are less intense and immediately traumatic than those which cause acute stress reactions and PTSD. The characteristics of acute stress disorders, PTSD and adjustment disorder are shown in Table 23.

Table 23	Three types of reaction to stressful experiences			
	Trigger	**Onset**	**Duration**	**Clinical features**
Acute stress disorder	Exposure to sudden and unexpected danger, eg an assault	Immediate	Brief: days	Anxiety Panics Autonomic arousal Denial Numbing
PTSD	Catastrophic event, eg natural disaster, transport disaster, torture and rape	Immediate or delayed	Prolonged: months/years	Hypervigilance Avoidance Increased arousal, intrusions and memories of that life event
Adjustment disorder	Major adverse life event, such as being informed of life-threatening illness, eg AIDS or cancer	Gradual	Prolonged: weeks/months	Anxiety Depression

AIDS, acquired immune deficiency syndrome; PTSD, post-traumatic stress disorder.

2.10.1 Acute stress reaction

Aetiology/psychopathology

By definition the necessary and immediate causative factor for this condition is an exceptionally stressful life event. Some individuals might be more prone to developing this disorder than others, and the reaction is more likely to occur in older people or if the person is physically exhausted. A previous history of psychiatric disorder also increases vulnerability.

Epidemiology

The prevalence of acute stress reactions depends on the severity of the trauma that instigates them and the degree of exposure to it. Thus, the incidence of acute stress reactions among the survivors of an industrial explosion and fire at a Norwegian paint factory was directly proportionate to the individual's proximity to the centre of the explosion and conflagration.
On the other hand, one-fifth of police officers who had to handle bodies after an aeroplane crash developed a severe stress reaction although there was no direct personal threat.

Clinical presentation and prognosis

This is a short-lived but severe disorder caused by an overwhelming, psychologically traumatic experience. The condition generally subsides within hours or days. Examples of such exceptional stressors include rape, assault, a life-threatening accident, a transport disaster, a domestic fire or multiple bereavements.

The symptoms of an acute stress reaction develop rapidly and tend to vary in character and fluctuate in intensity during the first few hours after exposure to the precipitating event (Table 24). The condition tends to resolve within a matter of days but some survivors will go on to develop PTSD (see Section 2.10.2). Some victims might withdraw into a dissociative stupor (see Section 2.1) or run away from the scene in a state of fugue.

Treatment

If there is persistent denial that the event has occurred, the survivor should be cautiously prompted to recall the facts. A very short course of a benzodiazepine tranquilliser and/or hypnotic is indicated for severe agitation or insomnia. Informal conversation with friends or family is often the most helpful course, but if there is a lack of social support the patient could be signposted towards counselling.

Table 24 Clinical presentation of acute stress disorder

Symptoms	Clinical presentation
Psychological	Feeling numb and detached, or dazed and disorientated
	Disbelief that the precipitating event has occurred
	Agitation and overactivity
	Fear, dejection, irritability and anger
	Hypervigilance and enhanced startle response
	'Action replays' of the incident in intrusive memories and dreams
	Withdrawal and avoidance of reminders of the incident
	Irrational guilt about surviving or failing to help others
	Poor concentration
	Loss of interest
Physical	Sweating
	Shakiness
	Rapid heartbeat
	Fatigue
	Insomnia
	Nightmares
	Loss of appetite
	Nausea and diarrhoea

2.10.2 Post-traumatic stress disorder

Aetiology/psychopathology

The individual is involved in or witness to a catastrophic event which is an extreme threat to themselves or others, such as a large-scale disaster (such as a terror attack or rail crash), or a personal trauma such a rape, torture or assault. The psychological impact of the traumatic event is known to be more severe when the stressor is 'man-made' rather than an 'act of God' such as a natural disaster.

Not all people exposed to the same trauma will develop post-traumatic stress disorder (PTSD), indicating personal predisposition must play a part. Factors thought to increase the risk include previous history of mood or anxiety disorder, previous trauma, lower intelligence, lack of social support and an anxious personality type.

Brain-imaging studies have shown hyperactivity in the amygdala, and hippocampal dysfunction likely interfering with memory processing.

Epidemiology

The incidence of PTSD is proportionate to the intensity of the psychological trauma. For example, 70% of rape victims are found to have PTSD at 9-month follow-up. In general about 25% of individuals exposed to traumatic events develop full-blown PTSD, but the frequency can vary. Thus, about 16% of London Underground train drivers who witnessed a train striking a person on the track developed PTSD, while careful psychological preparation of the police officers who handled the bodies of the Piper Alpha oil rig victims prevented the occurrence of any post-traumatic illness. Women develop PTSD more often than men.

Clinical presentation

PTSD is a protracted psychological and behavioural reaction to an exceptionally threatening or catastrophic event that immediately induces intense fear, horror and/or helplessness. The onset is typically after a few days, but may be delayed for several months following a trauma. Symptoms are shown in the following 'Key point'.

> **Key point**
>
> **Symptoms of PTSD**
>
> > reliving the incident in the form of flashbacks – recurrent, distressing and intrusive images of the event
>
> > dreams and nightmares which do not necessarily depict the incident
>
> > avoidance of reminders of the trauma
>
> > detachment and numbness
>
> > hyperarousal, anxiety, insomnia, poor concentration, hypervigilance, enhanced startle response and irritability.

The patient may also experience survivor guilt (defined as the irrational sense that one's life was purchased at the cost of another's), phobic avoidance of any situation that resembles the original traumatic event, depression, generalised anxiety disorder or substance misuse. Some patients become aggressive while others (perhaps surprisingly) behave recklessly.

Treatment

Psychological – where symptoms are severe or chronic, trauma-focused cognitive behavioural therapy (CBT) is often used, with remission rates of about 50–60% following treatment. Eye-movement desensitisation and reprocessing (EMDR) has an increasing evidence-base of similar efficacy.

Pharmacological – both serotonergic tricyclic antidepressants (eg clomipramine) and selective serotonin reuptake inhibitor antidepressants may help to suppress flashbacks and nightmares, as well as reducing the frequency of panic attacks, in addition to their specific antidepressant effect. Second-line treatment can include different classes of antidepressant, followed by augmentation with atypical antipsychotics. There may be a role for brief courses of hypnotics, eg zopiclone.

Prognosis

This has not yet been clearly established. About one-quarter of rescuers involved in an oil rig disaster were found to have PTSD almost 12 months after the event. There was still a high rate of PTSD in severely abused former prisoners of war 50 years after their release. Prevalence rates for PTSD can range from about 30% among Australian firefighters to over 80% among Cambodian refugees.

Prevention

Remind the survivor that it is perfectly normal to react emotionally to an abnormal event. Gently encourage the survivor to talk about the traumatic event rather than sweep it under the carpet: go at their pace and without intrusive pressure. Advise them to avoid using alcohol to suppress symptoms because it can delay resolution. Encourage them to keep up their usual routine activities.

Psychological debriefing following trauma is no longer recommended as there is no evidence it prevents PTSD and in some individuals may worsen their condition. Ensuring the patient has social support or access to counselling agencies is important.

2.11 Puerperal disorders

Psychiatric disorders associated with childbirth are maternity blues, postnatal depression and puerperal psychosis, but existing mental health conditions can worsen due to physiological changes and psychosocial stressors associated with childbirth and the future mothering role.

2.11.1 Maternity blues

Aetiology/psychopathology

> more common in first pregnancy

> more common in those with history of premenstrual tension

> not related to complications at delivery

> modestly associated with marked postnatal fall in progesterone levels.

Epidemiology

It occurs in 50–70% of women, mainly on the third to fourth day after delivery.

Clinical presentation

The midwives or partner might report lability of mood, tearfulness and irritability. Mood changes are usually sudden, fleeting and unexpected, with lows and highs on a background of euthymia. Symptoms tend to peak at 3–5 days, with spontaneous resolution of these problems within days to weeks.

Treatment

Provide support and reassurance.

2.11.2 Postnatal depressive disorder

Aetiology/psychopathology

Predisposing factors:

> previous depression

> family history of depression / postnatal depression

> recent adverse life events

> marital conflict

> lack of social support

> younger age

> poor relationship with own mother

> anxiety and poor sleep in late pregnancy.

Epidemiology

Occurs in 10–15% of women.

Clinical presentation

Diagnostic and statistical manual of mental disorders (DSM)-V states that the onset may be during pregnancy (50% of cases begin prior to delivery) or within 4 weeks of delivery. The clinical picture is as in non-psychotic depression.

Treatment

> psychosocial interventions including developing and involving the mother's social networks or via mother and baby groups, group work, guided self-help, psychotherapy and cognitive behavioural therapy (CBT)

> antidepressants for severe symptoms, history of severe episodes or persistent symptoms (see below).

Prognosis

Hazard
Outcome of postnatal depression

> Minor changes in mental state have potential for significant neglect of the child, particularly in the neonatal period.

Untreated postnatal depression can last for up to 2 years with damage to:

> relationships, including attachment bonds with child

> emotional and cognitive development of the baby

> any other children.

Risk of further episode is one in six.

2.11.3 Puerperal psychosis

Aetiology/psychopathology

> Genetic – if there is a strong family history of an affective disorder.

> Environmental – social stress is not implicated (unlike postnatal depression).

> Hormonal – postpartum fall in oestrogen causes supersensitivity of dopamine receptors.

Epidemiology

The frequency is one in every 500 births in the general population. Risk factors are a past history or family history (particularly in mother and sisters) of mood disorder, primipara, older age, and giving birth by caesarean section.

If there is a history of puerperal psychosis the risk of recurrence in future pregnancies is 50%, increasing to 50–90% in bipolar disorder. The puerperal trigger for psychosis relates to severe mood disorders including bipolar affective disorder, schizoaffective disorder and severe depression with psychotic features. Other psychiatric disorders in the puerperal period are predominantly triggered by psychosocial stressors.

Clinical presentation

Usually an affective (especially manic) disorder with psychotic symptoms, but 20% of incidences are schizophrenia-like. Onset tends to be abrupt and in the first 2 weeks postpartum.

Hazard
Ensure patient has assessment and appropriate investigations to rule out medical causes of delirium, such as postpartum infection.

Treatment

The key principles are shown in the following 'Key point'.

Key point

Management of puerperal psychosis

This should include:

> antenatal identification of high-risk mothers

> an assessment of risk to the mother, baby (or unborn baby), other children and partner

> moving those identified to a specialist mother and baby unit with nurses trained in both mental health and baby care

> an attempt to preserve mother–child bonding

> conventional treatment of depression, mania or schizophrenia, including electroconvulsive therapy if necessary

> breastfeeding (see below)

> assessment of mother–baby interaction before discharge

> monitoring the mother carefully during subsequent child bearing.

Psychiatric drug treatments in the perinatal period

Key point

All medication treatment decisions should be made with consideration not just of risks of action (eg potential teratogenic effects) but also the risks of inaction (eg untreated mental illness). There is growing evidence that untreated mental illness (even mild depression and anxiety) can also have teratogenic effects via increased inflammatory mediators and stress hormones which can lead to developmental delay, prematurity and low birth weight.

Hazard

Perinatal psychiatric drug treatments

> Lithium – avoid in pregnancy and after delivery if possible because:

> in the first trimester it can cause atrialisation of the right ventricle (Ebstein's anomaly)

> the renal clearance of lithium falls abruptly after delivery, causing a dangerous rise in serum lithium, which is secreted in breast milk such that toxic levels of lithium can develop rapidly in the infant, particularly if they become dehydrated.

However, there is an up to 70% risk of relapse postpartum if mood stabilisers are discontinued pre-conception. If possible, it is recommended to switch to a safer mood stabiliser such as an antipsychotic, but in severe cases or where there is a recent relapse, it may be felt best to continue with lithium after discussion of the risks.

> Carbamazepine, valproate and lamotrigine – avoid in pregnancy if possible due to risk of neural tube defects. High-dose folic acid treatment can reduce these risks.

> Antidepressants – exposure to antidepressants in the first trimester is associated with a small increased risk of preterm labour, and in the third trimester may cause withdrawal effects in the neonate. Tricyclic antidepressants such as amitriptyline or imipramine were often traditionally used as there was more data regarding their safety than selective serotonin reuptake inhibitors

(SSRIs). However, there is growing evidence of relative safety of certain SSRIs in pregnancy. Sertraline has the lowest level of placental transfer and expression in breast milk and has therefore become a first-line SSRI. Paroxetine and clomipramine are associated with fetal heart defects and are less safe than other SSRIs and should be avoided. It is not known whether venlafaxine and mirtazapine are safe, and hence they should be avoided.

> Antipsychotics – there is uncertainty about the risk of antipsychotic use and major fetal defects, but studies suggest any risk is small. Atypical antipsychotics are unlikely to be teratogenic, but may be associated with preterm labour, small birth weight and gestational diabetes. There is most experience with chlorpromazine, haloperidol, olanzapine and quetiapine.

Key point

Psychotropic drugs of choice when breastfeeding

> Use sertraline or tricyclic antidepressants (amitriptyline or imipramine, because more data are available about their effects).

> Use chlorpromazine, trifluoperazine and olanzapine (for the same reason).

Psychotropic drugs and breastfeeding

When giving a mother psychotropic drugs remember:

> All psychotropic drugs are secreted in breast milk, therefore use the lowest effective dose.

> Time feeds to avoid peak levels of drugs.

> Avoid use of more than one psychotropic drug.

> Monitor for development, sedation and irritability in the baby.

> Check the baby's hepatic and renal function.

> Citalopram and fluoxetine have highest levels of expression in breast milk and should be avoided if possible.

Prognosis

The prognosis is good for immediate recovery, but there is a risk of recurrence in 30–50% of patients if they have subsequent deliveries and 50% of patients develop non-puerperal depression.

Risks of puerperal psychosis

> suicide

> neglect of child (and of other children)

> harm to the baby if the mother holds delusional ideas about the child, and of infanticide followed by suicide

> harm to other children and partner.

2.12 Depression

Aetiology/psychopathology

Impaired neurotransmission in depression has been explained by the monoamine hypothesis, ie low mood is associated with reduced synaptic noradrenaline (NA) or 5-hydroxytryptamine (5HT; serotonin). Reserpine, a monoamine-depleting drug can cause depression. Conversely, tricyclic and monoamine oxidase inhibitors (MAOI) antidepressants increase the synaptic availability of NA and 5HT in the synaptic cleft.

However, there is a delay between the antidepressant-induced rise in synaptic NA and 5HT in an individual and any improvement in their mood. Furthermore, depressed patients do not have decreased levels of NA, 5HT or the metabolites of either in their blood, urine or cerebrospinal fluid. There is an excess of 5HT reuptake receptors in the frontal cortex of people who have committed suicide.

Some common exogenous causes of depression are shown in Table 25.

Vulnerability factors in women are:

> being responsible for the care of young children

> lack of a confiding relationship

> lack of a job outside the home

> separation from their own mother before the age of 11.

These vulnerability factors sensitise the individual to major adverse life events which are characterised by loss or threat of loss, eg redundancy, physical illness. There is a sixfold increase in adverse life events in the months before the onset of depression.

Table 25 Common exogenous causes of depression		
Psychosocial factors (mainly loss)	**Medical conditions**	**Drugs**
Bereavement	Cerebrovascular accident	Reserpine
Unemployment	Carcinoma of pancreas and bronchus	Beta-blockers
Divorce/separation	Hypothyroidism	Calcium antagonists
Mutilating surgery	Cushing's disease	Oral contraceptives
Disability	Systemic lupus erythematosus	Corticosteroids
	Parkinson's disease	Alcohol
	Multiple sclerosis	Cocaine withdrawal
		Amphetamine withdrawal

Other aetiological factors are:

> genetic – identical twins reared apart show 60% more concordance than dizygotic twins

> endocrine – loss of cortisol circadian rhythm, ie overactivity of hypothalamic–pituitary–adrenocortical system, which might be primary or secondary

> immunological – growing evidence of increased cytokine levels and raised acute-phase proteins

> psychological – learned helplessness, based on the model of harnessed dogs subjected to recurrent aversive stimuli who become apathetic and fail to escape when restraints are removed.

In contrast to vulnerability, there is a factor known as 'resilience' where due to favourable genetics and early developmental experiences, some people are less likely to develop depression, despite exposure to psychosocial stressors in later life.

Epidemiology

Of the general population, 5% will experience an episode of moderate to severe depression. Prevalence is 2–3% of men and up to 9% of women. It is commoner in lower socio-economic groups because of chronic adversity.

Clinical presentation

Key point
The commonly seen mood disorders are depression or bipolar disorder. Depression is much commoner than bipolar disorder. The features of each are:

> Bipolar disorder – there are episodes of persistent lowering of mood interspersed with bouts of sustained elation and overactivity.

> Depression – there are only downward mood swings.

Common
A mixture of psychological and biological symptoms present most days for at least 2 weeks (Table 26). At least two core symptoms, plus at least two other symptoms, are required for diagnosis according to *International statistical classification of diseases and health-related problems*, 10th edition (ICD-10), with severity (mild, moderate, severe) dependent on degree and number of symptoms. Patients may be agitated or retarded (Table 27).

Uncommon
Psychotic depression – severe depression can develop psychotic features with mood-congruent delusions and hallucinations. Examples of delusions include delusional convictions of disease, putrefaction, poverty, contaminating others, causing evil, and derogatory or humiliating themes. There may also be hallucinations, usually in the second person, with similar mood-congruent themes, especially accusing or derogatory voices.

Table 26	Clinical presentation of major depression (ICD-10)
Symptoms	Clinical presentation
Core	Persistent low mood
	Reduced energy levels
	Loss of interest and enjoyment (anhedonia)
Psychological	Reduced self-esteem
	Ideas of guilt and/or worthlessness
	Pessimistic views of the future (hopelessness)
	Helplessness
	Poor concentration and attention
	Thoughts of death, self-harm and/or suicide
Biological	Insomnia with early morning wakening (occasionally hypersomnia)
	Diminished appetite with weight loss (occasionally increased appetite)
	Loss of sex drive
	Lack of drive, energy and motivation

Table 27	Signs of psychomotor agitation and retardation
Condition	Signs
Psychomotor agitation	Pacing and hand wringing
	Repetitive and futile activity
	Quest for reassurance
Psychomotor retardation	Avoidance of company
	Self-neglect
	Mutism
	Slowed movements

Seasonal affective disorder – depression tends to occur in the winter months and is often accompanied by oversleeping and overeating. There is a female to male ratio of 6:1. Onset is in the mid-20s. Can be treated with antidepressants and phototherapy, which artificially lengthens the day and maintains biological rhythms.

Dysthymia is a chronic depression of mood, lasting at least several years, which is not sufficiently severe, or in which individual episodes are not sufficiently prolonged, to meet criteria for mild, moderate or severe depression.

Key point

Anxiety and depression often coexist.

Treatment

Treatment depends on the severity of the illness. Mild or subthreshold depression should initially be treated using low-intensity psychological therapy (guided self-help and group therapy). Where this is unsuccessful, or in moderate to severe depression, consider high-intensity psychological therapy (eg individual cognitive behavioural therapy (CBT)) or antidepressants.

> psychological – self-help, group therapy, cognitive behavioural therapy

> pharmacological – selective serotonin reuptake inhibitors (SSRIs) are first-line treatment. Add antipsychotic drug for delusions and/or hallucinations. Electroconvulsive therapy in very severe cases.

Key point

Management of severe depression

> Assess the patient for suicide risk (see Sections 1.2.2 and 1.3.2); if the risk is high then admission to a psychiatric unit is indicated, if necessary under the enforcement of the Mental Health Act (see Section 2.14).

> Social isolation, severe self-neglect and failure to eat or drink also require hospital admission.

> Mobilisation of support from carers and mental health professionals is required, especially community psychiatric nurses.

> Electroconvulsive therapy (ECT) may be used in very severe cases, such as where the patient is not eating or drinking, where a quicker response than using an antidepressant is desired.

Antidepressants

These tend to be more effective in severe depression and where biological symptoms are prominent. Drugs used include the following:

> SSRIs, eg fluoxetine, sertraline

> combination reuptake inhibitors (NA and 5HT), eg mirtazapine and venlafaxine

> tricyclics, eg lofepramine (less cardiotoxic) and amitriptyline

> MAOIs – these inhibit the reuptake of NA and 5HT, thereby increasing the amount of available neurotransmitter at the synapse.

Hazard

Monoamine oxidase inhibitors (MAOIs)

These carry a risk of tyramine response ('cheese reaction'), which causes a dangerous rise in BP. Clear dietary advice is essential prior to initiation. They are also incompatible with opioids, especially pethidine.

Hazard

Side effects of tricyclics

> anticholinergic, eg dry mouth, blurred vision, constipation, ileus, precipitation of glaucoma, urinary retention and delirium in older people

> α-adrenergic, eg postural hypotension

> cardiac dysrhythmias

> lowering the seizure threshold

> cardiotoxicity in overdose

> weight gain

> sexual dysfunction.

SSRIs – these have fewer cardiovascular effects than tricyclics and are less sedative. They also have no anticholinergic side effects, but they can cause gastrointestinal problems, agitation, insomnia and headache, which are common during initiation of treatment and usually subside within a week. They may also cause sexual side effects (but this can also be a feature of the underlying depression). All antidepressants can cause hyponatraemia but SSRIs have a greater propensity. SSRIs are used as first-line treatment as they have similar efficacy but are safer in overdose than other classes.

Tricyclics and SSRIs are probably of equal efficacy. In depression of psychotic intensity, an antipsychotic should be added to the antidepressant.

Antidepressants may take up to 3–4 weeks to exert their effects, though in many cases begin to work within 1–2 weeks. Antidepressant dosage needs titrating every 2–4 weeks towards the maximum, according to response and tolerability. If despite this there is little or no response, or the initial drug cannot be tolerated, then switching the class of antidepressant is recommended. After that, augmentation may be considered with appropriate specialist advice. National Institute for Health and Care Excellence (NICE) guidelines recommend continuing an antidepressant for 6 months after remission for a first episode of depression, and for 2 years for a history of recurrent depressive episodes.

Key point

Electroconvulsive therapy

This is the treatment of choice in instances of:

> severe depression

> refusal to eat or drink

> grave suicide risk

> failure of other treatment methods.

Electroconvulsive therapy is applied under general anaesthetic with muscle relaxants. The usual course is six to eight applications, with two applications per week. Major risk factors are those of the general anaesthetic. Side effects include headache, transient and persistent memory problems, seizures between treatments, delirium in older people and cardiovascular complications.

Prognosis

Most episodes of depression remit within 6 months. Of sufferers, 15% experience chronic symptoms. There is a high risk of recurrence if recovery from a particular episode is incomplete. The risk of recurrence increases with age. Mortality due to suicide is 15%.

Prevention

Cognitive behavioural therapy reduces the risk of further episodes. Also consider the continuation of treatment with antidepressants and mood stabilisers (see Section 2.13).

2.13 Bipolar affective disorder

This consists of recurrent episodes of mania and depression. Episodes of elevated mood are called mania if they are severe and/or have psychotic features (delusions and hallucinations). Less severe cases are labelled hypomania. Minimum duration of symptoms is 7 days for mania, and 4 days for hypomania.

Aetiology/psychopathology

There is a concordance rate of about 75% in monozygotic twins and about 54% in dizygotic twins. A cyclothymic personality (subclinical mood swings) is a predisposing factor.

Mania might be secondary to the following: antidepressant treatment, thyrotoxicosis, head injury, stroke, amphetamine or cocaine use, exogenous steroids.

Epidemiology

The lifetime risk of mania is 0.6–1%. The mean age of onset is 20, although diagnosis may be delayed. The incidence is the same in men and women. The age of onset of bipolar disorder is earlier than in depressive disorder.

Clinical presentation

Mania is characterised by features shown in the following 'Key point'.

Key point

Symptoms of mania

> sustained elevation of mood or irritability

> abundant energy

> disinhibition

> reckless behaviour with extravagant spending, fast driving and promiscuity

> pressure of speech

> increased self-esteem

> grandiose and self-important ideas

> sometimes a sense of special mission

> acceleration of thinking and flight of ideas

> reduced need for sleep

> poor concentration

> distractibility

> lack of insight

> sometimes delusions of grandeur

> auditory hallucinations in the second person (ie talking to the patient).

Key rating scales of manic symptoms include:

> Young Mania Rating Scale – for inpatient setting

> hypomania checklist (HCL-32) – for retrospective evaluation of hypomanic symptoms in the primary care setting.

Key point

Mixed affective states (ie co-occurrence of depression and manic symptoms) can occur in at least 16% of bipolar patients, usually while the mood is shifting between poles (during a mood episode that differs markedly from the normal baseline). This is not to be confused with mood instability in emotionally unstable personality disorder, which is persistent, pervasive and present in different situations throughout life.

Schizoaffective disorder – this diagnostic category is used for manic or depressive symptoms and schizophrenic symptoms occurring with equal prominence and sometimes independently during the course of the illness, but can also coexist within the same episode or within a few days of each other.

Rapid-cycling bipolar affective disorder – in this uncommon condition there are more than four episodes of severe depression or mania in a year. It is more common in women and in those taking antidepressants.

Differential diagnosis

Differential diagnosis of hypomania and mania in bipolar disorder is:

> drug-induced overactivity and euphoria – amphetamines, cocaine and ecstasy

> organic states – thyroid dysfunction, HIV, general paralysis of the insane and multiple sclerosis.

Treatment

Acute episodes of mania or hypomania

These are typically treated with:

> atypical antipsychotics, eg olanzapine, risperidone and quetiapine

> valproate or lithium.

Adjuncts may be useful to control agitation in the short term, including:

> benzodiazepines

> promethazine

> z-drugs (zolpidem, zopiclone, etc).

Key point

For mania, admission to hospital (which is compulsory if necessary) is usually indicated to prevent personal and social damage due to frenetic and reckless behaviour. Hypomania might be contained at home provided the patient can be supervised and is prepared to take regular medication.

Hazard

Watch for severe depressive downswing with risk of suicide.

Treatment of bipolar depression

Antidepressants as monotherapy may precipitate iatrogenic mania. They may only be given if depression is severe and persistent despite other options being tried. They can be combined with an antimanic for greater protection, and should only be given with careful monitoring and withdrawn as soon as the mood becomes euthymic again. Therefore, in bipolar depression recommended treatments include:

> combining fluoxetine and olanzapine

> an atypical antipsychotic, eg olanzapine or quetiapine

> mood stabilisers – lithium or lamotrigine.

Prophylaxis

Lithium is first-line treatment. Check renal and thyroid function, and an electrocardiogram (ECG) because of the risk of cardiac dysrhythmias in older patients. Monitor serum lithium levels, aiming for a level of 0.6–1.0 mmol/L. Watch for hypothyroidism (treat with L-thyroxine), nephrogenic diabetes insipidus and monitor renal function (long-term risk of chronic kidney disease).

Other options include quetiapine (which protects against both mania and depression) and lamotrigine (which only protects against depression without precipitating mania, but does not protect against mania), hence lamotrigine may need to be combined with an antimanic agent to give all-round protection.

Complications

> risk of death from suicide in a depressive phase

> risk of death from exhaustion after weeks of untreated mania

> manic stupor.

Prognosis

Untreated episodes might last between 3 and 6 months. Over 50% of sufferers will have further episodes if the disorder begins before the age of 30. Approximately 40% of patients with bipolar disorder have initially been misdiagnosed as having unipolar depressive disorder.

The duration of onset prior to correct diagnosis of bipolar illness is a prognostic indicator for future illness severity and response to medication. This duration is increased when depression is the first clearly identifiable mood episode. Always be mindful of the possibility of an underlying bipolar illness, even when the episode being considered is presenting as depression.

2.14 The Mental Health Act 1983

The Mental Health Act (MHA) deals with the compulsory detention and treatment of people suffering from mental disorders of a nature (type and history of illness) and/or degree (severity of the illness now) who are considered to be:

> a danger to themselves and/or

> a danger to others and/or

> at risk of deterioration of their health.

Key point

A patient with a mental illness may be detained under the Mental Health Act (MHA) on the grounds of health alone, ie the patient does not necessarily have to constitute an active danger to themselves and/or others.

The term 'mental disorder' is defined in the Act as 'any disorder or disability of the mind', and includes all the psychiatric disorders described in this book, with the following exceptions:

> Substance abuse or acute intoxication with drugs and/or alcohol – note that

psychiatric disorders arising out of substance misuse, such as alcoholic hallucinosis or drug-induced psychosis, are covered by the Act.

> An individual with a learning disability may not be detained under the Act solely because of their learning disability, unless it is accompanied by abnormally aggressive or irresponsible conduct.

> Personality disorders are covered by the Act, but careful thought has to be given as to whether inpatient treatment would be available and/or effective. Sometimes short-term admission can be harmful, resulting in the person feeling let down or abandoned when the admission ends, with no less ongoing risk of self-harm, whereas boundaried, consistent and ongoing holistic community treatment can be more helpful.

The least restrictive option must also be considered, which might include things like 'crisis resolution' or 'home treatment' teams who visit every day at home, and can provide help with eg monitored medication.

Physicians only need to be familiar with a limited number of Sections ('Sections' referring to main paragraph numbers of the Act). These key Sections are shown in Table 28.

Physical treatments and the MHA

The MHA allows for the compulsory assessment and/or treatment of a mental disorder. This treatment may include physical treatments where this is part of the treatment package relating to the mental disorder (eg a clozapine blood test, or nasogastric (NG) feeding in anorexia). However, where a physical treatment is required for a separate physical disorder the MHA does not allow for compulsory treatment, even if the patient also has a mental disorder or is detained under the Act. In these situations, consent must be obtained in the same way as for any other individual.

If the patient lacks capacity to consent to treatment of a physical health problem, treatment can be given if it is in their best interests according to the Mental Capacity Act. Where this might constitute a deprivation of liberty, a Deprivation of Liberty Safeguard (DoLS) authorisation should be sought. Recent case law has clarified that there is a deprivation of liberty in circumstances where a person is under continuous control and supervision, would not be free to leave, and lacks capacity to consent to these arrangements. This applies regardless of the relative normality of the situation, or whether or not the person actually attempts to leave, thus encompassing a large proportion of acute hospital inpatients.

Table 28	Key sections of the MHA relevant to physicians	
Section	**Applied by**	**Allows**
5(4)	Registered mental health or LD nurse	Hold patient on inpatient ward for up to 6 hours
5(2)	Doctor (with full GMC registration)	Hold patient on inpatient ward for up to 72 hours
2	AMHP, with two independent medical recommendations	Detention to hospital for assessment and treatment, for up to 28 days
3	AMHP, with two independent medical recommendations	Detention to hospital for treatment, for up to 6 months
CTO	Doctor (responsible clinician) and AMHP	Upon discharge from hospital the Section 3 is put on standby provided certain conditions are met by the patient. If conditions are breached then patients can be recalled to hospital for assessment
136	Police officer	Person to be removed from public place and taken to place of safety, for up to 72 hours

AMHP, approved mental health professional; CTO, community treatment order; GMC, General Medical Council; LD, learning disability.

Mental Capacity Act or MHA?

Where a patient has capacity to consent to an admission for psychiatric assessment or treatment, they can agree to a hospital admission informally. If they have capacity to consent but refuse, then only the MHA can be used for compulsory admission.

If the patient lacks capacity to consent to psychiatric admission or treatment, the key factor is whether the patient is objecting to psychiatric admission or treatment. If they are not objecting, this could take place in their best interests under the Mental Capacity Act with consideration of a DoLS authorisation. If they are actively objecting, the MHA should be used.

Holding powers

Doctors who are in charge of the care of a hospital inpatient (or their deputies) have holding powers under Section 5(2) of the MHA. It is important to note this only applies to inpatients – Section 5(2) cannot be used in outpatient departments or in emergency departments. In addition it does not allow for any powers of compulsory treatment, simply that the patient can be legally held on the ward if they are attempting to leave. It should be used when the doctor concludes that an application should be made under the MHA (because they have a mental disorder and pose a risk to themselves, others, or risk of deterioration) and allows the patient to be legally held in hospital for up to 72 hours for a full psychiatric assessment to take place.

Section 5(4) confers similar powers to mental health or learning disability nurses. This allows the patient to be held for up to 6 hours on an inpatient ward. It should only be used in cases where it is not possible for a doctor to attend the ward in a timely fashion.

Key point

Section 5(2) allows a doctor to legally hold an inpatient on the ward for up to 72 hours for a psychiatric assessment. It does not allow any compulsory treatment and does not apply to outpatients (including the emergency department).

Assessment for Sections 2 or 3

If a patient is held under Section 5(2), an MHA assessment must take place within the 72-hour time limit; and if a patient is held under Section 136, an MHA assessment must happen within 24 hours. An MHA assessment may also be requested directly, most commonly by a psychiatrist or mental health team.

Section 2 allows compulsory admission for assessment and any necessary treatment of a mental disorder for up to 28 days.

At this point the Section lapses so that prior to this a further application must be made for a Section 3 if needed. Section 3 allows for compulsory admission for treatment of a mental disorder for up to 6 months, with extensions of up to 1 year at a time if necessary.

The process is coordinated by an approved mental health professional (AMHP), who has particular training for this role. The patient must be examined by two doctors, at least one of whom must be approved as having special experience in the diagnosis and treatment of mental disorders. Ideally, one of the two doctors should also have had prior contact with the patient. Typically the two doctors would be psychiatrists or GPs.

If both doctors recommend detention under Section 2 or Section 3 of the MHA, the AMHP may then follow this recommendation (although they are not obliged to and the final decision rests with the AMHP). The AMHP has a duty to consult with the patient's nearest relative. The patient must be detained to a named hospital, whether this be medical or psychiatric. Patients can be transferred between hospitals (such as from a medical ward once medically fit for psychiatric admission) under other sections of the MHA.

Patients have the right to appeal against both Section 2 and Section 3 to an MHA tribunal. The nearest relative may also apply to hospital managers for the patient to be discharged.

Psychiatry: Section 3

3 Self-assessment

3.1 Self-assessment questions

MRCP(UK) Part 1 examination questions

Question 1

Clinical scenario

An 86-year-old man who had lived alone since his wife's death 1 year previously was found wandering in the street in the middle of the night after falling down a step. He was bewildered and frightened, and showed signs of self-neglect. He was disorientated and his speech was very hesitant. He described visual hallucinations that had started 6 months previously.

Question

What is the most likely diagnosis?

Answers

A dementia with Lewy bodies

B depressive pseudodementia

C dissociative fugue

D mania

E obsessive–compulsive disorder

Question 2

Clinical scenario

A 50-year-old woman had accidentally caused a small fire in her home when she forgot to switch off the oven. Her family reported that she had become increasingly forgetful over the last 6 months or so, also that she had suffered a severe head injury 1 year previously. She had been incontinent of urine and her balance was poor. Physical examination of her central nervous system was unremarkable.

Question

What is the most likely diagnosis?

Answer

A dementia with Lewy bodies

B Huntington's disease

C normal pressure hydrocephalus

D prion disease

E vascular dementia

Question 3

Clinical scenario

A 20-year-old university history student was not allowed to continue with his course because of poor attendance. For several months his written work had been characterised by bizarre, detailed and complex theories about the influence of intergalactic aliens on political events. He had smoked up to eight 'joints' of cannabis a day since he was 16. At interview his speech was slow and hesitant, and he constantly reverted to the theme of being controlled by trans-planetary visitors, who communicated with him and influenced his feelings and actions.

Question

What is the most likely diagnosis?

Answers

A antisocial personality disorder

B cannabis-induced psychosis

C dissociative disorder

D obsessive–compulsive disorder

E post-traumatic stress disorder

Question 4

Clinical scenario

A diagnosis of schizophrenia was made in a 28-year-old woman, which led to discussion of the use of an antipsychotic drug and its potential side effects.

Question

Which is a recognised side effect of antipsychotic medication?

Answers

A galactorrhoea

B hypoglycaemia

C hypotension

D menorrhagia

E weight loss

Question 5

Clinical scenario

A 28-year-old woman presented to the emergency department after she swallowed half a dozen zopiclone tablets in front of her boyfriend. She was drowsy but able to communicate. On taking the history you learned that she had taken many previous overdoses, and she reported fleeting paranoid ideas and visual hallucinations. She had never been able to settle for long with one partner or at any job. On examination she had numerous scars on her wrists.

Question

What is the most likely diagnosis?

Answers

A anxiety disorder

B depressive disorder

C drug use disorder

D personality disorder

E schizophrenia

Question 6

Clinical scenario

A 78-year-old man with carcinoma of the pancreas was admitted to a general medical ward because of abdominal pain and weight loss. He appeared miserable and preoccupied, and he barely talked to the other patients or staff.

Question

Which symptom would be helpful in deciding whether he has a severe depressive illness that requires treatment with an antidepressant?

Answers

A difficulty sleeping

B loss of appetite

C loss of energy

D loss of interest

E loss of libido

Question 7

Clinical scenario

Following her first pregnancy, a 23-year-old woman had delivered a healthy baby boy a week ago. She was distressed and low in her mood and would not let anyone touch her baby. She was convinced that the attending midwives want to take her baby from her, which was not true.

Question

What is the most likely diagnosis?

Answers

A delusional disorder

B maternity blues

C postnatal depressive disorder

D puerperal psychosis

E schizophrenia

Question 8

Clinical scenario

A 40-year-old woman was referred to a medical outpatient clinic with breathlessness on exertion and palpitations. On examination she appeared to be pale and you suspected that she was anaemic, but she refused to have any blood tests.

Question

Which feature would confirm the diagnosis of blood/injection/injury phobia?

Answers

A bradycardia when you show her a syringe

B hypertension when talking about blood tests

C paranoia that phlebotomists would try to kill her

D phobia of spiders

E vasovagal faints in biology lessons as a schoolgirl

Question 9

Clinical scenario

A previously well 74-year-old woman was brought to the emergency department by her daughter. She had been robbed in the street 2 days before. The robber threatened her with a knife, ripped her bag off her shoulder and pushed her over as he ran away. Other than some bruising she was not physically injured. Since then she had been agitated and irritable, with poor concentration and loss of interest in her usual activities, and she would not leave her flat. She said she was not affected by the robbery, but felt physically unwell with sweating, shakiness, rapid heartbeat and insomnia, and she was concerned about her heart.

Question

What is the most likely diagnosis?

Answers

A acute stress reaction

B generalised anxiety disorder

C panic disorder

D phobic anxiety disorder

E post-traumatic stress disorder

Question 10

Clinical scenario

A 47-year-old man with a history of recurrent depression presented with a further episode of depression that started 2 months previously. His mood was very low and he could no longer derive any pleasure from his usual activities. He felt hopeless about his future and wished he was dead. He had last been depressed 3 years previously when he responded to citalopram, which he had stopped taking 6 months ago because he felt well.

Question

Which would be the most appropriate management?

Answers

A amitriptyline

B citalopram

C electroconvulsive therapy

D lithium

E venlafaxine

MRCP(UK) Part 2 examination questions

Question 11

Clinical scenario

A 30-year-old unemployed woman was brought to the emergency department by the police after being arrested in a large department store for shoplifting. She had been in the store for about an hour, hurrying between various departments grabbing items of clothing and accessories, and talking loudly in an over-familiar way with other customers and staff. She had been apprehended when she tried to leave the store without paying, and she had been incensed by this, saying she did not need to pay because she owned the store and all the other shops on that street.

Question

Which would be the most appropriate treatment to start once she is admitted to a psychiatric ward?

Answers

A electroconvulsive therapy

B lithium

C lorazepam

D quetiapine

E valproate

Question 12

Clinical scenario

A 41-year-old man was brought to the emergency department by his wife. He had been sent home from work the previous day because he had been unplugging all the computer screens in the office, and had become threatening and angry when his work colleagues turned them back on. His wife said that over the past 5 months he had been drinking more, and becoming increasingly preoccupied about terrorists gaining information about him by using computers. He felt very threatened and believed that they were going to kill him by setting off an explosive device. He was not hallucinating and his thoughts were coherent.

Question
What is the most likely diagnosis?

Answers
A alcohol use disorder
B bipolar affective disorder
C obsessive–compulsive disorder
D persistent delusional disorder
E schizophrenia

Question 13
Clinical scenario
A 24-year-old man was admitted to a general medical ward for treatment of cellulitis of his arm. He said that he had been a heroin user for 3 years and was attending a drug treatment unit in another city where he was being prescribed 40 mg of methadone per day, although he could not provide a contact number for you to corroborate this information. He had no clear signs of opioid withdrawal.

Question
What would be the most appropriate next step?

Answers
A administer intravenous naloxone
B perform urine drug testing for opioids
C prescribe methadone 10 mg as needed
D prescribe methadone 40 mg daily
E prescribe methadone 10 mg twice daily

Question 14
Clinical scenario
A 22-year-old woman in the emergency department waiting room has started shouting abuse and kicking at the furniture. She is known to have a psychotic illness.

Question
What should you do first?

Answers
A arrange an urgent Mental Health Act assessment
B call hospital security services
C remove other patients, visitors and staff from the area
D tell her to calm down
E tell her to leave the emergency department

Question 15
Clinical scenario
A 30-year-old schoolteacher has been on sick leave for 7 months since she had a bout of gastroenteritis. Her diarrhoea and vomiting had stopped after 2 days, but she had felt exhausted ever since and spent increasing amounts of time resting in bed. She slept badly, her concentration was poor and she was worried about swollen glands in her neck. A nutritionist had advised her to eat no dairy or wheat products, while her reflexologist had recommended a course of trace elements and other dietary supplements to correct an alleged post-viral imbalance of her adrenal function. Extensive medical tests and investigations had failed to demonstrate any significant abnormality.

Question
Which would be the best treatment option?

Answers
A citalopram
B cognitive behavioural therapy
C immunotherapy
D joining an 'ME' self-help group
E watchful waiting

Question 16
Clinical scenario
You are called urgently to see a 65-year-old man on a cardiology ward. He has recently had cardiac surgery under general anaesthetic, with no perioperative complications, and has been recovering well. He has become acutely agitated and is talking about his beliefs that the ward nurses are plotting to blow up the hospital. He is not known to have a previous psychiatric history.

Question
What aspect of the history is most important to ascertain?

Answers
A alcohol use
B details of the cardiac surgery
C further details of his ideas about the bomb plot
D nature of the onset of symptoms
E whether he is having hallucinations

Question 17
Clinical scenario
A 32-year-old man with a history of schizophrenia was admitted to the medical ward. He was well known to the community mental health team, and had been on oral risperidone for many months. He had presented with acute confusion and agitation.
On examination, vital signs included temperature of 38.4°C and pulse 120 beats per minute. Neurological examination revealed increased tone throughout all four limbs.

Question
What is the most important diagnosis to consider?

Answers
A encephalitis
B epilepsy
C extrapyramidal side effects of antipsychotic
D neuroleptic malignant syndrome
E relapse of schizophrenia

Question 18
Clinical scenario
A 45-year-old woman returned to a medical outpatient clinic for review. She complained of difficulty swallowing, which had recently been investigated by the gastroenterology service. Multiple investigations, including an endoscopy

and computerised tomography (CT) scan, had all been normal. Her history had not changed since her previous appointments, but she was visibly anxious, and said that she was sure she must have throat cancer as she had looked it up online. She was not reassured by her normal investigations and demanded further tests to look for cancer. When you suggested that she might have a functional cause for her symptoms, she said that she was not 'mad' and absolutely did not need to see a psychiatrist.

Question
What is the most appropriate course of action?

Answers
A discharge her from the medical clinic

B reassure her, decline any further tests, and arrange to see her again

C refer for another gastroenterology opinion

D refer for a repeat endoscopy and CT scan

E refer to psychiatry

Question 19

Clinical scenario
You are asked to review a 72-year-old woman on a care for older people ward because she had stopped eating or drinking for 72 hours. She told you she was very low and did not want to live. She said that she had no interest in food, and believed that her insides were slowly dying. Her daughter said she had stopped responding to her.

Question
Which would be the best treatment option, in conjunction with psychiatric input?

Answers
A refer for cognitive behavioural therapy (CBT)

B refer for electroconvulsive therapy (ECT)

C start an antipsychotic

D start a selective serotonin reuptake inhibitor (SSRI)

E start lithium

Question 20

Clinical scenario
A 22-year-old woman with known depression and a history of substance misuse had been admitted following an overdose of her antidepressant. She was medically stable but required observation. She continued to have suicidal ideation and stated that she had no regret about the overdose, other than it not working. She claimed to have more tablets stashed at home, where she lived alone. A psychiatric nurse had reviewed her shortly after her admission to the medical ward and written in the medical notes that she may need psychiatric admission.

You have been called to the medical ward because she now says she wants to self-discharge, and when you arrive she is standing near the door to the ward.

Question
Which would be the best course of action?

Answers
A allow her to leave the ward

B call psychiatry services to attend the ward

C detain her under Section 5(2) of the Mental Health Act

D do a capacity assessment

E tell the nurses not to let her leave under Common Law

3.2 Self-assessment answers

Answer to Question 1

A: dementia with Lewy bodies

Dementia with Lewy bodies is responsible for approximately 10–20% of dementia occurring in older people. In addition to the cognitive impairment, which is often fluctuating, the diagnostic features also include parkinsonism, hallucinations, repeated falls due to syncopal episodes, sensitivity to antipsychotic medication and rapid eye movement sleep disorder.

Answer to Question 2

C: normal pressure hydrocephalus

The symptoms described above are typical of normal pressure hydrocephalus. In addition to severe head injury the common causes of this include subarachnoid haemorrhage and previous meningitis, but often no cause is apparent. The absence of any involuntary movements make Huntington's disease and prion disease unlikely. In vascular dementia ischaemic changes are usually seen on computerised tomography (CT) scan. Dementia with Lewy bodies commonly presents with Parkinsonism and psychosis along with the cognitive impairment.

Answer to Question 3

B: cannabis-induced psychosis

The highest risk period of inducing psychosis by smoking cannabis is in childhood and adolescence. It has been suggested that cannabis may precipitate psychotic symptoms in a person with a predisposition to developing schizophrenia. However, because cannabis is more potent in its currently available form ('skunk') due to a higher tetrahydrocannabinol (THC) to cannabidiol ratio, with heavy use it can produce a clinical picture indistinguishable from schizophrenia in a person without a genetic predisposition to it.

Answer to Question 4

A: galactorrhoea

Since antipsychotic drugs act by blocking dopamine receptors in the brain, they increase prolactin levels. This results in secondary amenorrhoea, galactorrhoea and impotence in men. A serious and often unrecognised side effect of antipsychotics is the metabolic syndrome, which includes weight gain, diabetes, hypercholesterolaemia and hypertension.

Answer to Question 5

D: personality disorder

This presentation is fairly typical in someone who has a borderline personality disorder, but beware that this diagnosis should never be made in an emergency department by professionals without expertise in this area. Antisocial personality disorder is characterised by a disregard and violation of the rights of others that results in frequent law breaking. People who have a schizoid personality disorder are socially very isolated, apparently self-sufficient and have a restricted capacity to express emotion. In obsessive–compulsive personality disorder the person is excessively perfectionist and inflexible. Dependent personality disorder is characterised by extreme dependency in relationships.

Answer to Question 6

D: loss of interest

Pain, nausea and discomfort caused by cancer or its treatment can result in symptoms that are indistinguishable from the biological symptoms of a depressive illness, ie loss of appetite, energy, libido and a sleep disturbance. The assessment therefore depends on the evaluation of mood, anhedonia, suicidal thinking and other psychological symptoms.

Answer to Question 7

D: puerperal psychosis

Puerperal psychosis is most likely from this list, but be aware of the need to rule out medical causes for delirium (eg postpartum infection). This is a high-risk situation because mothers with puerperal psychosis may harm themselves and/or their baby. Disruption of mother-and-baby bonding due to early separation should be avoided as this will impair the psychological development of the infant. In a specialist mother and baby unit adequate supervision is provided ensuring the safety of both the baby and the mother.

Answer to Question 8

A: bradycardia when you show her a syringe

Blood/injection/injury phobia is unusual and is counterintuitive in its autonomic nervous system response in that it is associated with bradycardia and hypotension. This can lead to fainting.

Answer to Question 9

A: acute stress reaction

Reassure the patient that this is a normal reaction to an abnormal event and that her symptoms should soon subside. To accelerate her recovery she should be encouraged, with the help of her daughter, to resume all her routine activities – especially those that take place outside her home, eg shopping – and ensure a healthy diet, exercise, good sleep. She should be followed up, and if her symptoms persist beyond 4 weeks she should be referred for psychological therapy, but evidence tells us that formal psychological therapy and 'debriefing' immediately after an event like this is harmful.

Answer to Question 10

B: citalopram

It is reasonable to re-prescribe the same antidepressant if someone has responded to it in the past. Lithium is used to augment antidepressants in the treatment of resistant depression, which is defined as a failure to respond to two antidepressants from different classes that have been taken in therapeutic doses for adequate periods. Venlafaxine increases both serotonin and noradrenaline, so would be a logical second-line treatment if selective serotonin reuptake inhibitors (SSRIs) had not worked. Amitriptyline is a very effective antidepressant but at treatment doses has worse side effects, and is more risky in overdose than SSRIs, hence it is rarely prescribed now for depression.

Answer to Question 11

D: quetiapine

This woman has mania, for which the treatment of choice is an atypical antipsychotic drug, eg olanzapine, risperidone or quetiapine. This may be augmented with a benzodiazepine or a mood stabiliser, eg valproate. Lithium can be given in acute mania but is also indicated for prophylaxis, usually after two severe episodes in 2 years.

Answer to Question 12

D: persistent delusional disorder

This is a description of persistent delusional disorder. The mean age of onset is 35–45 years. The clinical picture is dominated by delusions, which are generally persecutory in content. There may also be hallucinations, but these are not prominent. The delusions tend to be encapsulated, ie the patient can generally function fairly well in areas unaffected by the delusions.

Answer to Question 13

B: perform urine drug testing for opioids

Giving methadone to someone who is not dependent on opioids can kill them. Also if a drug user exaggerates their methadone or heroin use and you use this dose to calculate the equivalent amount of methadone, you can kill them. Look for the objective use of opioids with urine drug screens. Also look for objective signs of withdrawal including lacrimation, runny nose, agitation, sweating, piloerection, tachycardia, vomiting, shivering, yawning and widely dilated pupils.

Answer to Question 14

B: call the hospital security services

In this situation a calm head is needed. You should not try to manage this on your own, hence your first action should be to call for help from the hospital security services. Think of the safety of other patients, visitors, staff and the abusive patient herself. It is important to bear in mind patients who are violent may also be at risk of self-harm. Attempt to find out what she is upset about. Do not assume that this is necessarily due to hallucinations or delusions.

Answer to Question 15

B: cognitive behavioural therapy

This is a fairly typical presentation of chronic fatigue syndrome (myalgic encephalomyelitis (ME)). The only treatments for which there is significant evidence of effectiveness are cognitive behavioural therapy and graded exercise treatment, and these are recommended in NICE guidelines. There is no evidence that medication is useful in chronic fatigue syndrome, although it may be used to treat associated conditions, eg depression.

Answer to Question 16

A: alcohol use

This is most likely delirium. While it may be due to the recent surgery, anaesthetic or medications (such as analgesia), the onset of delirium in a hospital inpatient should always prompt you to consider the possibility of alcohol withdrawal and delirium tremens. Take a collateral history from a relative or carer. Remember to administer parenteral vitamin B_{12} if there is a risk of Wernicke's encephalopathy.

Answer to Question 17

D: neuroleptic malignant syndrome

This is classical presentation of possible neuroleptic malignant syndrome, which is an idiosyncratic reaction to antipsychotic medication. Features include an altered mental state, stiffness and rigidity of the limbs, autonomic instability and hyperthermia. It is the most important diagnosis here because if unrecognised and untreated it has a mortality as high as 20% in some studies. Pertinent investigations include plasma creatine kinase (CK) and full blood count (FBC). The most immediate treatment is to stop the antipsychotic medication, and provide supportive care.

Answer to Question 18

B: reassure her, decline any further tests, and arrange to see her again

This is illness anxiety disorder, where the patient has a persistent concern about having a particular disease. These patients tend to struggle to accept normal investigations or any psychological explanation of the difficulty. Discharging her from the clinic will most likely result in her re-presenting elsewhere. Further investigations will expose her to iatrogenic risk without good justification. Referral to liaison psychiatry may be appropriate, but she may need to form more of a rapport with you, over a short period of time, before she will accept a referral.

Answer to Question 19

B: refer for electroconvulsive therapy (ECT)

This sounds like a severe depressive episode with psychotic symptoms (her beliefs are typical of nihilistic delusions). The patient has stopped eating or drinking and is now physically compromised as a result. Due to the severity, and the desire for a quick response to ameliorate her physical compromise, electroconvulsive therapy (ECT) should be considered. Antidepressants and antipsychotics may both be indicated, but there is likely to be a delayed clinical response, and ECT is more likely to be effective in this case.

Answer to Question 20

C: detain her under Section 5(2) of the Mental Health Act

In this case, the patient has a known mental disorder and is presenting with ongoing suicidal ideation, planning and intent, which is a significant risk to self. She is likely to require a psychiatric admission and is clearly opposing this by attempting to self-discharge. Therefore, regardless of her capacity, she is liable to be detained under the Mental Health Act. Section 5(2) allows her to be legally held on the ward for up to 72 hours, so that a full psychiatric assessment can take place, and she may then be detained under Section 2 or 3 for a compulsory hospital admission. Calling psychiatry may be helpful, but does not deal with the fact the patient is about to leave. Common Law can be used in an acute situation, such as to prevent someone leaving the emergency department prior to a psychiatric assessment, but should not be relied upon for continued restraint over a longer period of time. Allowing her to leave the ward would not be advisable: if she were to abscond, you should inform hospital security and the police.

Index

Note: page numbers in *italics* refer to figures, those in **bold** refer to tables.

brainstem death 88, **89**
brainstem encephalitis 144
brain tumours
   age distribution, by site *139*
   chemotherapy 142
   classification *139*
   clinical presentation 140, *140*, **141**
   differential diagnosis 141
   disease associations 142
   epidemiology 139
   investigation 141
   neurocutaneous syndromes as part
       of **143**
   pathology 139
   prognosis 142
   treatment 141–2
branch retinal vein occlusion (BRVO)
       192, *193*, 193–5
   fluorescein angiography in 194, *194*
British Society of Haematology 194
bulbar dysarthria 42
bulimia nervosa 219, 220

C

CAA (cerebral amyloid angiopathy)
       135
cancer-associated retinopathy 144
carbohydrate metabolism, disorders of
       (glycogen storage diseases)
       98–100, *99*
carnitine palmitoyltransferase (CPT)
       deficiency 15, 100
carotid Dopplers 76, 130–1, 154, *155*
carotid surgery 131
carpal tunnel syndrome 92
cataplexy 18
catechol-*O*-methyltransferase (COMT)
       106, 107
cavernous sinus syndrome 47
central nervous system 21, 144
central retinal vein occlusion (CRVO)
       192, *193*, 193–5
central sleep apnoea 17

cerebellar disease 69
   gait disturbance in 29
   tremor of 39
cerebellar speech 54
cerebellar syndrome **30**, 30–1
cerebral amyloid angiopathy (CAA)
       135
cerebral biopsy 141
cerebral herniation, post-lumbar
       puncture 149
cerebral oedema 78
cerebrospinal fluid (CSF) examination
   Guillain-Barré syndrome 95
   in memory impairment 13
   multiple sclerosis 112
   numb toes 66
   paraneoplastic syndromes 145
   peripheral neuropathies 93
   subarachnoid haemorrhage 79, 137,
       138
cerebrovascular disease
   intracerebral haemorrhage 134–7
   stroke 127–32
   subarachnoid haemorrhage 137–9
   transient ischaemic attacks 132–4
cervical myelopathy 36
channelopathies 102
Charcot–Marie–Tooth disease 21
chemotherapy
   brain tumours 142
chest X-ray
   status epilepticus 82
   stroke 75
chorea 14–15
chronic fatigue syndrome 223
classical migraine 3
clinically isolated syndrome (CIS) 111
Clinical Skills for PACES 169
clonidine 236
clozapine 245, 246
cluster headache 5, 6, 8, 118–19
Cochrane review 77
codeine 4
cognitive behavioural therapy (CBT) 241,
       254, 266

cognitive estimates, neuropsychological
       assessment 146
cognitive function 229
cognitive impairment 11, 12
cognitive signs
   in hemiplegia 37
coma 85, 86, **86**, 87, **87**, 88
comprehension
   speech disturbance and 54–5
computerised tomography angiography
       (CTA) 150, 152
computerised tomography (CT) 5
   brain tumours 141
   contraindications 152
   facial pain diagnosis 7
   indications 150, 152
   intracerebral haemorrhage 135,
       135–6
   memory impairment 13
   principle 150
   stroke 75
   subarachnoid haemorrhage 79, *80*,
       137
concrete thinking, neuropsychological
       assessment 146
constant facial pain 6, **6**
conus lesion, of spinal cord *26*
conversion disorder 59–60
cortical dementias, assessment 147
corticosteroids 4
Costen's syndrome 6, 8
cotton-wool spots 170, *172*
cranial nerves
   examination
       in acute ischaemic stroke 75
       in subarachnoid haemorrhage
           79
       in multiple sclerosis 112
       neurological examination 35
Creutzfeldt–Jakob disease 241
CSF *see* cerebrospinal fluid (CSF)
CTA *see* computerised tomography
       angiography (CTA)
CT *see* computerised tomography
       (CT)

episodic headache 3–6
episodic memory 146
Epworth Sleepiness Scale 18, *19*
European Cooperative Acute Stroke
Study III (ECASS III) 130
evoked potentials 149–50
excessive daytime sleepiness 16, 17
see also insomnia; non-restorative sleep
executive dysfunction 241
extrapyramidal disorders *see* Parkinson's
disease
eye
examination 169–73
in ptosis 43–4
in unequal pupils (anisocoria) 42
paraneoplastic syndromes involving 144

F

facial nerve palsy 48
facial pain 6–8, **6**, 7
facial weakness
Bell's palsy 50–1
bilateral facial palsy 49–50
clinical examinations **46**, 47–50, *50*
differential diagnosis 47
upper motor neurone 49, *50*
facioscapulohumeral dystrophy 50, 102
familial fatal insomnia 18
fatigue
in multiple sclerosis, treatment for
114
femoral nerve lesion 25
fingolimod 114–15
flare 186
fluency, speech disturbance and 54
fluorescein angiography 201, 204,
206
in BRVO 194, *194*
retinal artery occlusion 192
flurbiprofen 189
focal or partial seizures **122**, 122–3
focal resections, in epilepsy 125–6

foot drop *see* numb toes and foot
drop
Froment's sign 33
'frontal apraxic' gait 29
frontal lobe dysfunction 146
frontotemporal dementia 110
frontotemporal lobar degenerations
(FTLD) 11
fugue **240**
functional imaging 154
functional MRI (fMRI) 243
functional neuroimaging
memory impairment 13
functional neurological symptom
disorder 241
funny turns/blackouts 8–11, 9

G

GAD *see* generalised anxiety disorder
(GAD)
gait 69
spastic 27, 29
ataxia in cerebellar syndrome 30
gait disturbance 27–30
GBS *see* Guillain–Barré syndrome (GBS)
generalised anxiety disorder (GAD)
251–4, **253**
generalised seizures 121–2
genetic tests/testing
chorea 14
for memory impairment 13
giant cell arteritis 6, 8, 177–80
ischaemic optic neuropathy in 196–8,
197
Glasgow Coma Scale (GCS) score 74, 78,
79, 86, **87**
glatiramer acetate (GA) 114
glaucoma 173
glycogen storage diseases
(carbohydrate metabolism
disorders) 98–100, *99*
gradual loss of vision 173–5

see also age-related macular
degeneration
Guillain–Barré syndrome (GBS) 50, 66
acute weakness of legs in 72, 73
clinical presentation 94–5
treatment 96

H

haemorrhagic stroke 74
hallucinations
hypnogogic 18
visual *see* visual hallucinations
headache(s)
cluster headache 118–19
migraine 115–17
optic disc swelling and 180–3, **181**
over-diagnosed causes of chronic
120
periodicity of pain in 3, 4
post-lumbar puncture 149
signs and symptoms 4
tension-type headache 119–20
trigeminal neuralgia *117*, 117–18
see also episodic headache; facial
pain
hemiballismus 14
hemiplegia 36–7, **38**
hemiplegic migraine 115
hereditary inclusion body myositis 100
hereditary motor and sensory
neuropathy
numb toes and foot drop in 21
heroin 236
high-risk patient recognition, self-harm
and 232
history taking
chorea 13–15, **14**
eating disorders 219–21
episodic headache 3–6, 4, 5
facial pain **6**, 6–8, 7
funny turns/blackouts 8–11, **9**
medically unexplained symptoms
222–4

postherpetic neuralgia 6, *7*, 8
post-lumbar puncture headache 149
postnatal depressive disorder 262
post-Sydenham's chorea 14
post-traumatic stress disorder (PTSD) 261
postural tremor 68
pregnancy
    epilepsy in, management of 126
    episodic headache and 4
    idiopathic intracranial hypertension in 6
    migraine in 117
presyncope 9
proliferative diabetic retinopathy 200,
    200–2
proverbs, neuropsychological assessment
    and 146
proximal muscle weakness 34–5
pseudobulbar/spastic dysarthria 42
pseudodementia 11, 12
pseudo-relapse 114
pseudoseizures 63
    see also seizure(s)
psychotic depression 265
ptosis 43–4, **44**, 44
PTSD *see* post-traumatic stress disorder
    (PTSD)
puerperal disorders 261–4
puerperal psychosis 262–4
pupils
    assessment 175
    dilatation 171, 172, **173**

R

radial nerve lesion 33
radicular lesions
    pain radiation in **23**
radiotherapy
    brain tumours 142
rapid-cycling bipolar affective disorder 264
rapid eye movement (REM) 18
rasagiline
    for Parkinson's disease 107
reading
    speech disturbance and 55

red eye 183–5
reduced vision in diabetes **176**, 176–7
    see also diabetic retinopathy
refractory status epilepticus 84–5
rehabilitation
    acute ischaemic stroke 77
relative afferent pupillary defect (RAPD)
    196
repetition
    speech disturbance and 55
respiratory failure
    myasthenia gravis and 104
respiratory function
    measurement in GBS 95
resting tremor 68
retinal artery occlusion 189–92
retinal migraine 116
retinal transient ischaemic attack (TIA) 178
retinal vein occlusion 192–5
retinopathy
    cancer-associated 144
    diabetic *see* diabetic retinopathy
right third nerve palsy 45, *46*
    causes **49**
root/radicular lesion 32, **32**

S

safe alcohol consumption 233
SAH *see* subarachnoid haemorrhage (SAH)
schizoaffective disorder 264
schizophrenia 243, 244, **244**
sciatic nerve lesion 22, 25
scleritis 186, 187, 188–9, *188*
screening tests
    visual hallucinations 20
seasonal affective disorder 266
sedatives 230
seizure(s) 78
    antiepileptic drugs 64
    classification **121**
    control, causes of deterioration
        in 62, **63**
    defined 120

focal or partial **122**, 122–3
generalised 121–2
increasing frequency of 62–5
neurological examination 64
recurrent, risk of **126**
see also epilepsy; pseudoseizures
selective serotonin reuptake inhibitors
    (SSRIs) 256, 266–7
selegiline (Deprenyl/Eldepryl)
    for Parkinson's disease 107
self-harm 225–6, 230–2
self-starvation 221
semantic memory 146
sensory/posterior dysphasia 55
sensory signs
    in hemiplegia 37
severe, non-proliferative diabetic
    retinopathy 200, *200*
sexual dysfunction
    in multiple sclerosis, treatment for
        114
simple phobias 256
single-fibre electromyography 103
single-photon emission computed
    tomography (SPECT) 154
    memory impairment 13
sleep apnoea 18
sleep disorders 16–19
small-fibre neuropathy 92
Snellen chart 174
social issues
    opioid use disorder 235
social phobias 256, 257
somatic symptom and related disorders
    240–1
somatosensory evoked potentials
    (SSEPs) 150
spastic gait 27, 29
spasticity
    in multiple sclerosis, treatment for
        113
spastic legs **26**, 26–7
specific (simple) phobias 256
SPECT *see* single-photon emission
    computed tomography (SPECT)